T0156175

RAND

Prostate Cancer Patient Outcomes and Choice of Providers: Development of an Infrastructure for Quality Assessment

Mark S. Litwin, Michael Steinberg,
Jennifer Malin, John Naitoh,
Kimberly A. McGuigan, Rebecca Steinfeld,
John Adams, and Robert H. Brook

Prepared for the Bing Fund

Contents

FIGURES

TABLES

EXECUTIVE SUMMARY

Prostate cancer is the most common solid malignancy diagnosed in American men. More than half of the new cases identified each year are localized prostate cancer, an early stage of the disease in which the tumor is confined to the prostate. The usual approach to localized prostate cancer includes radical prostatectomy, radiation therapy, or watchful waiting. Unfortunately, clear evidence about the comparative efficacy of these treatments is lacking; and, even untreated, most men with early stage prostate cancer have a life expectancy comparable to similarly aged men without prostate cancer.

The most common potential long-term complications after treatment include urinary incontinence, impotence, and bowel dysfunction. The rates of these complications reported by different researchers and institutions in the scientific literature vary substantially. Although this variability may simply reflect differences in the patients included (case-mix) or the ways in which the data were collected, it does raise concern that widespread variation exists in the quality of treatment provided for men with prostate cancer across the United States.

Given the large number of men diagnosed and treated for prostate cancer each year, it is essential to determine how variations in quality of care affect treatment outcomes. This report presents the results of a RAND study conducted to develop the infrastructure necessary to begin evaluating the quality of care provided to men with early stage prostate cancer.

- We review and summarize the medical literature on both surgical and radiation treatment of localized prostate cancer.
- We report the results of interviews with physician experts in both surgical and radiation treatment of prostate cancer about what they consider essential to providing excellent quality care.
- We describe the findings of focus groups conducted with patients and spouses to understand what information is most needed by men who face treatment decisions for newly diagnosed early stage prostate cancer.
- We report the recommendations of an expert consensus panel convened to rate

the clinical validity and feasibility of draft quality indicators and potential case-mix adjusters, developed by the RAND research team.

The central outcome of this study is a list of candidate indicators of quality of care, endorsed by our RAND consensus panel as appearing to be valid, feasible, and appropriate for further testing in a population-based sample. These candidate indicators include measures of structure, process, and outcome, as well as a list of covariates which must be controlled for in quality-of-care studies. Detailed in Chapter 8, this list comprises the following. The four endorsed measures of structure include (1) volume (number) of patients treated; (2) availability of conformal therapy (radiation oncology facilities); (3) availability of psychological counseling resources; and (4) knowledge of treating institution outcomes. The twelve endorsed measures of process include (1) pre-treatment assessment with DRE, PSA, and Gleason grade; (2) documentation of pre-treatment urinary, sexual, and bowel function; (3) assessment of family history of prostate cancer; (4) documentation that the patient was presented with alternative treatment modalities; the opportunity to consult with a provider of an alternative treatment modality; and the risk of treatment complications in the experience of the practitioner or facility; (5) evidence of institutional adherence to practice protocol of College of American Pathologists Cancer Committee for management of pathology specimens; (6) for conventional external beam radiation therapy: use of CT during treatment planning; use of patient immobilization during treatment; delivering recommended doses (68-72 Gy isocenter [ICRU]); (7) For conformal external beam radiation therapy: use of CT during treatment planning, use of patient immobilization during treatment, appropriate protection of rectal mucosa during high-dose conformal treatment, and delivering escalated doses (70-80 Gy ICRU); (8) for radiation therapy: use of high energy linear accelerator (>=10 MV); (9) at least 2 follow-up visits by treating physician during the first year post-treatment; (10) documentation or evidence of communication with patient's primary care physician or provision of continuing care; (11) operative blood loss; and (12) use of clinical and pathological TNM staging by treating physicians. The six endorsed measures of outcome include (1) primary treatment failure indicated by 3 consecutive rising PSA values after radiation therapy or any confirmed detectable PSA value after radical prostatectomy; (2) following primary treatment by radiation therapy: hospitalization or medical or surgical treatment for cystitis, proctitis, hematuria, or rectal bleeding; (3) following primary treatment by radiation therapy or radical prostatectomy: hospitalization or medical or surgical treatment for bladder neck contracture / urethral stricture; (4) acute surgical complication rate (death, cardiovascular complications, deep vein thrombosis, pulmonary embolus, blood loss necessitating transfusions, etc.); (5) patient assessment of urinary, sexual, and bowel functioning following primary treatment by radiation therapy or radical prostatectomy, using a reliable, validated survey instrument; and (6) patient satisfaction with treatment choice, continence, and potency. Endorsed covariates for which various quality measures should be controlled include age, life expectancy, pre-treatment PSA, clinical stage, Gleason grade, family history of prostate cancer, history of other cancer, use of neoadjuvant or adjuvant hormone therapy, co-morbidity indicators, insurance, education, and income.

Based upon the results of this study, we make the following recommendations for further research:

1. Field-test the candidate quality indicators in a national sample of institutions to empirically test their validity and demonstrate their feasibility.

2. Identify which aspects of structure and process of care are important to producing excellent outcomes in early stage prostate cancer.

3. Determine which patient characteristics among those endorsed by the expert panel must be adjusted for when comparing institutions, so that quality measurement will not be confounded by differences in patient populations and factors beyond providers' control that affect outcomes (case-mix).

4. Develop an education program for men newly diagnosed with early stage prostate cancer to help them interpret scientific data and use information on treatment outcomes in their decision about which treatment to pursue.

Chapter 1

INTRODUCTION

Background and overview of the study

The problem: High incidence of prostate cancer, no consensus about treatment

Prostate cancer is the most common non-cutaneous malignancy in American men. In 1999, more than 179,300 cases are expected to be diagnosed, and more than 37,000 men are projected to die from this disease (Landis et al. 1999). Adoption of prostate-specific antigen (PSA) testing (Potosky et al. 1995) has increased the probability of detecting prostate cancer in its early stages. In 1993, before PSA testing became widespread, 165,000 new cases of prostate cancer were identified in the United States. With the August 1994 FDA approval of PSA testing, it became possible to diagnose and treat tumors before they became palpable. As a result, the number of detected cases has grown substantially, though it has begun to decline in the past two years.

More than half of the new cases identified each year are localized prostate cancer, an early stage of the disease in which the tumor is still confined to the prostate. The approach to localized prostate cancer can include surgery (radical prostatectomy), radiation therapy (external beam, conformal radiation therapy, or brachytherapy), or watchful waiting, in which the cancer is treated only when it spreads and produces symptoms.

Unfortunately, clear evidence about the comparative efficacy of these treatment modalities is lacking. The scientific evaluation of the effect of treatment on survival is extremely challenging – even untreated, many men with early stage prostate cancer can expect to live for at least ten to fifteen years without becoming symptomatic from the spread of the disease. They may even enjoy a life expectancy comparable to men their age without prostate cancer.

These challenges and the absence of data from randomized controlled trials have proved insurmountable to two national attempts to develop guidelines for the treatment of localized prostate cancer. At the 1987 National Institute of Health Consensus Conference, no consensus was reached regarding the optimal therapy for localized prostate cancer (National Institutes of Health 1988). The American Urological Association's (AUA) Prostate Cancer Clinical

Guidelines Panel, after performing a systematic review of the literature, determined that differences in significant patient characteristics, including age, tumor grade, and pelvic lymph node status, did not permit valid comparisons of outcomes from clinical case series (Middleton et al. 1995). The AUA panel recommended that "patients with newly diagnosed, clinically localized prostate cancer should be informed of all commonly accepted treatments."

Although long-term survival is the main concern for many men as they decide which treatment modality for localized prostate cancer to pursue, treatment-related complications, which are frequent and can vary with the mode of treatment, become important considerations as well. Risks associated with treatment include urinary incontinence and strictures, impotence, and bowel dysfunction. Potency and urinary continence are impaired more often with surgery (Litwin et al. 1995, Shrader-Bogen et al. 1997, Talcott et al. 1998), while bowel function is affected most by radiation. Thus, the decision of which treatment to choose for localized prostate cancer is generally individualized, based on the size, grade, and stage of the tumor, the patient's age and life expectancy, and his personal preferences.

The complication rates after treatment of localized prostate cancer reported in the literature vary substantially. The American Urological Association reports widespread variation in the reported rates of treatment-related complications, even when stratifying by treatment modality: surgery, external beam radiation, or brachytherapy (Middleton et al. 1995). Following radical prostatectomy, rates of stress incontinence range from <10% to 50%, and impotence rates range from 25% to 100% across series reports. Complications following external beam radiation included proctitis, with rates ranging from <10% to over 50%; cystitis, ranging from 0% and 80%; and impotence, ranging from <10% to nearly 40% or higher. Similarly, complication rates reported for brachytherapy range from 0% to 75% for proctitis, <10% to 90% for cystitis, and from <10% to 75% for impotence (Brandeis et al. 2000). Although this variability may simply reflect differences in the patients included (case-mix) or the ways in which the data were collected, it does raise concern that widespread variation exists in the *quality* of treatment provided for men with prostate cancer across the United States.

A number of research projects are studying these variations in prostate cancer outcomes. Two notable studies are the Prostate Patient Outcomes Research Team (PORT) and the National Cancer Institute's Prostate Cancer Outcomes Study (PCOS). The PORT has been using Medicare claims data and patient surveys to describe variations in outcomes following radical prostatectomy and radiation therapy (Lu-Yao et al. 1996). The objective of PCOS is to evaluate recent diagnostic and treatment practice patterns among men diagnosed with prostate cancer in order to evaluate the prevalence of long-term urinary, bowel, and sexual function complications subsequent to initial treatment (Gilliland et al. 1999). However, while these patterns-of-care studies will provide valuable information about the range of experience of men with prostate cancer, they will not inform us about the quality of care provided for prostate cancer in the United States. In order to be able to describe the quality-of-care for prostate cancer, outcomes must be risk-adjusted and information is needed about processes of care. To date, no such information comparing the quality of care for men with early stage prostate cancer exists.

Much is written about how to chose the type of treatment for localized prostate cancer, both in the medical literature and the lay press (Desch et al. 1996, Mazur and Hickam 1996, Mazur and Merz 1995, Mazur and Merz 1996). Some two-hundred entries on Amazon.com, the online bookstore, provide information and advice for the man faced with a diagnosis of localized prostate cancer about how to choose a treatment. For the patient diagnosed with localized prostate cancer, there is currently little guidance about how to choose the *best place* to be treated, even though this may be as, if not more, important a decision.

Building an infrastructure for assessing quality of care for prostate cancer

In their recently issued report *Ensuring Quality Cancer Care*, the Institute of Medicine's National Cancer Policy Board (NCPB) concluded that "for many Americans with cancer, there is a wide gulf between what could be construed as the ideal and the reality of their experience with cancer care" (National Cancer Policy Board, Institute of Medicine 1999). Although this report was not specific to prostate cancer, five of its recommendations are of particular relevance:

1. Patients undergoing procedures that are technically difficult to perform and have been associated with higher mortality in lower-volume settings should receive care at high-volume facilities.
2. Providers should use evidence-based guidelines.
3. The quality of care should be monitored and measured using a core set of quality measures.
4. A cancer data system should be established to provide quality benchmarks.

5. Research sponsors should support studies of patterns of care and factors associated with the receipt of good care.

The NCPB's recommendations have focused national attention on quality-of-care research and a monitoring system for cancer patients. RAND conducted the Prostate Cancer Patient Outcomes and Choice of Providers Study to provide the necessary infrastructure for assessing the quality of treatment for men with localized prostate cancer.

The study, and this report, comprised four separate but interdependent projects: (1) literature reviews; (2) expert interviews; (3) focus groups with patients and spouses; and (4) an expert consensus panel. Each of these four pillars was necessary to create a solid foundation for further work in evaluating the quality of early stage prostate cancer care.

Review of the medical literature. The literature reviews consisted of summaries of available information from the medical literature on structure, process, and outcomes of early stage prostate cancer care. We searched MEDLINE for clinical trials or single- or multi-institutional case series of outcomes of localized prostate cancer treatment. We identified all articles in English indexed by MESH subjects Prostatic Neoplasms and Therapy/Surgery or Treatment/Surgery or Prostatectomy or Radiotherapy, limited by one the following subject headings: Treatment Outcome or Outcome Assessment or Treatment Failure or Recurrence or Outcome and Process Assessment (Health Care) or Process Assessment (Health Care) or Mortality or Quality of Health Care or Quality of Life. We retrieved articles on surgical outcomes published between January 1980 and September 1997. For radiation therapy, we limited our search to articles from 1985 onward to reflect more recent practices in standard care. We supplemented this database with additional studies as they became available. We reviewed and abstracted data on the study population, treatment, outcomes, and other relevant variables, and entered the data into a computer spreadsheet.

In Chapter 2, we review and summarize the medical literature on surgical treatment of localized prostate cancer. This summary includes many items that pertain to the structure and process of care, as well as treatment outcomes, which may be considered for potential quality measures of surgical treatment. Appendix A summarizes the variation in outcomes after surgical treatment for localized prostate cancer reported in the medical literature.

In Chapter 3, we review and summarize the medical literature on radiation treatment of localized prostate cancer. Like the review of surgical treatment, this summary includes many items that pertain to the structure and process of care, as well as treatment outcomes, which may be considered for potential quality measures of radiation therapy. Appendix B summarizes the variation in outcomes after radiation therapy for localized prostate cancer reported in the medical literature. Chapter 4 illustrates some of the challenges we encountered in interpreting the available literature.

Interviews with experts. Because most of the medical literature on early stage prostate cancer is focused on the efficacy of treatment and not on quality assessment, we went directly to physician leaders in both the surgical and radiation treatment of prostate cancer to learn what they consider essential to providing excellent quality care. In addition, we wanted to learn whether the information these leading institutions provide to patients about the outcomes of treatment reflects their own institutional experience or that reported in the literature. Chapter 5 summarizes the recommendations of these experts in prostate cancer treatment.

Focus groups with patients and their partners. To understand the types of information most needed by men newly diagnosed with early stage prostate cancer facing a treatment decision, we conducted focus groups with patients who had undergone radiation therapy or radical prostatectomy, as well as their partners. Chapter 6 summarizes these focus groups and specifically addresses the following important questions:

- What information is currently available to men with localized prostate cancer about the various treatment options and their side-effects as they make their treatment decisions?
- How do patients select facilities and providers for the treatment of localized prostate cancer?
- Do patients report that their physicians communicate the outcomes of treatment for early stage prostate cancer?
- Do patients see a need for information about the quality of prostate cancer treatment?

Because one of the goals of developing a national system to evaluate and monitor the quality of early stage prostate cancer treatment is to inform patient choice about where to get treated, Chapter 7 examines important issues that affect patient decision-making. In particular, we review the scientific literature on communicating risk and apply it to the challenge of communicating to patients about localized prostate cancer.

Expert consensus. In Chapter 8, we present candidate quality indicators for early stage prostate cancer and describe the method used to develop them:

- Using the data obtained in Chapters 1-3, the RAND research team developed draft quality indicators to be considered for use in evaluating the quality of early stage prostate cancer care across the three domains of structure, process, and outcomes.

- Relying on the evidence reviewed in Chapters 1 and 2, the RAND research team also developed a list of potential variables to be used to adjust for differences in the baseline characteristics of patients when attempting to compare quality of care across facilities or providers.

- A panel of experts in the treatment of localized prostate cancer was convened at RAND to rate the draft quality indicators and potential case-mix adjusters on their clinical validity and feasibility.

Recommendations. In the final section of this report, we summarize RAND's recommendations for further research needed to measure and report the quality of prostate cancer treatment nationally.

In the remainder of this chapter, we briefly review the types of measures used to assess quality.

How is quality of care measured?

In order to evaluate and compare the quality of treatment for men with prostate cancer across health systems, facilities, or physicians, we must have a way to measure it. To measure quality, health care is often stratified into three components: structure, process, and outcome (Donabedian 1980).

Structural measures. Structure encompasses the human, technical, and financial resources needed to provide medical care. Organizations such the Joint Commission on the Accreditation of Healthcare Organizations (JCAHO) and the American College of Surgeons have generally relied on structural measures in their accreditation procedures. Important structural attributes for quality of care may include clinician characteristics (e.g., percentage of physicians who have board certification, average years of experience, distribution of specialties), organizational characteristics (e.g., staffing patterns, reimbursement method), patient characteristics (e.g., insurance type, illness profile), and community characteristics (e.g., per capita hospital beds, transportation system, environmental risks). Structural measures specific to prostate cancer quality could include the presence of a particular type of equipment or psychological support services.

Although certain structural characteristics may be necessary to provide good care, they are usually insufficient to ensure quality of care. Therefore, the best structural measures are those that can be shown to have a positive influence on the process of care and on patient outcomes (although this relationship has not been confirmed) (Brook et al. 1990). One structural measure that is positively associated with outcomes is the volume or number or cases treated by a particular physician or institution (Grumbach et al. 1995, Hannan et al. 1997, Kitahata et al. 1996, Luft et al. 1990). Lu-Yao et al. (1996) found that patients treated at facilities that performed fewer radical prostatectomies reported more surgical complications than patients treated at facilities with a higher volume of the surgeries. Ellison et al. (2000) have reported similar results. It is not clear what characteristics of hospitals that perform many prostatectomies contribute to better outcomes; however, high volume appears to be an important predictor of good quality care.

Process of care measures. Process of care is the set of activities that goes on between patients and practitioners and is often divided into interpersonal process and technical process. *Interpersonal process* refers to way in which the clinician relates to the patient and includes issues such as whether the clinician supplied sufficient information in a clear enough manner for the patient to make an informed choice regarding his treatment. Patient survey data are generally used to assess quality of interpersonal process.

Technical process refers to whether the medically appropriate decisions are made when diagnosing and treating the patient and whether care is provided in an effective and skillful manner. One way to evaluate the appropriateness of medical treatment is to determine if the care provided is consistent with current medical knowledge and adheres to the professional standard. This assessment can be done by developing *quality indicators* that describe a process of care that should occur for a particular type of patient in a specific clinical circumstance. In order to be

7

valid, these quality indicators should be based on the evidence in the medical literature and on current professional standards of care. Determining the latter often requires an expert panel in order to achieve consensus. The performance of physicians and health plans is then assessed by calculating rates of adherence to the indicators for a sample of patients.

Using quality indicators to evaluate appropriateness of care is relatively straightforward. However, assessing the effectiveness or skill of technical process of care is much more difficult. Indeed, direct observation may be necessary to assess quality of technical process of care. Alternatively, we may have to rely upon measuring outcomes to evaluate whether care was provided in a skillful manner. For example, measurement of surgical blood loss or number of specimens with positive margins, both surgical outcomes, may be indicators of the quality of surgical technical process.

Outcomes measures. Outcomes include changes in patients' current and future health status, including health-related quality of life, as well as patient satisfaction (consumer satisfaction). Cancer researchers have generally used survival or progression-free survival as the main outcome measure in clinical studies. Sometimes proxy measures (also called surrogate end points or intermediate outcomes) are used that do not measure the outcome directly but are thought to be correlated with it. When a proxy measure is used as a quality indicator, we must have evidence that the proxy measure is truly a substitute for the outcome we are trying to measure. For example, a rising PSA after treatment of localized prostate cancer appears associated with cancer recurrence, so PSA-free-survival may be a reasonable proxy for disease-free-survival. However, it is controversial and may not necessarily be a good proxy for overall survival. In fact, not all biochemical failures are associated with clinically significant recurrences (Pound et al. 1999b). For proxy measures to be useful as quality measures, intervention should affect both the measure and the cancer itself (Schatzkin et al., 1996).

Another important outcome is health-related quality of life, a multidimensional construct that includes somatic symptoms, functional ability, emotional well-being, social functioning, sexuality and body image, as well as overall well-being (Cella 1995; Cella and Bonomi 1995). Quality of life assessment provides a comprehensive evaluation of how the illness and its treatment affect patients. Quality of life for cancer patients is measured using validated patient surveys such as the Cancer Rehabilitation Evaluation System (CARES) (Ganz et al. 1992, Schag and Heinrich 1990) or the Functional Living Index-Cancer (FLIC) (Schipper et al. 1984). The UCLA Prostate Cancer Index is a survey instrument specifically developed and validated to evaluate men's treatment-related symptoms and quality of life after treatment for prostate cancer (Litwin et al. 1998a).

Patient satisfaction outcomes measure patients' perceptions of the quality of care they received and are usually assessed by patient survey. A limitation of satisfaction ratings is that patients are not necessarily able to evaluate the technical quality of their care. In fact, studies have found no consistent relationship between patient satisfaction and technical quality of care (Cleary and McNeil 1988, Davies and Ware 1988, Hayward et al. 1993). That is, a physician who interacts with patients in a warm and open way may provide care that is technically poor (Aharony and Strasser 1993). In addition, patients' satisfaction ratings may vary with their expectations. As such, unless used in conjunction with other measures, data about patient satisfaction may or may not not provide useful information about overall quality of care.

There are many challenges to using outcomes to evaluate quality of care.

First, adverse outcomes may be uncommon events, so large samples of patients may be needed when using outcome measures to detect differences in quality among health systems or hospitals. For example, to detect a two percentage point difference in the rate of post-operative wound infections between two hospitals (e.g., five percent for one and seven percent for the other), each hospital would need to have at least 1900 patients who had the surgery.

Second, a single outcome may be affected by many different factors, making it difficult to establish accountability. For example, when comparing differences in surgical outcomes across hospitals, one does not know if the differences in outcomes are related to the skill of the surgeon, the competence of the surgical team, the post-operative care, or the case-mix. And the more time that elapses between the intervention and the outcome, the more difficult this problem becomes. For example, when comparing 10-year survival of men treated for localized prostate cancer at different facilities, what is more important – the quality of the initial treatment or the quality of care for relapsed cancer?

Third, patient characteristics may also influence treatment outcome. For example, older patients may be more likely to experience complications after surgery. If this fact is not considered when comparing surgical complication rates across hospitals, evaluators may erroneously conclude that a hospital with an older patient population is providing poorer quality care. To use outcomes to measure quality of care, we need to adjust for these other factors, including baseline patient characteristics and intervening treatments. This adjustment (referred to a case-mix adjustment or risk adjustment) can be extremely complex, and the selection of factors must be done carefully so that outcomes can be interpreted accurately (Iezzoni 1996, Iezzoni et al. 1996).

Outcomes can also be measured for more than one purpose. Although we are interested in developing outcome measures for evaluating the quality of care received by men with prostate cancer, outcomes are also used clinically to track a patient's progress and, in clinical trials, to measure the efficacy or effectiveness of a new drug or intervention. The same measures can sometimes be used for both purposes, but certain measures are better suited for one purpose or the other. For example, five-year survival rates are a standard measure used in studies of new cancer treatments. However, when measuring quality of care for purposes of accountability or quality improvement, we generally need a shorter time horizon than five years. If we compared the 5-year survival of men with early stage prostate cancer at two institutions, we might indeed find that one institution had higher survival rates, suggesting that it had better quality of care. However, during those five years, staff changes, revamped procedures or new technology may have improved or weakened the quality of care at the hospitals, thereby making the comparison of historical but not practical value.

Implicit measurement of quality. In addition to the Donabedian model, other approaches to measuring quality of care rely upon implict review or assessment without explicit criteria. This typically involves having an acknowledged expert carry out a formal evaluation of the episode of care by reviewing the medical chart without the establishment of specific criteria for quality. The evaluator makes an implicit judgment of whether or not the care rendered was of high quality. This approach is de facto qualitative and may not yield valid and reproducible results.

Summary. Given the large number of men diagnosed and treated for prostate cancer each year, we need to understand how variations in quality of care affect outcomes of prostate cancer treatment. To accurately measure the quality of prostate cancer care, we must develop reliable and valid quality indicators for prostate cancer. In addition, we need to measure and report the quality of prostate cancer treatment nationally so that patients and their physicians have the information as they consider where and how to be treated. To accurately report quality of care at the facility or provider level, we must identify the patient characteristics that affect our ability to obtain reliable measurements and develop methods to mathematically neutralize their effect on our results.

Chapter 2

REVIEW OF THE MEDICAL LITERATURE
ON RADICAL PROSTATECTOMY

This chapter summarizes information from the medical literature on the structure, process, and outcomes of radical prostatectomy for early stage prostate cancer. Most conclusions in this literature are based on case series, retrospective case-controls, and expert opinion. Only a few conclusions are based on data derived from prospective trials. As a consequence, the reported links between process, structure and outcome in the radical prostatectomy literature are often based on inference and conventional wisdom.

Pre-treatment workup

The standard pre-treatment evaluation of the patient with clinically localized prostate cancer involves testing to determine the resectability of the tumor (staging) as well as the patient's life-expectancy. Unfortunately, while current modalities are generally able to detect the presence of advanced (stage T3, T4 or N+) cancer, they lack the sensitivity to detect microscopic spread. In addition, even though an integral part of the pre-treatment evaluation involves evaluating co-morbidity to determine anesthetic risk and life expectancy, there is a paucity of data in the literature that actually discuss how these parameters are measured in clinical practice.

The following tests are advocated as potentially useful for staging patients prior to surgery: the digital rectal examination, transrectal ultrasound, prostate specific antigen (PSA), prostate acid phosphatase (PAP), ProstaScint scanning, pelvic computerized tomography scan (CT) or magnetic resonance imaging scan (MRI), and bone scan (Epstein et al. 1996, Kupelian et al. 1996, Stein et al. 1992, Winter et al. 1991, Zietman et al. 1994). However, despite the widespread availability of these imaging and serological tests, their utility in pre-operative staging is limited by two factors. First, the poor sensitivity and specificity of these tests limit their utility in staging patients. Second, although factors such as a high PSA level or high Gleason grade are associated with a poor outcome from surgery (such as a tumor that is not completely resectable or a detectable PSA level following surgery indicating residual cancer), unfavorable results on tests used in the pre-treatment evaluation do not necessarily imply that the patient will die from prostate cancer. Nor can they reliably predict clinically significant cancer recurrence following surgery (Yang et al. 1998).

For a variety of reasons, the clinical utility of staging studies for locally advanced cancer has yet to be demonstrated. In particular, prostate tumors behave in heterogeneous ways; more than 50% of patients who have a biochemical relapse do not appear to develop a detectable cancer recurrence on X-ray, bone scan, or biopsy; and we do not know how surgery affects the natural history of a given tumor (i.e., whether surgery improved the overall survival of a patient, or whether the tumor would take an indolent course, impacting neither the quality nor quantity of life). However, despite these limitations, the standard staging studies used in men with prostate cancer include the digital rectal examination (DRE), PSA, bone scan (in selected patients), and CT scan (in selected patients).

Digital rectal exam. The DRE has been the mainstay of clinical prostate cancer staging modality because it is inexpensive, rapid, and relatively noninvasive. However, the DRE is limited by significant inter-observer variability, limited diagnostic accuracy, and poor sensitivity. Overall, there is a tendency for the DRE to understage prostate cancer (Table 2.1) (Ennis et al.1994, Narayan et al. 1995) . Given these results, the DRE is unreliable for determining whether or not the tumor is confined to the prostate.

Table 2.1 Digital rectal examination tends to understage prostate cancer (Catalona 1990)

Clinical Stage Based on DRE	Pathological Stage T3 or Higher
Stage A1 (found on TURP)	0%
T1C (normal examination)	40%
T2A (induration < 1/2 of 1 lobe)	20%
T2B (Induration > 1/2 of 1 lobe)	60 - 76%

Prostate-specific antigen testing. With an improved understanding of the biology of PSA, this serum marker has also been used to stage patients prior to surgery. Although there are many benign conditions that can cause an abnormal elevation of serum PSA, the degree of PSA elevation is proportional to the volume of cancer, and pre-treatment PSA roughly correlates with the pathologic stage that is determined at the time of radical prostatectomy, as well as the risk of failure following radiation therapy (D'Amico et al. 1997, O'Dowd et al. 1997). In studies of surgically treated patients, relapses of prostate cancer in men with pre-operative PSA levels less than 4 ng/mL treated with radical prostatectomy were exceedingly rare (Lerner et al. 1996). In contrast, when the PSA is greater than 10 to 20 ng/mL, the chance that the tumor will be confined to the prostate at the time of surgery is markedly decreased, and there is a markedly increased risk of subsequent cancer recurrence (Blackwell et al. 1994, D'Amico et al. 1996, D'Amico et al. 1997, Narayan et al. 1995, Winter et al. 1991, Zietman et al. 1994). Similar data have been shown for patients undergoing radiation therapy, where a pre-treatment PSA greater than 20 to 30 ng/mL is thought to be a reflection of occult metastatic disease (Zagars 1993).

These data notwithstanding, the utility of PSA as a staging tool is limited in the majority of patients who have clinically localized prostate cancer (Winter et al. 1991). PSA has not performed well when used alone as a staging tool because (1) most patients who undergo surgery have only mild elevations in their PSA (between 4 and 10) and (2) the absolute PSA level may not reflect the patient's actual tumor burden or stage due to the confounding influences of prostatitis and BPH (Douglas et al. 1997b). However, although the serum PSA alone has limited ability to discriminate between organ-confined and advanced prostate cancer, studies have shown that the PSA level can be used to identify patients who will benefit most from further evaluation with imaging tests such as bone scan, CT scan, or the ProstaScint scan. For example, patients with a pre-treatment PSA less than 10 ng/mL have an extremely low risk of bone metastases, and therefore do not need a staging bone scan prior to treatment (Lee and Oesterling 1997; Oesterling 1993). Similarly, in patients with small, low-grade prostate tumors and a low PSA, the incidence of pelvic lymph node metastases is so low as to make a staging pelvic lymphadenectomy unnecessary (O'Dowd et al. 1997). Furthermore, when used in combination with the Gleason score of the biopsy and with DRE findings, the pre-treatment PSA can be used to identify patients for whom the staging pelvic lymphadenectomy can be deferred.

Radionuclide bone scan. The radionuclide bone scan is also often included in the staging evaluation for the patient with localized prostate cancer. Given the propensity of prostate cancer to spread to the axial skeleton, bone scans can identify patients who have metastatic disease in their bones and thereby exclude some patients who will not benefit from surgical treatment. Unfortunately, bone scans lack both sensitivity and specificity for detecting metastases from prostate cancer. Other diseases such as healing fractures, degenerative joint disease or Paget's disease yield false positive results, and MRI or plain radiographs are often needed to confirm the diagnosis (Levy and Resnick 1997). Furthermore, as discussed previously, a bone scan is of little value in patients whose pre-treatment PSA is less than 10 ng/dl. However, the risk of bony metastasis is markedly increased when the PSA is greater than 20 ng/dl, making a bone scan useful to rule out the presence of bone metastases in these patients (Levy and Resnick 1997).

Other imaging – transrectal ultrasound, CT scanning, MRI. Although use of the bone scan in the pre-treatment evaluation of selected patients with prostate cancer is widely accepted, use of other imaging studies is more controversial. The development of *transrectal ultrasound* (TRUS) in the 1980s changed the way prostate biopsy is done, making it possible to perform ultrasound-guided biopsies of the prostate. Initial studies suggested that TRUS could also be useful in detecting the presence of extracapsular disease or seminal vesicle invasion; however, more recent studies found TRUS of limited value in staging, since cancer has no characteristic appearance on ultrasound and the resolution of the ultrasound images is limited (Pontes et al. 1985).

CT scanning has also had limited utility in cancer staging due to limited resolution. Recent advances in technology have improved the resolution of the CT, and some experts have suggested that modern (spiral or thin cut) CT scanning may be a more sensitive imaging modality for detecting nodal metastasis (Seltzer et al. 1999). CT scanning is limited by a lack of specificity (inflammatory, non-cancerous nodes can also be detected on CT scan), its inability to provide information about the local extent of the primary tumor, and its inability to detect micrometastatic disease. At a minimum, as was the case for bone scans, patients who have a PSA less than 10 do not need a CT scan prior to surgery. The risk of metastatic disease is markedly increased once the pretreatment PSA is greater than 20 to 30, and a spiral CT scan in this circumstance may prove useful. However, current evidence is insufficient to recommend its routine use.

Other authors have proposed that *MRI* may be valuable in staging patients with early stage prostate cancer, especially in patients where the clinical staging and PSA testing are inconclusive (D'Amico et al. 1994, D'Amico et al. 1997). A few case series have shown that MRI (especially endorectal coil MRI) may provide additional staging information about the presence of capsular penetration and seminal vesicle invasion in patients where the PSA and DRE yielded ambiguous results. In addition, D'Amico et al. (1997) showed that MRI findings can independently predict the occurrence of PSA relapse following radical prostatectomy. However, these results have yet to be replicated, and endorectal coil MRI is available at only a few centers. Thus, for the moment, endorectal MRI must still be considered an experimental technique.

Other serum markers – prostate-specific membrane antigen and prostatic acid phosphatase. Another potentially useful staging test is the *Indium-111 Capromab Pendetide* scan (*ProstaScint scan*: Cytogen Corporation, Princeton, NJ). This test is based on the discovery of an antibody to a prostate specific protein called prostate-specific membrane antigen (PSMA). PSMA is a relatively new tumor marker for prostate cancer. Although the functional significance of the PSMA protein is unknown, the protein appears to be a 100 kd molecular weight protein that has an extracellular domain, a transmembrane region, and an intracellular domain (Israeli et al. 1997). Immunohistochemical studies have shown that the expression of PSMA is largely restricted to tissues of prostatic origin, although low levels of this antigen can be found in the brain, salivary glands, and small intestine (Israeli et al. 1994). Some investigators have reported encouraging results with markers such as PSMA and RT-PCR (Katz et al. 1995).

Unlike PSA, the expression of PSMA is increased primarily in poorly differentiated and metastatic tumors (Abdel-Nabi et al. 1992). Thus a novel staging technique has been developed based on the 7e11-c5.3 antibody, which binds to PSMA, tagged with the radioisotope indium-111 (ProstaScint). Extraprostatic sites of prostate cancer are supposed to be recognized by ProstaScint, making them detectable on a nuclear medicine gamma camera (Abdel-Nabi et al. 1992). However, the 7e11-c5.3 antibody can only recognize and bind to an intracellular epitope of PSMA (Troyer et al. 1997). Thus, in the best case scenario, the ProstaScint scan will have limited ability to detect prostate cancer because the cells must be dead for the antibody to gain access into the cell and bind to its target. In addition, background accumulation of the tracer in the blood and bowel obscures the resolution of the test and accumulation of the tracer into the bladder hinders visualization of the lymph nodes. These factors pose major threats to the sensitivity and specificity of this test, as well as the inter- and intra-observer variability in the interpretation of test results. Data on the validity and efficacy of the ProstaScint scan are not available.

Because of the limitations just described and the limited resolution of the images, modifications in the technique of ProstaScint scanning have been proposed to improve its performance and are currently being evaluated. The modifications include using more imaging cameras to improve resolution and combining the ProstaScint with a tagged red blood cell scan to allow for subtraction of the blood-pool artifact.

In spite of the lack of information regarding the accuracy of the ProstaScint scan, it is FDA-approved and has already entered clinical practice. However, the efficacy of the ProstaScint scan still must be demonstrated before it can be included as a part of the standard staging evaluation. ProstaScint scanning should not be considered standard care since (1) the sensitivity and specificity of the test remain unproven and (2) some studies have shown that spiral CT scanning might be more a more sensitive indicator of metastatic disease (Seltzer et al. in press).

Prostatic acid phosphatase (PAP), another serum marker that can identify disseminated prostate cancer, was the first prostate-specific serum marker that was widely used for prostate cancer staging (Huggins and Hodges 1941). Besides its use as a diagnostic marker, many studies have shown that PAP levels can be directly correlated to the stage of prostate cancer, and can also be correlated to treatment response following hormonal manipulation (Foti et al. 1977, Huggins and Hodges 1941). Although it was classically believed that an elevated PAP (based on the Roy enzymatic assay) was an insensitive indicator for the presence of advanced cancer, it has also been reported that an elevated enzymatic PAP is very specific for the presence of micrometastatic disease (Bauer and Schmeller 1984, Lowe and Trauzzi 1993, Oesterling et al. 1987, Paulson et al. 1990). More recently, a PAP radio-immune assay has allowed the detection of lower levels of PAP, but it cannot reliably discriminate between the presence or absence of micrometastatic disease (Stamey et al. 1987, Wilson et al. 1983). Thus, while the presence of an elevated Roy enzymatic PAP is indicative of metastatic cancer and can predict the failure of local therapy, a normal PAP does not exclude the existence of an advanced tumor.

Because surgery and radiation therapy are contra-indicated in the patient who has an elevated enzymatic PAP due to the presumed presence of metastatic disease, some clinicians advocate the use of the old Roy enzymatic PAP in the staging of a patient where the suspicion of advanced cancer is high and needs to be confirmed. However, PSA and other staging modalities (pelvic CT, bone scan, and MRI) have largely eradicated PAP from modern prostate cancer diagnostic and staging algorithms because it rarely adds unique staging information (Gao et al. 1997).

Wrap-up. Standard prostate cancer staging includes a pre-treatment PSA and a digital rectal examination. In patients who have small prostate nodules and a PSA less than 10 ng/dl, no further evaluation is needed. In contrast, patients with a PSA greater than 10 should have a bone scan. PAP, CT scanning, MRI, or ProstaScint scanning can also be used in selected circumstances, although the data supporting the use of these tests are more limited.

Standards for surgical care

Surgical treatment for localized prostate cancer involves removing the cancer-containing prostate gland as well as the pelvic lymph nodes using one of two surgical approaches: through the perineum (perineal prostatectomy) or through an incision above the pubic bone (radical prostatectomy). The perineal prostatectomy has the advantage of a shorter post-operative course. However, since perineal prostatectomy is associated with a (1) higher risk of rectal injury (Boeckmann and Jakse 1995; Lassen and Kearse 1995), (2) a lower chance that potency will be preserved, (3) a higher risk of positive margins (Wahle et al. 1990), and (4) the necessity of performing separate procedure to examine the pelvic lymph nodes (Lerner et al. 1994), the surgical standard has moved away from the perineal prostatectomy towards the radical retropubic prostatectomy.

Radical prostatectomy. The method by which radical prostatectomy is performed is highly variable. Since the first description of radical prostatectomy in the 1980s by Dr. Patrick Walsh, numerous modifications to the surgical technique and peri-operative care have been devised with the goals of decreasing the length of surgery, blood loss, and surgical complications. Retropubic, perineal, nerve sparing, modified apical dissections, and bladder neck sparing represent some of the variations that have been used.

Unfortunately, beyond a single identified report that used validated methods to correlate improved urinary outcomes to a change in the surgical technique (Klein 1993), the scientific literature lacks well-designed studies demonstrating that these new approaches result in better outcomes. However, despite the limitations of the medical literature, several conclusions may be drawn about the technique of radical prostatectomy; these are detailed below.

Several authors have published the following observations about the *nerve-sparing* technique. (1) Nerve-sparing surgery can be performed in selected patients (specifically, in those men who have small palpable tumors away from the edge of the gland) without compromising the ability to remove all of the cancer (Oesterling 1993); (2) potency rates as high as 60-70% can be expected following radical retropubic prostatectomy if bilateral nerve sparing is performed by experienced surgeons in carefully selected young patients (Lee and Oesterling 1997, Quinlan et al. 1991); (3) patients who have only unilateral nerve sparing have lower potency rates than men who had bilateral nerve sparing, (Bigg et al. 1990); (4) if a patient has a high-grade, bulky tumor, or if the nerves are adherent to the prostate, nerve sparing should not be performed (Bigg et al. 1990, Catalona 1990); (5) older patients have a lower chance of retaining sexual function, (Quinlan et al. 1991); and (6) nerve sparing and preservation of potency are less feasible in a perineal than in a retropubic approach (Wahle et al. 1990).

Evaluations of surgical outcomes have demonstrated that variations in surgical technique can affect *preservation of bladder control*. Specific modifications in the apical dissection and urethral anastomosis can improve the return of continence following surgery (Klein 1993). The method used to incise the bladder neck and the number of sutures connecting the urethra to the bladder do not appear to be important in preserving continence. However, since bladder neck contractures result in a higher risk of incontinence (Licht et al. 1994), employing "bladder neck sparing" dissections, which lower the risk of stricture without compromising the ability to eradicate the tumor, helps to preserve continence. In addition, the "Vest" procedure for connecting the bladder to the urethra results in a higher stricture rate and should be avoided (Berlin et al. 1994).

The remainder of the literature that discusses modifications in surgical technique in an effort to improve continence rates (for example, the use of endoscopes or urethral balloons to improve suture placement) lacks valid data documenting advantages to these modifications

(Douglas et al. 1997a). Some studies provide no outcome data at all; others fail to use validated methods to measure post-operative bladder function, or do not have a long enough post-operative follow-up period to draw conclusions about outcomes.

Additional controversies regarding the surgical approach to prostate cancer revolve around the use of *epidural or general anesthesia* to decrease blood loss, the routine banking of autologous blood prior to surgery, and the use of hemodilution techniques (Goodnough et al. 1994b). Although in case series the type of anesthesia used does not appear to impact overall complication rates, evidence from a prospective, randomized study indicates that epidural anesthesia results in less blood loss (Shir et al. 1995). Nevertheless, epidural anesthesia has not become the practice standard, and most radical prostatectomies continue to be performed under general aneasthesia. The majority of surgical series report autologous storage of 2 units of blood in most patients to decrease patients' need for donated blood, even though this practice has been shown not to be cost-effective.

A final issue in trying to improve surgical outcomes involves implementing *clinical care pathways*. By standardizing post-operative care, these pathways aim to improve the quality and decrease the cost of surgical treatment. Through the use of such pathways, the average hospital stay following radical retropubic prostatectomy can be decreased from 7 days to 2 days without an increase in post-operative complications, re-admissions for complications, or a decrease in patient satisfaction (measured prospectively with validated instruments) (Klein et al. 1996, Koch and Smith 1995, Litwin et al. 1997, Litwin et al. 1996). With these reductions in hospital stay, the post-operative course following perineal prostatectomy and radical retropubic prostatectomy are now comparable, further establishing the latter as the standard for prostate cancer surgery. Despite these observations, other intervening factors may also be responsible for the effect on hospital stay thought to be related to the implementation of clinical care pathways.

Wrap-up. No randomized controlled trials have evaluated the surgical treatment for prostate cancer. The standard surgical approach to the patient with localized prostate cancer is based upon surgical case series and anecdotal experience. Radical retropubic prostatectomy has become the standard surgical treatment for localized prostate cancer. In selected potent patients who have small tumors and no nerve fixation at the time of surgery, the nerve-sparing technique may be appropriate. In patients who are already impotent or in whom the erectile nerves are fixed to the prostate, nerve-sparing surgery does not appear to have any benefits. Bladder neck preservation is preferred, but numerous other modifications to the surgical technique remain unproven in their ability to improve the results of surgery (Schellhammer et al. 1997). Despite evidence to suggest that it can decrease blood loss during surgery, epidural anesthesia is not in widespread use, and most surgeons continue to offer patients autologous blood donation even though it is not cost-effective. Clinical care pathways are being used to decrease the cost of surgery while attempting to maintain or even improve outcomes.

Post-operative follow-up

Appropriate follow-up for patients who have undergone radical prostatectomy for prostate cancer is undefined. The goals of follow-up are to monitor patients for treatment complications and to detect cancer recurrence. As these are also the important outcomes of treatment, monitoring patients for events after radical prostatectomy or radiation therapy is extremely important for both clinical research and evaluating quality of care.

Monitoring PSA. Identifying and treating late complications is a primary reason for patient visits after surgery or radiation. Follow-up is also done to detect cancer recurrence. The most sensitive way to detect cancer recurrence involves the use of PSA (Ferguson and Oesterling 1994). For patients who have undergone radical prostatectomy, the PSA should be undetectable if all PSA-producing tissue was removed. Similarly, the PSA following radiation therapy should also be very low if all the cancer was destroyed by the treatment, although it can take up to a year for the PSA to reach its nadir value (in brachytherapy, there is some evidence that it can take up to 5 years for the PSA to reach its lowest point) (Schellhammer et al. 1997). In these patients, the persistence of PSA in the bloodstream is usually indicative of residual prostate cells, although it is not necessarily indicative that there are residual *cancer* cells.

Due to the power of serum PSA to detect the presence of PSA-producing cells and its ability to detect recurrent cancer many months before symptoms or radiographic evidence of cancer recurrence occurs, PSA has become the intermediate end point by which the success of different prostate cancer treatments has been measured and compared (Malkowicz 1996). Recent development of an ultrasensitive assay for PSA has lowered the biological detection limit to 0.02 ng/mL (the biological detection limit is defined as the PSA level that the assay can reliably discriminate from a level of zero); however, the utility of this ultrasensitive assay is controversial (Witherspoon 1997, Yu et al. 1995).

The utility of detecting asymptomatic cancer recurrence is questionable in a disease process where there is no effective salvage therapy. Although androgen deprivation therapy can significantly reduce tumors, this response may be only temporary. Recently, new evidence has appeared that suggests a potential salutory role for early hormone treatment in men with advanced disease and with positive lymph nodes (Messing et al. 1999). The clinical usefulness of detecting asymptomatic cancer recurrences based on the existence of an elevated PSA remains controversial, but this is an area of rapidly changing opinions.

The use of PSA as an intermediate end point to determine success or failure following surgery or radiation treatment must also be questioned (Stein et al. 1992) . Historically, a rising PSA following surgery or radiation was considered to be a harbinger of the inevitable events of cancer progression, metastatic cancer, and subsequent death from the tumor. On average, PSA relapse precedes clinically detectable cancer recurrence (based on physical examination or bone scan) by between 6 to 48 months, with the development of assays that can detect even smaller amounts of PSA theoretically increasing this lead time (Lange et al. 1989, Yu et al. 1995).

The importance of the doubling time of PSA. More recent evidence suggests that a PSA relapse does not necessarily indicate that clinically measurable cancer recurrence will ever occur (Pound et al. 1999). Partin and associates showed that information about the rate of change and the time that PSA relapse occurs can separate patients who have a relapse in the pelvis versus distant relapse following radical prostatectomy, and therefore could identify patients who could benefit from adjuvant pelvic radiation therapy (Partin et al. 1994). However, in this series, the majority of patients had a relapse based on PSA alone, with no other detectable signs of recurrent cancer. Patel et al. further studied the utility of PSA velocity and patterns of cancer recurrence in patients following radical prostatectomy. Based on an average follow-up of 4 years, these investigators showed that patients who have a rapidly rising PSA (doubling time less than 6 months) had a high probability of developing a clinically detectable, distant relapse. In contrast, patients who have a slowly rising PSA (doubling time of more than 14 months) had a low probability of developing any other signs or symptoms of cancer recurrence. Thus, patients who have a rapidly rising PSA have a significant chance of developing symptomatic distant metastasis. These patients are probably best treated by immediate hormonal therapy. In contrast, patients who have a PSA that is taking more than a year to double in size are likely to have tumor recurrence in the prostate fossa. In fact, the tumor may not ever become clinically apparent during the patient's life. For such patients, either adjuvant radiation therapy to the pelvis or observation are reasonable management alternatives.

Despite the controversies that surround the utility of PSA as a predictor of eventual death from prostate cancer, post-treatment PSA monitoring is a widely accepted practice and a valued outcome. In the asymptomatic patient, post-operative follow-up usually consists of a history, a physical examination with digital rectal examination, a serum PSA measurement, and some sort of assessment of post-operative bladder and sexual function.

Most physicians rely on the history and physical exam to evaluate patients' post-treatment urinary tract function and quality of life, both in clinical practice and in research studies. However, research suggests that physician assessments do not always accurately reflect patients' experiences (Litwin et al. 1998b). Therefore, although it is not yet standard practice, a more accurate way to evaluate patient outcomes is having the patient complete a validated survey instrument. Such instruments, which allow quantitative assessment of factors such as quality of life, potency, and continence, are necessary to obtain accurate data for research studies, but they would probably also be useful in clinical practice (Reifel and Ganz, 1998).

Outcome measures following surgery

In general, the goals of surgery are curing cancer, prolonging the patient's life, and preserving quality of life. Thus, the standard outcomes that have been measured following surgery include (1) freedom from clinical relapse, (2) freedom from biochemical (PSA) relapse, (3) survival, (4) peri-operative complications, (5) post-operative sexual function, (6) post-operative bladder control, and (7) health-related quality of life. However, despite the existence of well-defined complications following surgery, controversy remains over the best way to measure these outcomes and to quantify the relative impact that these individual factors have on the patient's overall sense of well being.

Disease-free survival. Following radical prostatectomy, there are two types of cancer recurrence. *Clinical recurrence*, defined as a recurrence that is detectable on physical examination or by radiologic evaluation, and *biochemical recurrence*, defined as a recurrence that is suggested by a rising PSA level after surgery. Earlier studies (before the discovery of PSA) used clinical recurrence as the outcome to assess, a particularly useful approach since clinical recurrence is a significant predictor of the cancer's progression and of eventual death. However, this definition was limited by clinicians' inability to detect cancer recurrence until it was advanced, and the variability in how often radiographic studies were performed to detect recurrence.

More recently, the PSA test has become the preferred surrogate marker for cancer cure following surgery because it (1) can provide objective data on cancer recurrence, (2) is relatively inexpensive and non-invasive, and (3) allows for the detection of prostate cancer recurrence many months to years before it becomes clinically detectable. After surgery, the PSA should remain undetectable. A detectable PSA level following surgery has been considered to be definitive proof that there are prostate cells growing somewhere in the patient, which implies that the cancer has recurred.

However, despite the apparent power of PSA to detect recurrent prostate cancer, the prognostic value of a PSA recurrence has recently come into question. Approximately 30% of men have a biochemical recurrence of their cancer following surgery (D'Amico et al. 1995). However, a PSA relapse following surgery does not necessarily imply that a clinically significant cancer relapse will follow, nor is death from recurrent cancer inevitable (Oesterling 1993). Up to 50% of patients with a PSA relapse, especially those in whom the post-operative PSA is rising very slowly, will remain free of any signs or symptoms of their recurrent cancer despite the presence of a detectable PSA (Kupelian et al. 1996, Lerner et al. 1996, Oesterling 1993). The majority of these patients will likely outlive their cancer recurrence, obviating the need for any additional treatment (Oesterling 1993). Furthermore, some of the other patients who have a PSA recurrence following prostatectomy may still enjoy a normal lifespan through the use of palliative treatments such as androgen deprivation, which can slow the tumor's growth.

Quality of life. In addition to cancer control and overall survival, there are other outcomes that are important to patients. The need for transfusions after surgery can expose the patient to infections, while rectal injury or bladder neck/urethral stricture formation can result in disability and the need for secondary surgical procedures. Furthermore, radical prostatectomy can have a significant impact on the patient's long-term sexual function and bladder function: some patients may be willing to exchange some quantity of life for improved quality.

The relative importance of cancer control, surgical risks, potency, and continence on an individual patient's overall satisfaction with treatment is unknown. Some studies have tried to measure the importance of sexual function relative to the cure. However, the main study based its assessment on responses of a group of men who did not have prostate cancer (Singer et al. 1991). The hypothetical nature of their responses may not reflect the decision-making process of patients who actually have cancer. In addition, many men who undergo prostatectomy are at an age where sexual function is already diminishing, and there are many treatments available that can restore sexual function following surgery.

Short-term complications: bleeding, rectal injury, stricture. The medical literature commonly reports certain outcomes following surgery. Some of the standard outcome measures involve the rates of complications that are directly attributable to the treatment, such as intra-operative bleeding, rectal injury, or bladder neck contracture (stricture). However, although many surgical series routinely report these complication rates, it is not always clear how the data were collected, since both prospective and retrospective case identification can result in underreporting of the true complication rate. The literature also contains scant information about how bladder neck contractures are defined and diagnosed: differences in stricture rates reported between different series maybe related as much to case identification as to actual differences in the incidence of this complication. Estimates of blood loss are relatively unreliable, especially since the fluid in the suction canister may contain both blood and urine. Inter-observer variability in estimating blood loss, and inter-individual variance in the criteria for transfusion also limit the utility of blood-loss data. However, despite these difficulties, the standard measures of peri-operative outcome that have been widely reported include operative mortality, deep vein thrombosis, pulmonary embolus, intra-operative blood loss, rectal injury, and stricture formation.

Based on an analysis of these outcome measures, we can draw some conclusions about standard intra-operative and peri-operative care of radical prostatectomy patients.

1. Blood loss can be decreased through maneuvers to control the dorsal vein complex, although objective data that can actually compare blood loss between different techniques are lacking (Davis and Fair 1994, Hrebinko and O'Donnell 1993).

2. Early results suggested that ligating the hypogastric arteries can also decrease blood loss, but this has not been confirmed in other studies.

3. Autologous blood donation is a common practice and remains prevalent despite the number of studies that show it not to be cost effective (Goh et al. 1997, Goodnough et al. 1994a).

4. There is some evidence that epidural anesthesia can lessen the amount of blood loss relative to general anesthesia, but these findings have not been replicated beyond the original reports from the initial prospective, randomized trial (Frank et al. 1998, Shir et al. 1995).

We can also draw some conclusions about short-term complications.

1. Although rectal injury is an uncommon complication, there is some evidence that perineal approaches are associated with a higher risk of rectal injury.

2. Bladder neck contracture is another post-operative phenomenon that can be attributed to differences in surgical technique.

3. Although the bladder neck-sparing approach appears to minimize this risk, the use of the Vest method to complete the vesico-urethral anastomosis results in a higher risk of post-operative stricture formation (Berlin et al. 1994).

Long-term complications: impotence and incontinence. Measurement of long term complications (continence and potency) are also standard outcome measures for prostatectomy patients. A recent study by Stanford and colleagues details for the first time the quality of life results of a population-based investigation of community patients in both the Medicare and non-Medicare age groups (Stanford et al. 2000). In terms of bladder function, most current series report that only 20% of patients who undergo radical prostatectomy will have any degree of stress urinary incontinence following surgery, with less than 1% having severe leakage (deKernion et al. 1998). However, other case series have reported much higher rates of post-surgical incontinence. At this time, it is unclear if these differences were due to differences in the skill of the surgeons or in the way that post-operative continence was measured (Fowler et al. 1995, Jonler et al. 1994). The most accurate way to measure continence appears to be through the prospective use of validated survey instruments or diaries. However, most of the studies that

27

reported post-operative continence rates collected the data in ways that were subject to significant biases (e.g., most of the data were based on the physician's assessment of the patient's bladder function).

Measurement of post-operative sexual function has also been limited (Mettlin et al. 1997). The technique of peeling the erectile nerves off of the lateral edge of the prostate has markedly improved sexual function following surgery, but the return of normal erections also depends on the pre-operative sexual function and the age of the patient. However, studies that focused on sexual function were largely based on physician-patient interviews, with baseline sexual function data often missing (Mettlin et al. 1997). In addition, while interviews of the spouse or the use of a validated survey instrument might provide a more accurate picture of pre-treatment and post-treatment function, most studies collected data via interviews, and had ambiguous definitions of potency and no clear cut method to measure this outcome.

Wrap-up. Outcome measures that have been widely used to assess patients who have undergone radical prostatectomy include disease-free survival (based both on PSA and on clinical grounds), short-term complications (bleeding, rectal injury, and stricture), and long-term complications (impotence and incontinence). Significant differences in these outcomes have been reported by different case series; unfortunately, differences in methodology do not allow us to distinguish variations that result from differences in patient selection, measurement, or the quality of care (Soh et al. 1997). Furthermore, the relative contribution of each of these many outcomes to the patient's well-being and satisfaction with treatment remains to be determined. We need to understand the relative effect of each outcome if we want to accurately assess important outcomes following surgery (Shrader-Bogen et al. 1997).

Definitions of high quality care

Although there has been a hesitation to use the term "high quality" in the literature that looks at surgery for prostate cancer, some papers clearly focus on modifications in the pre-operative evaluation, surgical technique, and peri-operative care that were intended to improve the outcome over the current standard of care (Berlin et al. 1994, Catalona 1990, D'Amico et al. 1997, Davis and Fair 1994, Douglas et al. 1997a, Frank et al. 1998, Gao et al. 1997, Goh et al. 1997, Goodnough et al. 1994a, Goodnough et al. 1994b, Hrebinko and O'Donnell 1993, Lee and

Oesterling 1997, Lerner et al. 1996, Licht et al. 1994, Malkowicz 1996, Oesterling 1993, Shir et al. 1995, Stamey et al. 1987, Yu et al. 1995).

In terms of the *staging evaluation*, the standard tests include the pre-treatment PSA and the DRE, with radiologic imaging using pelvic CT scan and bone scanning applied in selected situations. However, the current modalities used for staging are limited by a tendency to underestimate the tumor stage and tumor grade. It has been suggested that spiral CT scanning, ProstaScint scanning, and endorectal MRI all represent improvements in the ability to stage prostate cancer prior to definitive therapy. However, the data for each of these tests are limited and need to be replicated at other centers before they can considered part of a higher standard.

In terms of the *surgical approach* to patients, numerous technical papers focus on subtle modifications of the original Walsh technique that are designed to minimize blood loss, improve potency, or improve continence (Bell 1993, Douglas et al. 1997a, Hanash 1992, Klein 1993, Maggio et al. 1992, Menon and Vaidyanathan 1995). Of all of these modifications, only three have been proven efficacious with adequate case numbers and appropriate methodology: they involve the suspending the urethra to the symphysis to permit an earlier return of continence (Eastham et al. 1996), modifying the apical dissection (Klein 1993), and sparing of the bladder neck muscle fibers, which can decrease the risk of stricture without affecting the surgeon's ability to completely remove the primary tumor (Gomez et al. 1993). Numerous other reports describe techniques to improve the dissection, improve suture placement in the anastomosis, or improve vascular control, but none of these reports provides empirical evidence of the technique's benefit (Bell 1993, Hanash 1992, Maggio et al. 1992, Petroski et al. 1996).

In terms of *peri-operative care*, the use of clinical pathways to standardize post-operative management may also be considered a measure of "high quality" since there is strong evidence based on valid measurements that (1) hospital costs and length of stay can be safely decreased and (2) the patients had a high degree of satisfaction despite the decreased amount of time spent in the hospital (Klein et al. 1996, Koch and Smith 1995, Litwin et al. 1997, Litwin et al. 1996).

Summary

Standard evaluation. The standard pre-treatment staging evaluation for patients with clinically localized prostate cancer is limited in its accuracy. The DRE and pre-treatment PSA are the cornerstones of the standard evaluation; conversely, up to 60% of patients will be understaged when bone scan and CT scan are used. Other tests such as MRI or ProstaScint scanning may be able to improve pre-treatment staging, although their utility still needs to be proven in large, prospective studies.

Surgical standards. The anatomic nerve-sparing radical retropubic prostatectomy, using a modified bladder neck dissection and modified urethro-vesical anastomosis, has been shown to yield optimal results in methodologically sound, statistically valid studies. Although many other modifications in the surgical technique and peri-operative care have been proposed, there is a paucity of data to prove that these modifications produce better outcomes than standard surgical approaches.

Outcomes. Few studies have used validated methods to measure the level of function or the degree of patient satisfaction following treatment. However, the standard outcome measures have included (1) cancer control, (2) peri-operative complications, (3) post-operative bladder function, (4) post-operative sexual function, and (5) resource utilization. Although we know that the surgical treatment of prostate cancer can have adverse effects on all of these parameters, we do not understand the relative importance of each.

Chapter 3

REVIEW OF THE MEDICAL LITERATURE
ON RADIATION THERAPY

In this chapter, we review the medical literature on radiation therapy for prostate cancer. Most conclusions in this literature are based on case series, retrospective case-controls, and expert opinion. Only a few conclusions are based on data derived from randomized, prospective trials. As a consequence, the reported links between process, structure, and outcome in the radiation therapy literature are often based on inference and conventional wisdom.

Pre-treatment evaluation of the radiation therapy patient

The goals of the pre-treatment evaluation of the radiation therapy patient are similar to those of the surgical patient. Identifying organ-confined disease is the most important prognostic factor that determines the success or failure of local treatment: patients who have more advanced disease need more extensive therapy (such as dose-escalation, field modifications, or adjuvant anti-androgen medications) (Hanks et al. 1996a). Patients who have markedly elevated pre-treatment PSA levels, clinical stage T2B-C tumors, and high-grade tumors all have a higher rate of cancer recurrence following radiation therapy (Ennis et al. 1994, Movsas et al. 1997, Pisansky et al. 1997a, Pisansky et al. 1997b, Roach et al. 1992).

Although it is assumed that such pretreatment factors can be correlated with increasing tumor volume and stage, it remains unclear if recurrent (or persistent) cancer following radiation treatment is due to inadequate treatment, the inherent resistance of some prostate tumors to radiation therapy, or the selection of patients who already have occult metastatic disease (Ennis et al. 1994, Hanks et al. 1996a). In any case, standardized determination of these critical pre-treatment variables is necessary for accurately stratifying patients for outcome analysis, and will allow for the improved study of the process variables (such as dose and treatment volume) that affect rates of cancer control and complications.

Important prognostic factors. The pre-treatment clinical stage, serum PSA level, and histologic grade are the most important prognostic factors, with imaging tests, surgical lymph node staging, and prostate acid phosphatase also having value in selected patients (Fukunaga-

Johnson et al. 1997, Geara et al. 1994, Russell et al. 1991). These factors have been previously discussed in relation to the evaluation of patients prior to radical prostatectomy. Of these factors, the *pre-treatment PSA* appears to be the most important prognostic factor based on univariate and multivariate analysis, where patients have a greater risk of relapse if the pretreatment PSA level is greater than 10 to 20 ng/dl (Fukunaga-Johnson et al. 1997, Leibel et al. 1996, Movsas et al. 1997, Ritter et al. 1992, Zagars et al. 1995c). Four years following treatment, approximately 50-60% of patients who had a pretreatment PSA > 20 ng/mL relapsed due to either persistent local disease or metastasis, while the 3-year survival with no evidence of disease (NED) has been reported to be 86% for patients who had pre-treatment PSA levels less than 15 ng/mL (Hanks et al. 1996a, Zagars and Pollack 1995,). Since the absolute PSA level is proportional to the overall volume of cancer, treatment failure in these patients could be due either to the inadequate eradication of bulky local disease or to selection of patients who have occult metastatic disease (Schellhammer et al. 1993, Zagars et al. 1995b).

The *Gleason score and clinical stage* are also important pre-treatment factors, although the accuracy of their measurement is less certain than PSA (Beyer and Priestley 1997). The accurate determination of the pre-treatment histologic grade is limited in radiation therapy patients because the determination of the Gleason score of the tumor is estimated from an analysis of a few small cores of tissue. Sampling error and distortion of the glandular architecture within the biopsy make interpretation of biopsies difficult, and variations in the number of biopsies obtained also affect the accuracy of the pre-treatment evaluation (Albertsen et al. 1999, Bostwick 1994). The exact number of biopsies that is optimal for accurate diagnosis is undefined (Eskew et al. 1998), although a mapping of the prostate with a 5-zone method appears to give more information than sextant biopsies, and sextant biopsies appear to yield more information than quadrant biopsies.

Many studies divided cancers into "low," "intermediate," and "high" grade categories. While older studies combined Gleason 5, 6 and 7 tumors together, more recent data suggested that Gleason 7 tumors, due to their behavior, should either be a separate category, or should be included with the high grade cancers (Russell et al. 1991, Tefilli et al. 1999, Zagars et al. 1995a, Zagars et al. 1995c). Additionally, recent data from Stanford suggested that the percentage of high-grade cancer in a specimen is the most important predictor of successful treatment following radical prostatectomy (Stamey 1995). At any rate, the prognostic stratification of tumors based on the Gleason score has been flawed in the past; however, despite these flaws, the stratification of tumors based on tumor grade or Gleason score has been shown to have prognostic value (Anscher and Prosnitz 1991, Lai et al. 1991, Lerner et al. 1991, Perez et al. 1989, Zietman et al. 1995).

Clinical stage is also valuable in pretreatment evaluation, although it cannot reliably detect extra-capsular disease, and is hampered by high inter-observer variability (Hanks et al. 1996a, Perez et al. 1993, Roach et al. 1992). Despite these limitations, the clinical tumor stage is independently correlated with the outcomes of biochemical relapse, clinical recurrence, NED survival, and overall survival (Arcangeli et al. 1995, Lai et al. 1992, Lai et al. 1991, Lerner et al. 1991). Although the finding of extra-capsular tumor is a very specific and clinically useful finding on DRE, the false-negative rate of DRE to predict organ-confined disease is 48% (O'Dowd et al. 1997). Furthermore, the definition of palpably normal glands (T1C), and the categorization of varying degrees of prostate induration, asymmetry, and nodularity can vary across examiners.

This variation can affect the accuracy of patient stratification based on pre-treatment variables (Smith and Catalona 1995). A comparison of clinical evaluations, done on the same patients by the same physician in the office and later in the operating room, showed that 50% of patients changed clinical stage after a more thorough DRE was done under anesthesia (Glick et al. 1990). However, given the ease of obtaining the data, and the lack of other modalities that can be used to evaluate the local extent of cancer (such as CT, MRI, or ultrasound), DRE will remain an important prognostic variable. At best, CT and MRI have only a 30-60% sensitivity for detecting extra-capsular disease (O'Dowd et al. 1997).

Beyond the use of PSA, DRE, and tumor grade, the use of other pre-treatment tests is more controversial (O'Dowd et al. 1997). Although pre-treatment evaluation of radiation therapy candidates involves determining the same factors that are measured in surgical patients, the main difference between radiation therapy and surgery is the lack of pathologic confirmation in irradiated patients that the tumor was truly organ-confined. When prostate and adjacent lymph nodes are removed, pathologic analysis of the specimen permits precise stratification of the cancer based on tumor grade, tumor volume, extra-capsular extension, and lymph node status.

33

Thus, in surgical patients the pathologic stage can be used both as a prognostic factor and as an outcome measure that indicates the success or failure of surgery to eradicate cancer. In contrast, the actual stage and grade of the cancer remain uncertain in the radiation therapy patient and can only be inferred from the pre-treatment staging evaluation, using a mix of objective and subjective measurements.

Besides local tumor factors, the juxta-regional lymph node status is one of the most powerful predictors of outcome following treatment, since it identifies patients who have nodal metastasis and therefore are at risk of distant tumor relapse and eventual death from prostate cancer (Arcangeli et al. 1995, Gervasi et al. 1989, Hanks et al. 1991, Lee and Sause 1994, Perez et al. 1989). Node-positive patients were found to have a 57%-78% chance of dying from prostate cancer 10-15 years following radiation therapy; the rate was only 15-17% for node-negative patients (Lee and Sause 1994, Lerner et al. 1991).

Determination of lymph node status is based on pathologic analysis, which implies either a percutaneous biopsy or formal lymphadenectomy. However, there is currently no standard approach to the pre-treatment evaluation of the lymph nodes prior to radiation therapy: CT scans and lymphangiography are clearly limited in their sensitivity and specificity, and surgical lymph node dissection potentially results in a higher complication rate following radiation therapy (Lee and Sause 1994, O'Dowd et al. 1997, Perez et al. 1988). The Radiation Therapy Oncology Group (RTOG) found that patients who were found to be free of nodal metastasis based on surgical staging had better overall and disease free survival when compared to patients who were staged by lymphangiography (Asbell et al. 1989). Additionally, pre-treatment lymphadenectomy is associated with a higher rate of complications following radiation therapy, although the effect of the confounding factor of tumor burden is unclear (Rosen et al. 1985).

Fortunately, in the modern era of PSA-based prostate cancer detection, rates of lymph node involvement have declined, and the status of the lymph nodes can be estimated based on other clinical parameters. For example, although the Partin tables have limitations, they can provide a probabilistic estimate that the lymph nodes will be involved with the tumor (for more details, see the discussion of the Partin tables in the surgery section) (Naitoh et al. 1997, Partin et al. 1997). Some of the other mathematical models that predict nodal status, tumor stage, and overall response to radiation therapy were nicely summarized by Movsas and colleagues (Movsas et al. 1997).

Side effects of therapy. In addition to tumor control outcomes, the adverse effects of therapy and the effects of treatment on quality of life are also important treatment endpoints. Radiation therapy can have adverse effects on bowel, bladder, and sexual function, with the patient's underlying prostate cancer and baseline lower urinary tract symptomatology potentially confounding outcomes analysis. Many radiation therapy patients tend to be older, with impaired bladder emptying, decreased sexual function, and bowel problems that existed prior to treatment. Differences in the study population can exist in baseline function, and these differences can have an adverse effect on outcome analysis independent of the factors due to the type of treatment. For example, older patients do worse than younger patients in terms of recovering bladder and sexual function following treatment (Talcott et al. 1998). Thus, measurement of baseline bowel, bladder, and sexual function is needed to establish a cause-and-effect relationship between side effects and different process.

The main challenge in assessing side effects is that there is currently no widely accepted way to measure bladder, bowel, and sexual function. The RAND 36-Item Health Survey (SF-36), the UCLA Prostate Cancer Index, the Functional Assessment of Cancer Therapy (FACT), and the Prostate Cancer Treatment Outcomes Questionnaire (PCTO-Q) are some of the instruments currently in use (Albertsen et al. 1999, Beard et al. 1997, Litwin et al. 1995, Shrader-Bogen et al. 1997, Talcott et al. 1998). Furthermore, retrospective determinations of baseline function have limited value due to recall bias in which the patient forgets pretreatment function and attributes all symptoms to the effects of treatment (Litwin and McGuigan 1999). The limitations of chart review and physician-reported adverse events have been previously discussed, with patients tending to under-report their symptoms and physicians tending to downplay the symptoms' severity (Talcott et al. 1998).

Thus, the best approach to measuring the side effects of therapy involves objective and prospective measurement of bladder, bowel, and sexual function using unbiased data collection methods. Although trained interviewers can be used to assess symptoms, validated survey instruments can also be used to measure function. These instruments can be cumbersome to use; however, the best way to measure function before and after treatment will involve prospective application of patient-centered instruments. As such, the RTOG recently established a Quality of Life Subcommittee that will oversee and facilitate quality of life research for future RTOG studies (Wasserman and McDonald 1995).

Although less critical, patient stratification by ethnicity and socio-economic status might also be important, since these pre-treatment variables affect reporting of adverse effects, access to health care, and the degree of bother associated with the toxic effects of treatment (Albertsen et al. 1999, Roach et al. 1992). In addition, there is some evidence that ethnicity may have some direct relation to the intrinsic aggressiveness of prostate cancer (Austin and Convery 1993).

Finally, the patient's age, health, and co-morbidity at baseline are important pre-treatment parameters if overall survival is to be used as an outcome measurement (Roach et al. 1992). Prostate cancer tends to be a slow growing tumor, and patients who undergo radiation therapy tend to be older and to have competing illnesses that reduce life expectancy. A previous study clearly demonstrated the importance of co-morbid disease on overall survival in prostate cancer patients; patients who had high co-morbidity and low-grade cancer had a greater chance of dying from intercurrent disease (Albertsen et al. 1995). Thus, given the potential differences of opinion that exist between physicians regarding the use of watchful waiting versus aggressive treatment in older or sicker patients, baseline medical status must be established so that a valid comparison of survival outcomes can be made independent of the co-morbidity of the study population. How to best quantify co-morbid disease remains a problem, but there are many validated instruments that allow for reliable and reproducible measurement, including the Index of Coexistent Disease (ICED) and the Charlson Index.

Outcome measures in the radiation therapy literature

The outcomes reported in the radiation therapy literature are similar to those reported in surgical series in that they usually involve controlling either the cancer or the adverse effects of treatment. The limitation in the literature lies in how these events are defined, how the outcomes are measured, the intensity of the search that is used to detect an adverse outcome, and the time points after treatment at which the outcome is measured.

Cancer control. Many definitions of cancel control are used, including clinical local recurrence, local failure, distant metastasis, biochemical failure, NED survival, cause-specific survival, and overall survival. All of these definitions can be useful, but there is currently no standard schedule that is used to follow patients following radiation treatment. As a consequence, comparing different case series is difficult. The rate of cancer recurrence is partly a function of the frequency with which the patient is examined and partly a function of the intensity of the search for recurrent cancer (Albertsen et al. 1999, Russell et al. 1991, Schellhammer et al. 1993, Schneider et al. 1996). Although most radiation oncologists would agree that a physical examination and a serum PSA should be obtained during follow-up, the frequency with which these parameters should be checked is debatable. Furthermore, the role of post-treatment prostate biopsy, bone scan, and CT scan to detect cancer recurrence is controversial.

Survival. The most important outcome measurement is survival. However, very few studies are adequately powered to look at overall survival as an endpoint, since doing so requires 10 to 20 year data (Albertsen et al. 1999, Kuban et al. 1993). Additionally, since prostate cancer grows slowly and occurs in older men with multiple competing causes of death, many men will die from causes other than prostate cancer during follow-up. Although some investigators have tried to compensate for this factor by comparing the Kaplan-Meier survival curves of their treated patients to an age-adjusted, population-based sample, there are limits to the validity of such an analysis (Hanks et al. 1991, Hanks et al. 1994b, Kaplan et al. 1994, Perez et al. 1989, Zagars et al. 1988, Zietman et al. 1995). Patients who undergo treatment tend to be healthier than age matched controls, since sicker patients tend to be steered towards watchful waiting or primary hormonal therapy. Thus, adjustments for baseline co-morbidity and the aggressiveness of the primary tumor have to be made if overall survival is used as the final outcome measure. Patient stratification along these parameters should then allow for valid comparisons of survival outcomes between different facilities and treatment processes (Albertsen et al. 1999).

To overcome the limitations and long follow-up required for overall survival calculations, cause-specific mortality is used as a surrogate end point in some studies, where patients are censored at the time of death based on the cause of death (Gervasi et al. 1989, Kaplan et al. 1994). However, while cause-specific mortality is a potentially powerful endpoint, an analysis based on it might be unreliable since the cause of death can be open to interpretation. Review of death certificates alone can be inaccurate, while formal review of medical records can be cumbersome and requires trained chart abstractors (Albertsen et al. 1999, Gervasi et al. 1989).

The RTOG Patterns of Care Study was unable to determine the cause of death in up to 44% of the patients they reviewed (Roach et al. 1992). So although cause-specific survival is potentially a useful outcome measure, it is also more prone to error than overall survival.

Cancer recurrence. Cancer recurrence is also commonly used as an outcome since it can occur many years before death, and it allows for shorter follow-up intervals to assess the efficacy of treatment. Two types of cancer recurrence are currently reported: clinical recurrence and biochemical (PSA-based) recurrence.

Clinical local recurrence is one of the most common outcomes in the literature, since it is an indicator of active cancer growth and predicts the development of metastasis and eventual death from prostate cancer (Fuks et al. 1991, Lai et al. 1992, Lerner et al. 1991, Sylvester et al. 1997). Unfortunately, there are many definitions of local recurrence, including finding a new or enlarging prostate nodule; development of voiding symptoms, hematuria or ureteral obstruction that requires treatment; a positive post-treatment prostate biopsy; or the need for secondary treatments to alleviate symptoms from tumor growth in the pelvis or elsewhere in the body (Gervasi et al. 1989, Kaplan et al. 1994, Kaplan et al. 1992, Roach et al. 1992, Rosen et al. 1985, Russell et al. 1991, Schellhammer et al. 1993, Schneider et al. 1996).

It is unclear at this time which definition of local recurrence is best, since the findings on DRE are subjective and the development of local symptoms requiring treatment could be due to recurrent cancer, re-growth of benign prostate enlargement, or radiation therapy-associated voiding dysfunction. In addition, the positive predictive value of the DRE to detect local tumor recurrence based on biopsy is as low as 25% (Forman et al. 1993). Furthermore, a study of selected patients who underwent biopsy showed that the presence of a palpable nodule alone was not predictive of a positive biopsy result, with almost one third of these patients having a negative post-treatment prostate biopsy (Egawa et al. 1992). However, despite these limitations, post-radiation therapy DRE as an outcome measure remains a standard of care because the information is so easy to obtain.

The meaning of post-treatment biopsies is also controversial, given the varying rates of positive biopsies that are reported, the variations in the clinical indications for biopsy that exist between centers, and the difficulty in the histologic interpretation of the irradiated prostate. Furthermore, the meaning of a positive biopsy is not uniformly accepted, with the argument made that post-treatment prostate biopsy results do not correlate with outcome. It has been shown that histologic evidence of prostate cancer can persist up to 18 months following treatment, and may represent not a metabolically active tumor but rather cells that are lethally damaged and cannot replicate (Kuban et al. 1993). In addition, while it is argued that post-irradiation biopsies can be difficult to evaluate because of the similar appearance of radiation atypia and malignancy, the use of basal cell specific, high molecular weight cytokeratin immunostaining may be helpful in this regard (Kuban et al. 1993, Ragde et al. 1997). Furthermore, studies requiring post-irradiation prostate biopsies may suffer from detection bias because patients receiving routine care typically do not have an opportunity to undergo such biopsies.

The main controversies surrounding use of post-irradiation biopsy relate to the varying rates of positive biopsy that are reported in the literature, and the relation of biopsy results to other outcomes such as biochemical relapse, disease-free survival, and overall survival (Kuban et al. 1993). The rate of positive biopsy ranges from 10% to 93% in the literature, with this range reflecting the time interval between treatment to biopsy, the number of core samples obtained, the biopsy technique, and the patient population who underwent biopsy (Hanks 1992, Kabalin et al. 1989, Kaplan et al. 1992, Ragde et al. 1997). In general, biopsies performed less than 18 months following treatment with external beam radiation therapy (or less than 24 months for brachytherapy) had little prognostic value, while positive biopsies that were positive 2 or more years after the biopsy directly correlated to the appearance of a positive DRE, metastasis, and eventual death from prostate cancer (Sylvester et al. 1997). Overall, positive post-treatment biopsies were associated with a 60-70% clinical recurrence rate, versus 20-35% if the biopsy was negative (Kabalin et al. 1989, Kaplan et al. 1992, Ragde et al. 1997).

However, in the majority of patients who have a positive biopsy, there were other signs of persistent/recurrent cancer, including a biochemically (PSA) defined treatment failure, a positive bone scan, or a lesion felt on digital rectal examination (Hanks 1992, Kabalin et al. 1989, Prestidge et al. 1992). Only 5% of patients who have PSA levels less than 4.0 ng/mL will have a positive ultrasound-guided biopsy two years following treatment; approximately two-thirds of patients with an elevated post-treatment PSA will have a positive biopsy (Forman et al. 1993).

The results of biopsy also depended on the process that was used to obtain the biopsy (finger guided vs. ultrasound guided), the number of cores obtained, and whether or not a systematic mapping of the prostate was done (Egawa et al. 1992, Kabalin et al. 1989, Prestidge et al. 1992). Additionally, when patients who had a positive post-treatment biopsy were compared to those who had a negative post-treatment biopsy, the patients with recurrence had higher pre-treatment PSA levels, more locally advanced tumors, and higher-grade tumors (Kuban et al. 1993). In other words, one can predict which patients would have a positive post-treatment biopsy based on the pre-treatment parameters (PSA, clinical stage, and Gleason score) that identify high risk patients. The prostate biopsy alone is rarely the sole indicator that the cancer recurred following radiation therapy (Hanks 1992, Kaplan et al. 1994, Kuban et al. 1993). Thus, beyond the research environment, the clinical importance of systematically obtained, ultrasound-guided biopsies in patients is limited.

Clinical recurrence can be used as an outcome measure if a standard definition of it can be widely accepted. Changes on digital rectal examination (despite substantial inter- and intra-observer variability) or the signs as described above appear to be the more widely accepted options, while tissue diagnosis of recurrence does not appear to be as important in the modern era of PSA-based follow-up. In addition, new lesions on bone scan or CT scan are also accepted definitions of recurrence, although the rate of positive findings depends in part on the frequency with which imaging tests are being obtained (Albertsen et al. 1999, Russell et al. 1991, Schellhammer et al. 1993, Schneider et al. 1996).

In the PSA era, clinical recurrence as an outcome measure may have limited validity due to PSA-based decision-making, where hormone therapy is initiated before the appearance of a clinically detectable cancer recurrence. Wide practice variations in the use of anti-androgen medications in both the adjuvant and neo-adjuvant setting will also affect the timing and rate of clinical recurrence. Although studies such as the Bolla trial are trying to define the role of anti-androgen therapy in the irradiated patient, the timing and duration of these hormonal manipulations are indiscriminate and not based on sound scientific evidence (Bolla et al. 1998). These differences in the application of hormone therapy will confound any outcome analysis that is based on clinical recurrence, because the therapy suppresses and delays the appearance of clinically detectable recurrent tumors.

Due to the potential pitfalls regarding clinical recurrence as an endpoint, the initiation of secondary hormonal treatments to treat recurrent cancer has also been used as an outcome measure following radiation therapy (Fukunaga-Johnson et al. 1997, Russell et al. 1991, Schellhammer et al. 1993). However, again due to the indiscriminate and undefined use of hormone therapy at this time, the validity of such an outcomes analysis will be limited until consensus can be reached regarding (1) the role of neo-adjuvant or adjuvant hormone therapy, (2) the duration of the hormone treatment, and (3) the indications for the use of hormone therapy for relapse based on either clinical criteria or PSA level.

Biochemical (PSA) recurrence has become a common definition of recurrence used in the radiation therapy literature (Geara et al. 1994, Kaplan et al. 1992, Shipley et al. 1999). The discovery of PSA and its relationship to tumor growth and tumor burden has revolutionized the follow-up of patients who have prostate cancer. The primary advantages of PSA-defined cancer control are its objectivity, its predictive value to indicate cancer remission if the post-treatment PSA level is low, and the fact that it provides a 4-5 year lead time over other cancer control end points (Geara et al. 1994, Lee and Sause 1994, Russell et al. 1991). High pre-treatment PSA levels are strong predictors of treatment failure following external beam radiation therapy since PSA roughly correlates with primary tumor volume in the prostate, as well as with the probability of systemic disease (Zagars et al. 1995b). However, besides being prognostic, PSA is a valuable outcome measure since low post-treatment PSA levels correlate to NED survival, metastasis-free survival, and cause-specific survival (Lee and Sause 1994).

Problematically, the literature mentions multiple definitions of "biochemical" cancer relapse, and the stringency of the definition affects the reported success rates of radiation therapy. Although PSA should be undetectable (and remain so) in the patient who has undergone radical prostatectomy, the behavior of PSA following radiation therapy is less well defined. Furthermore, the relationship between biochemical recurrence and clinical recurrence is variable due to the heterogeneous clinical course of patients who have an elevated PSA after treatment (Pollack et al. 1994). However, despite these limitations, three commonly accepted definitions of biochemical cancer control have emerged: *normalization of PSA* (bringing the value of PSA to below the normal reference range), *stable PSA* (where the PSA remains unchanged or is

41

decreasing on serial evaluation), and *PSA nadir* (the point to where PSA reaches its lowest value after therapy).

Numerous papers have used *normalization of PSA* as an outcome measure, with correlation seen between the failure of PSA to normalize within 6 – 12 months of therapy and the later development of a clinical relapse (Beyer and Priestley 1997, Ritter et al. 1992, Russell et al. 1991, Schellhammer et al. 1993, Schneider et al. 1996). PSA normalization at 6 months was correlated to an 80 - 94% clinical disease free rate versus an 8 - 36% disease-free rate for those patients whose PSA levels did not normalize (Russell et al. 1991, Schneider et al. 1996).

The advantage of using normalization of PSA as an outcome is that it is applicable independent of the PSA assay used, but it is limited by its ability to identify patients who will remain clinically NED over the long term. With a median follow-up of 2 years, approximately 20% of patients who had normalization of their PSA after treatment already had signs of clinical recurrence (Ritter et al. 1992). In addition, this definition is invalid in the increasing numbers of patients with very low PSA levels who are being diagnosed with prostate cancer.

Although the rate of PSA decline following treatment was not a factor that predicted outcome (Kavadi et al. 1994, Ritter et al. 1992), a *stable PSA* following treatment is perhaps a more useful definition, since a rising PSA indicates biologically active recurrence. The majority of patients who fail clinically will have a rising PSA from 6 to 24 months prior to the occurrence of clinical relapse (Kavadi et al. 1994, Russell et al. 1991). The percentage of patients who will eventually progress clinically following a rising PSA has ranged from 63% to 91%; the variation is most likely due to variations in the number of PSA tests that were checked during follow-up, the heterogeneity in the velocity with which PSA rises after treatment, and variations in the overall length of follow-up (Geara et al. 1994, Kavadi et al. 1994, Pollack et al. 1994, Schneider et al. 1996). A recent large series from the Fox Chase Cancer Center showed that approximately 75% of patients will develop clinical evidence of cancer recurrence 5 years after the PSA began to rise; patients who have a rapidly rising PSA are more likely to develop distant metastasis (Lee et al. 1997).

The definition of a rising PSA has varied in the literature, and is also subject to the test-retest variation that exists within the PSA assay itself (Ragde et al. 1997). Definitions have included two consecutive rises above the normal range, two rises once the PSA is greater than

1.5, three consecutive rises of PSA greater than 10%, or two rises above the nadir value (Fukunaga-Johnson et al. 1997, Lee et al. 1997) . Although the best definition has yet to be determined, ASTRO has suggested that the following definition should be used for PSA failure: three consecutive rising PSA values, with the time of failure defined as the midpoint between the date of the nadir value and the date of the first rising PSA value (ASTRO 1997).

Nadir PSA following treatment has emerged as potentially the simplest way to measure cancer control following radiation therapy. Extrapolating from the data that showed the value of PSA normalization as an endpoint, other investigators recently found that the nadir PSA (which occurred within 12 months of treatment) is also a good indicator of complete tumor ablation, and is one of the most powerful independent predictors of disease outcome (Kavadi et al. 1994). Patients who remained NED had a median PSA nadir of 0.9, while patients with local and distant recurrence had median nadirs of 2.8 and 9.2, respectively (Ritter et al. 1992).

Early studies suggested that a PSA nadir less than 1.0 ng/mL was able to discriminate between patients who remained NED versus those who did not (Kavadi et al. 1994, Zagars et al. 1995c). However, later studies have shown that a lower nadir value (<0.5) was a better indicator of complete tumor eradication (Schneider et al. 1996). 90% to 95% of patients who had a nadir of < 0.5 ng/mL remained biochemically and clinically NED at 5 years, while only 29% to 34% were NED if the nadir was greater than 1.0 (Critz et al. 1996, McNeil 1996, Zietman et al. 1996). In these studies, PSA nadir was the most powerful predictor of treatment outcome. A stable PSA following nadir has also been shown to be a potentially useful endpoint, with one study showing that 100% of patients who had an undetectable PSA at two years following treatment remained NED for 5 years after treatment (Crook et al. 1998, Johnstone et al. 1998).

Current data regarding nadir PSA are suggestive, but there are insufficient long-term data to suggest which nadir value will best predict long-term disease-free survival, although few patients with a nadir less than 0.5 relapse (Kavadi et al. 1994, Zietman et al. 1996). However, while the PSA nadir of 0.5 is more strict and therefore a better absolute predictor of disease-free status, the stricter definition may not affect survival in the population of patients who are treated by radiation therapy because of their age and co-morbidity. In fact, a strict PSA endpoint might not be relevant in the patient population that undergoes radiation therapy, since *clinical* control of cancer might be more important relative to longevity than *biochemical* cancer control

43

(Schellhammer et al. 1993). Some definition of PSA nadir could be used as an outcome measure to permit comparison among different measures of structure and process. Although not all patients need to reach the nadir to have a good outcome, types of treatment where lower proportions of the treated patients reach the accepted PSA nadir can be identified for further study.

Measured treatment morbidity. Measured treatment morbidity is also an important outcome to analyze. Some studies have suggested that the methods by which radiation is delivered to the prostate can have a profound influence on treatment-related side effects. The classic late effects of prostate irradiation include urinary frequency, urgency, dysuria, hematuria, incontinence, fecal urgency, diarrhea, tenesmus, frequent bowel movements, rectal bleeding, rectal ulceration, necrosis, and erectile dysfunction (Roach et al. 1996, Rosen et al. 1985). Most of the radiation therapy studies in the literature have derived complication rates from chart reviews or physician notes. Based on these data, the severe complication rates associated with radiation therapy are relatively low. Collection of these data is relatively simple and rapid, and the standardization of data collection is helped by the RTOG morbidity system, which categorizes the severity of the event relative to the need for treatment (Pilepich 1988, Ragde et al. 1997).

Unfortunately, there are methodologic limitations to this retrospective approach that affect the validity of these reports. It is known that there can be inadvertent bias in the way that the complication rates are measured in retrospective studies (Talcott et al. 1998). Because patients under-report complications and physicians underestimate them, the results of abstracting medical records for complication rates can be misleading (Albertsen et al. 1999, Talcott et al. 1998). In addition, some studies that used survey instruments had limited value because they did not use tested instruments, or did not have pre-treatment data to establish baseline status (Roach et al. 1996, Shrader-Bogen et al. 1997).

When validated survey instruments were used to assess quality of life and side effects of radiation therapy, the reported adverse event rate was much higher than previously reported (Beard et al. 1997, Fowler et al. 1996, Talcott et al. 1998). Of course, patient population and baseline function remain factors, which emphasizes the need for baseline assessment of functional status. However, validated surveys paint a very different picture of complications than emerges from simple chart review.

Another factor that must be defined for outcome measurement is the time between treatment and the measurement of long term sequelae. Although the side effects of surgery diminish over time, the effect of radiation therapy on normal tissues may only become manifest after a year or more has passed. For example, reports of post-therapy potency will not be accurate if assessment is done shortly after radiation therapy because erectile dysfunction continues to decrease over a long time course following radiation treatment (Talcott et al. 1998).

Wrap-up. There are many ways to define successful radiation therapy for localized prostate cancer. Although the goal of radiation therapy is to eradicate the cancer with few side effects or complications, the definitions of what those outcomes should be and how best to measure them remain unclear. The literature suggests that the optimal cancer control outcome is a patient who has no evidence of disease based on rectal examination and has a PSA that remains low and stable following treatment. Prospective use of validated survey instruments, in conjunction with determination of pre-treatment functional status, is the most accurate way to measure treatment-related side effects. Assessment of the long term sequelae of radiation treatment should be done at least 1 year following treatment because erectile dysfunction and bowel damage have a delayed presentation following radiation therapy. Finally, to allow for valid comparisons of different structures and treatment processes, evaluations of side effects need to be done in a standardized manner, and at similar time points following treatment (Schneider et al. 1996).

Quality indicators, process, and standards of care for the delivery of external beam radiation therapy

Radiation therapy can vary in a number of ways that can affect outcomes. Even in Canada, where health care is provided by a single insurer, a 1985 review of radiation therapy practices showed significant differences between regional referral centers in terms of patient selection, pre-treatment evaluation, and the type of radiation treatment that was used (McGowan and Hanson 1985). Through the efforts of the Radiation Therapy Oncology Group (RTOG), some of these factors were studied in a prospective manner in an attempt to determine which factors are important for cancer control.

External beam radiation therapy is delivered to the prostate by a machine that produces high-energy particles (usually photons) that are aimed at the prostate target using fixed ports or rotational arcs. How the radiation is delivered to the target tissue varies among radiation oncologists. In the United States, daily doses between 1.8 and 2 cGy are given over a period of 6 to 9 weeks, with doses ranging from 6,000 cGy to over 8,000 cGy used in dose escalation conformal protocols. The volumes of treatment can cover the whole pelvis and regional nodes or may be limited to the prostate and a 5 mm to 3 cm margin of normal surrounding tissue. Thus some of the process variables that can affect outcome include total dose, duration of treatment, the number of fields used, the volumes of treatment, and the nature of treatment planning.

Structural factors. There is some evidence that radiation therapy departments with a high ratio of patients to treatment staff have worse outcomes and lower compliance rates with generally accepted quality processes such as the obtainment of treatment portal films (Diamond et al. 1991, Leibel et al. 1984). This outcome may represent the staff's inability to provide adequate treatment planning because they lack time, or it might be a sign that the radiation therapy department is short on physical resources and therefore does not have state-of-the-art equipment or treatment processes.

Other studies have also looked at structure in relation to outcomes and compliance with the Patterns of Care "Best Current Patient Management" type guidelines (Leibel et al. 1984). Early reports from the Patterns of Care Study showed that in 1983 approximately half of the patients who were retrospectively reviewed received a sub-optimal dose of radiation, and about one quarter were treated with a volume that was smaller than recommended. In addition, the study found that linear accelerators gave better cancer control rates than cobalt machines, that perineal fields and parallel opposed ports had worse outcomes, and that use of parallel-opposed fields or perineal fields for boosting the prostate dose was associated with an increased frequency of bowel side effects. Larger centers with full-time radiation oncologists had better outcomes than small centers with only part-time radiation oncologists. In addition, smaller centers were also less likely to be compliant with the Patterns of Care guidelines and were less likely to do treatment portal films: however, despite these apparent differences in treatment quality, no difference in cancer recurrence was seen between different types of treatment facilities (Leibel et al. 1984).

In the years since the first report, compliance with the Patterns of Care Guidelines has improved. Serial surveys based on the Patterns of Care methodology showed increased compliance with the guidelines for the treatment of prostate cancer, cervical cancer, and Hodgkin's disease. Between 1973 and 1989, fewer patients were treated with suboptimal doses, and there was increased use of dedicated simulators, routine port films, linear accelerators versus Cobalt machines, individually shaped blocks, and CT scans for treatment planning (Hanks et al. 1994b, Hoppe et al. 1994, Komaki et al. 1995). It can be inferred that such organized efforts can result in improved outcomes by identifying and eliminating therapeutic outliers. However, a direct cause-effect relationship between the efforts of the Patterns of Care study group and improved treatment quality cannot be proven.

Treatment process. The RTOG has examined treatment processes and their relation to outcomes (Pilepich 1988). Early studies suggested that protracted treatment of prostate cancer with radiation resulted in a higher failure rate because of the potential for re-population of the prostate with more radioresistant cells (Amdur et al. 1990). But later prospective randomized studies by the RTOG showed that variations in *treatment duration* had no impact on outcome. When controlled for tumor stage, treatment duration less than 7 weeks versus more than 9 weeks did not affect overall survival, NED survival, local recurrence, or complications (Lai et al. 1991).

The *total amount of radiation* delivered to the prostate appears to affect cancer control rates and side effects. Those receiving doses below 6,000 cGY had a higher failure rate, and this dose appears to be insufficient (Hanks et al. 1988b, Leibel et al. 1984, Perez et al. 1989, Perez et al. 1993, Perez et al. 1988). For conventional radiation therapy in so-called low risk patients (Gleason < 6, stage T1/T2, and PSA < 10), doses between 6,600 and 7,000 cGY appeared to be adequate, especially since higher doses markedly increased side effects (Hanks et al. 1996b, Hanks et al. 1985, Hanks et al. 1988b, Leibel et al. 1996, Teshima et al. 1997, Zietman et al. 1996). In multiple case series, for patients who have T1 or T2 tumors and pre-treatment PSA levels less than 10 ng/mL, doses between 6,600 and 7,200 cGY provided equivalent degrees of cancer control outcomes (Hanks et al. 1996b, Hanks et al. 1988b, Leibel et al. 1984, Leibel et al. 1996, Teshima et al. 1997, Zietman et al. 1996). With the use of traditional, 4 field box non-conformal radiation therapy, the incidence of major side effects increased from 3 - 6% to 7 - 11% when the dose was increased to > 7,000 cGY (Hanks et al. 1988a, Hanks et al. 1985, Hanks et al. 1988b, Leibel et al. 1984, Zagars et al. 1988).

In contrast to the low risk patients, doses > 7,000 cGy produced better cancer control for more advanced tumors (bulky T2B/T3), higher pre-treatment PSA levels (between 10 and 20), and higher grade tumors (Gleason > 6). However, those receiving these higher doses also had higher complication rates (Hanks et al. 1996a, Hanks et al. 1985, Perez et al. 1989, Perez et al. 1988, Rosen et al. 1985). For patients who had pre-treatment PSA levels greater than 10 ng/dl, treating at doses greater than 7300 cGy resulted in a 81% disease-free survival rate at 2 years, compared to 60% when lower doses were used (Hanks et al. 1996b).

From such data, the concept of dose escalation for prostate cancer has evolved. With the advent of better treatment planning using CT scans, computer-based dosimetry, and conformal radiation delivery that minimizes exposure of critical structures, it is now possible to safely deliver doses > 7,000 cGy to the prostate. The benefit of dose escalation is clear for high risk patients, but for patients who have clinical stage T1/T2 disease with either higher pre-treatment PSA levels or higher grade tumors, it is unclear if doses > 7,000 cGY will improve cancer control (Perez et al. 1993). Ongoing studies are examining the role of dose escalation for these intermediate-risk patients.

Radiation treatment volume may also be a significant factor. Prospective, randomized trials showed that pelvic node radiation and extended field (peri-aortic) irradiation did not improve cancer control (Asbell et al. 1988, Perez et al. 1993, Pilepich et al. 1986, Zagars et al. 1988). The efficacy of irradiating the juxta-regional obturator nodes is uncertain, although the treatment of these tissues is a commonly accepted practice. However, it is known that patients who underwent whole-pelvis irradiation had delayed rectosigmoid and intestinal complication rates and decreased quality of life in comparison to patients who had treatment of the prostate alone (8.7 - 11% versus 1.6 - 5%) (Perez et al. 1994, Rosen et al. 1985). Data from validated survey instruments showed that whole-pelvis radiation was associated with a 22% rate of obstructive voiding symptoms, compared to 8% in patients who had prostate-only treatment. Erectile dysfunction also appeared to be higher in patients who were treated with larger fields (Beard et al. 1997).

Reducing the field size too much also caused problems when traditional methods were used to target the prostate (Leibel et al. 1996). In the pre-CT scanning era, using the older methods of AP:PA and lateral fields with standard 8 x 8 field size, the majority of larger prostates were under-treated (Sandler et al. 1992). The smaller field is also correlated with a higher local recurrence rate, possibly due to the failure of the 8 x 8 field to cover the seminal vesicles and bladder base (Rosen et al. 1985).

Three-dimensional conformal therapy was designed to overcome some of the limitations of therapies that used plain X-rays for treatment planning and standardized field sizes. The underlying concept behind conformal therapy is the use of multi-planar imaging where the treatment is designed to conform the radiation to the prostate while providing shielding to critical structures (Sandler et al. 1992, Suit et al. 1988). The key processes for CT-based conformal radiation therapy involve immobilizing the patient to minimize set-up variation between treatments, CT-guided treatment planning, customized blocking of normal tissues (using either cerrobend blocks or multi-leaf collimators), and follow-up evaluation of treatment dosimetry (Fukunaga-Johnson et al. 1997, Soffen et al. 1992). With conformal methods, CT scans are used to localize the prostate and techniques such as Beam's Eye View (BEV) are used to create customized treatment portals that target the prostate and spare the adjacent bladder and rectum (Leibel et al. 1996, Soffen et al. 1992).

The initial reports of 3D conformal techniques have shown that it is effective, and based on retrospective case series, it has few short-term complications (Fukunaga-Johnson et al. 1997, Hanks et al. 1994a, Soffen et al. 1992). Other studies have focused on the advantages of conformal therapy over standard external beam radiation therapy. These studies showed that a 40% volume error occurs when traditional anatomic landmarks are used to plan treatment instead of CT-defined treatment fields (Sandler et al. 1992). Furthermore, it has been shown that bladder and rectal exposure can be decreased by up to 50% when patient immobilization and conformal treatment are used; patient immobilization decreases set-up variation of the delivered dose between treatments by 67% (Soffen et al. 1992, Soffen et al. 1991, Ten Haken et al. 1989). In addition, the acute side effects of 3D conformal treatment appear to be less, as does the negative effect of treatment on quality of life, relative to older treatment processes (Beard et al. 1997).

Because of the initial success with standard dose 3D-conformal treatment, higher doses – with dose adjusted to the grade and stage of the tumor, are now being used in an attempt to improve cancer control outcomes (Bolla et al. 1997, Fukunaga-Johnson et al. 1997, O'Dowd et al. 1997, Sandler et al. 1992). At this time, the outcomes of such dose escalation protocols are known from only a handful of centers. Thus far, a few investigators have increased the dose to between 7,380 cGy and 8,100 cGy, with few moderate or severe (grade 3 or 4) RTOG side effects observed (Hanks et al. 1994a, Leibel et al. 1996). One recent study noted a 50% reduction in short-term side effects despite an 8% increase in the radiation dose that was used for therapy when conformal treatment was used (Hanks et al. 1994a).

The process of dose escalation is still evolving and further refinements are being developed as new long-term side effects are encountered with these higher doses. Teshima et al. noted that the incidence of long-term grade 2 and 3 rectal bleeding increased once the rectal wall dose increased to above 7,400 cGy; only 1.7% had RTOG Grade 3 rectal bleeding if the dose was less than 7,400 cGy, while the rate increased to 7% if the dose was above this (Teshima et al. 1997). This center has now modified its treatment process by using blocks to decrease the dose to the rectal wall, but how this technical adjustment will affect outcomes is unknown.

It is also unknown if the majority of patients who have clinically localized prostate cancer will benefit from dose escalation, since cancer persistence/recurrence following radiation therapy might be due either to sub-optimal local control that can be improved with dose escalation or to the selection of some patients who have occult metastasis at the time of treatment (Zietman et al. 1996). Increasing the intensity of the local treatment appears to improve cancer control in higher grade and bulky tumors (T2B/T3). Higher doses that yield better local control might be critical in some patients but not in others. Patients who have low grade tumors and stage T1 and T2 tumors are becoming the focus of future prospective, randomized trials (Sandler et al. 1992).

Another process related factor that is correlated to outcome is the use of *neo-adjuvant hormone therapy*. In an effort to decrease target volume along with the potential synergy that can be seen in combining radiation therapy with androgen deprivation therapy, the goal of combination therapy was initially to improve the outcome for advanced prostate cancer (Bolla et al. 1997). Multiple prospective studies, including recent large multi-center, prospective randomized trials, demonstrate the advantages of neo-adjuvant hormone deprivation therapy in combination with external beam radiation therapy in terms of local cancer control, disease-free survival, and overall survival for patients who have T2B/T3 tumors (Pilepich et al. 1997, Pilepich et al. 1995).

At this time, it is unknown if these benefits can be extrapolated to patients who have lower risk disease (pre-treatment PSA < 10, clinical stage T1/T2a, and Gleason grade < 7). In addition, the impact of neo-adjuvant hormone therapy on complications and quality of life remains poorly documented, although hormone therapy can cause hot flashes, gynecomastia, leukopenia, osteoporosis, and impaired sexual function (Bolla et al. 1997, Pilepich et al. 1995). Computer modeling of treatment dosimetry before and after hormone treatment showed that the exposure of the bladder and rectum is decreased by 15 - 20% due to a 37% decrease in the size of the prostate (Forman et al. 1995). As part of its process, Memorial Sloan Kettering Cancer Center has used pre-treatment dosimetry calculations to determine the need for neo-adjuvant hormone therapy: patients where the rectal or bladder exposure is excessive are given 3 months of pre-treatment hormone therapy (Leibel et al. 1996). Although these results are interesting, more data are needed to see if the hypothesized effects of neo-adjuvant hormone therapy (cytoreduction, geometric size reduction, and synergistic induction of apoptosis) will actually improve outcomes by increasing the cancer cell kill ratio as well as decreasing the long-term side effects. The use of neo-adjuvant hormone treatment or extended post-radiation therapy hormonal ablation further confounds future analysis of outcomes of care.

Brachytherapy for localized prostate cancer

The concept of implant therapy (brachytherapy) for prostate cancer is not new. Because radioactive implants can deliver a high dose of radiation to a very well defined area, it was hoped that brachytherapy would result in high cancer control rates with few complications (Ragde et al. 1997, Sylvester et al. 1997). At this time, there are two methods for implant therapy. High-dose-rate brachytherapy involves temporarily placing radioactive needles in the prostate; permanent methods involve implanting small radioactive seeds permanently (Duchesne and Peters 1999).

As originally performed, the procedure was done via a retropubic approach using a "freehand technique" for seed placement (Weyrich et al. 1993). This approach was combined with pelvic lymphadenectomy to allow for more accurate tumor staging. However, seed placement was done by palpation; thus the seeds could be unevenly distributed in the gland. Eventually, this approach fell out of favor due to poor patient selection and uneven dosimetry, both of which resulted in a high local failure rate (Ragde et al. 1997, Sylvester et al. 1997, Weyrich et al. 1993).

Recent technical advances have stimulated renewed interest in brachytherapy. The technical advances of new isotopes (palladium 103), transrectal ultrasound, CT-based treatment planning, and the use of perineal templates have improved the ability to place the implants uniformly in the prostate (Ragde et al. 1997, Sylvester et al. 1997). Early data show that these techniques allow permanent seed implantation that provides excellent cancer control rates for low grade, low stage prostate cancer (Beyer and Priestley 1997, Ragde et al. 1997, Ragde et al. 1998). For higher stage or higher grade disease, the results so far have been less successful for implant monotherapy (Beyer and Priestley 1997, D'Amico et al. 1998b). Due to the higher cancer recurrence rate that is seen in high grade and bulky tumors, neo-adjuvant hormonal therapy and adjuvant external beam radiation therapy are now used in selected patients (Stone and Stock 1999).

The main factors that appear to determine successful tumor eradication with permanent implant therapy involve patient selection, uniform seed placement, and routine evaluation of post-treatment dosimetry to confirm that the treatment was done correctly (Beyer and Priestley 1997). In terms of outcome measures, the same parameters that were described for external beam radiation therapy are applicable, except that the PSA nadir might take up to 2 years to be reached, given the slower rate of tumor eradication that is seen following brachytherapy. However, an additional outcome measure that can be used in permanent seed implantation is post-treatment dosimetry, since precise seed placement is critical to a good outcome because of the limited tissue penetration of the palladium 103 and iodine 125 pellets. This post-implant dosimetry may serve as a measurable quality indicator of the patient's implant.

Although the side effects appear to be low, the effect of permanent implant therapy on erectile function has not been extensively described. However, it has been reported to be in the range of 21 - 53% (Beyer and Priestley 1997, Stock et al. 1996, Weyrich et al. 1993, Zelefsky et al. 1999). Besides the standard side effects of cystitis, urinary incontinence, and proctitis, the need for secondary interventions for post-implant urinary retention is used as another endpoint, with 1 - 11% of patients needing a TURP or medical intervention following treatment due to persistent voiding dysfunction (Beyer and Priestley 1997, Ragde et al. 1997, Sylvester et al. 1997, Weyrich et al. 1993). There is currently no quality of life instrument shown to measure irritative voiding symptoms in this population with good reliability and validity.

Because seeds need to be placed precisely, some centers have chosen to use high dose rate brachytherapy, where interstitial needles are temporarily implanted in the prostate and are used to robotically deliver radiation to the prostate in a controlled manner. The advantage of this approach is that precise placement of the implant is not as critical, and homogeneous conformal doses can more easily be achieved. The scientific literature about this method is limited (Sylvester et al. 1997), but some recent literature suggests that this technique may be radiobiologically superior to other implant techniques.

Wrap-up. Many questions remain regarding the process of brachytherapy and its relation to outcome. The relative efficacy of high dose rate versus permanent implants has not been studied in a randomized, prospective manner. Peripheral loading of seeds (Parker-Patterson method) versus an uniform loading of seeds (Quimby method), the use of intra-operative fluoroscopy versus open coil MRI imaging to identify cold spots during implantation, the use of palladium 103 versus iodine 125, and the roles of neo-adjuvant hormone therapy and adjuvant external beam therapy all need further study to see if they are critically related to either cancer control or quality of life (Ragde et al. 1997, Sylvester et al. 1997). The complication rate for brachytherapy appears to be low (Beyer and Priestley 1997), but long-term side effects (especially in regards to sexual function) need to be studied using validated survey instruments with prospective data collection. A recent report used the FACT-G and the I-PSS instruments to measure overall quality of life and urinary symptoms following permanent seed implantation. This prospective study showed short-term decreases in quality of life and voiding function following brachytherapy, but this study was flawed because it did not separately examine sexual and bowel function; it used the I-PSS, which has not been validated in this patient population; and it studied patients who had only 3 months of follow-up (Lee et al. 1999).

Chapter 4

CHALLENGES IN INTERPRETING THE LITERATURE

When we reviewed the available literature, we encountered substantial challenges that prevented us from pooling data from different studies in order to measure variations in treatment outcomes across institutions. First, studies reported different end-points. Second, disease severity varied substantially across studies. Third, differences in the methods used to assess patient-focused outcomes limited their utility. We summarize and illustrate our results below.

Heterogeneity in the evaluation of outcomes across studies is a significant challenge to pooling results. Some studies evaluated survival while others used disease-free survival, and the methods used to determine disease-free survival vary as well. Disease-free survival is extremely sensitive to the method used to determine cancer recurrence. Further complicating matters, the assessment of disease-free survival has changed dramatically over the last decade with the adoption of the tumor marker test prostate-specific antigen (PSA) in the early 1990s. The PSA blood test provides an earlier indication of treatment failure than older methods, such as physical exam or radiographic studies. For example, in Figure 4.1, disease-free survival is presented for the same patients using two different measures of recurrence. The curve to the right indicates the 5-year disease-free survival rate using clinically-assessed recurrence while the curve to the left indicates the 5-year disease-free survival rate when biochemical failure (PSA) is used. Disease-free survival appears better with clinically-assessed recurrence that with PSA-determined recurrence. In order to compare outcomes across facilities, identical measures must be used.

Survival is less subject to measurement variation than disease-free survival, but long survival rates in prostate cancer make this an unsuitable outcome for evaluating quality of care. Most case series using survival as an endpoint reported 10- or 15-year follow-up data. Such long follow-up times, coupled with the time lags for scientific publication, mean that the results reported in 1998 reflect the quality of care provided in the late 1980's or earlier – hardly relevant to variations in care today.

The patients treated at different U.S. institutions are extremely heterogeneous with respect to disease severity. Baseline differences in disease severity are an important determinant of disease recurrence, regardless of treatment. Patients with lower Gleason scores and with smaller tumors (earlier stage) will have better rates of disease-free survival.

Figure 4.2 (radiation therapy) and 4.3 (surgery) illustrate outcomes for localized prostate cancer patients without stratifying for stage of disease. In Figure 4.2 the curves for a number of the series do not overlap, suggesting significant differences in outcomes across the radiation therapy series. There is somewhat less variation across series when controlling for stage of disease, one of several factors that must be controlled for when making comparisons across facilities.

Although recurrence is the most salient disease-specific outcome, other patient-focused measures may be important outcomes when trying to assess variation in the quality of treatment provided. Treatment-related complications are common following either surgery or radiation therapy, and rates of urinary incontinence, impotency, and bowel functioning problems experienced by localized prostate cancer patients can vary considerably across series (e.g., Middleton et al. 1995).

Four issues create substantial challenges to pooling these data across studies. First, many case series do not report these outcomes at all. Second, differences in methods used to assess the outcome may contribute importantly to variation. Many studies report the physicians' assessments of complications while others obtain this information directly from patients. Physicians' assessments of treatment-related complications generally differ from patients' self-report, with patients more likely to identify problems. Also, as with other outcome measures, it is important to have a common method for reporting, to rule out the possibility that observed variations may be due to differences in methods of measurement. Third, many men may experience problems in these domains even prior to treatment (Litwin et al. 1995) so it is important to have baseline measures to control for differences in pre-treatment rates across facilities.

Different endpoints, variation in disease severity, and differences in methods used to assess outcomes proved to be insurmountable challenges to pooling data from medical literature for purposes of evaluating variation in prostate cancer treatment outcomes across institutions. Although statistical methods can be used to control for some variation in populations when trying to pool data from different studies, the incredible heterogeneity among studies in the prostate cancer literature made such analysis infeasible. Our results are consistent with previous attempts to summarize outcomes across case series in the medical literature (Wasson et al. 1993, Middleton et al. 1995). Perhaps the most important limitation to using the medical literature to assess variations in outcomes is the fact that most of the series reports represent only a small subset of facilities that treat localized prostate cancer. These series typically report the experience (and patients) of large, academic hospitals and therefore may not represent variation in outcomes that would be observed across all prostate cancer providers in the United States.

Figure 4.1. Disease-free survival in the same patients, assessed clinically or by PSA

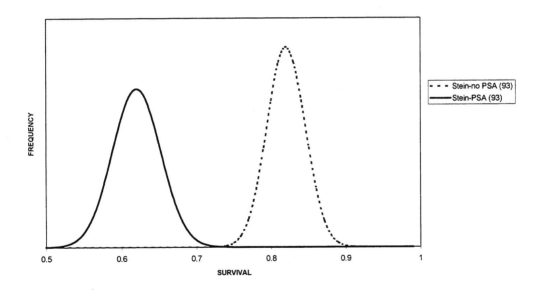

Figure 4.2. 5-year disease-free survival following surgery – studies of T1 and T2 cancers combined

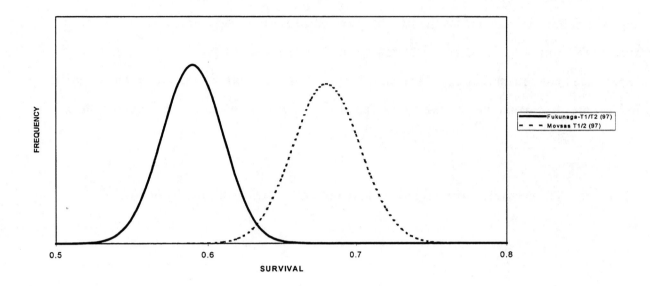

Chapter 5

INTERVIEWS WITH PROSTATE CANCER EXPERTS

Introduction

Most of the medical literature we reviewed focused on efficacy of treatment, not quality of care. To fill this information gap, we interviewed physician leaders in both surgical and radiation treatment of prostate cancer to learn what they considered to be essential to providing excellent care.

We wanted to learn what kind of *information was available* to both patients and physicians and how this information was communicated. Specifically, we investigated:

- What information sources were available to prostate cancer patients
- How physicians inform patients about the nature of the treatment and its expected outcomes
- What kind of information physicians provided to patients
- What physicians saw as patients' most important concerns
- What information resources physicians used, including medical literature, tabulated data, and their personal experience.

To gain information about factors in the *structure and process* of care that could be indicators of quality outcomes, we asked detailed questions about:

- Elements of the patient work-up before treatment
- Elements of the process of treatment and care that the experts felt were necessary to ensure good outcomes.

In terms of *outcomes*, we asked the experts:

- Which factors they thought were most important in determining outcomes
- Which elements of follow-up care were important to ensure and measure successful treatment outcomes.

Methods

We conducted a series of structured interviews with 14 experts who have experience in diagnosing and managing early stage prostate cancer. The goal of the interviews was to provide clinical perspective for the subsequent development and evaluation of quality-of-care indicators. Each interview was conducted face-to-face by two members of the research team, at least one of whom was a physician. Interviews were recorded and transcribed to facilitate qualitative analysis. We created an interview protocol to structure the interviews and to ensure that common issues were discussed. The protocol appears in Appendix C.

To identify candidates for the interviews, we asked the major professional organizations in urology (American Urological Association) and radiation oncology (American College of Radiology, American Society of Therapeutic Radiology and Oncology, American College of Radiation Oncology) to nominate a list of clinicians with expertise and experience in treating patients with localized prostate cancer. If nominees were interested in participating in the interviews, we asked them for a resume. From this group, the research team selected eight academic and community-based radiation oncologists and six academic urologists who represented geographic diversity, as well as a cross-section of training and known clinical approaches. In most cases, the experts see patients for consultation or management after previous diagnosis elsewhere.

Table 5.1 shows the characteristics of these physicians and their practices and provides a demographic profile of the prostate cancer patients whom they treat.

Table 5.1 Characteristics of experts interviewed

Practice variables

	Expert Urologists		Expert Radiation Oncologists	
	Mean	Range	Mean	Range
Years in practice	24	(16-29)	22	(10-35)
New patients seen per year	390	(180-800)	363	(200-700
Prostate cancer patients treated per year	235	(100-600)	172	(45-500)

Demographics of localized prostate cancer patients

Age					
	Under 65	64%	(40%-85%)	30%	(20%-50%)
	65-74	30%	(15%-60%)	54%	(50%-65%)
	75 or older	6%	(0%-20%)	16%	(10%-30%)
Ethnicity					
	African-American	5%	(5%-6%)	12%	(3%-35%)
	Hispanic	4%	(1%-15%)	4%	(0%-20%)
	Caucasian	88%	(80%-95%)	77%	(45%-95%)
	Other	2%	(0%-8%)	1%	(0%-5%)
Education level					
	< High school	3%	(0%-10%)	15%	(5%-30%)
	High school	25%	(15%-50%)	39%	(15%-70%)
	Some college	72%	(50%-85%)	61%	(20%-80%)
Insurance coverage					
	Medicare	33%	(10%-60%)	47%	(15%-75%)
	Medicaid	1%	(0%-3%)	1%	(0%-5%)
	Fee-for-service	37%	(15%-62%)	12%	(10%-20%)
	Managed care	21%	(0%-50%)	32%	(10%-70%)
	Self pay	7%	(0%-15%)	2%	(0%-5%)
	Indigent	2%	(0%-10%)	3%	(0%-10%)

Summary of interviews with radiation oncology experts

Information provided to patients. Almost all of the eight radiation oncologists whom we interviewed said that they give patients newly diagnosed with prostate cancer information about the three conventional options for management: radiation therapy, surgery, and watchful waiting. In addition, the interstitial implant options of permanent seed or high-dose-rate were offered either by the expert, within the expert's group, or by referral. All the respondents mentioned hormone ablation therapy as a possible adjunct, but only half the physicians generally advised it to all their patients. This response is interesting since there is no published evidence that hormone ablation therapy combined with radiation therapy improves outcome in patients whose tumor characteristics give them a good prognosis. One expert radiation oncologist who performs brachytherapy but not external beam radiation therapy reported that he routinely discussed only the implant modality and its morbidity with his patients.

When asked about information they provided to the patient regarding alternative treatment facilities, the majority of the experts said they would consider referral to "people they know," but most would volunteer information in this regard only when asked. When the experts were asked in what circumstances they would recommend surgery rather than radiation therapy, six said they would do so when the patient is afraid of radiation therapy, three said they would do it if the patient had inflammatory bowel disease (these respondents considered this co-morbidity an absolute contraindication to radiation treatment), and one in each group responded he would recommend surgery when the patient does not understand the radiation option and when the patient is young.

To explain treatment outcomes to their patients, seven of eight respondents said they use probabilistic language (i.e., odds or percentages). Six respondents used numbers (e.g., "one in ten men"), five used words (e.g., "might" or "should not expect"), and three used numbers and words together. Physicians frequently tailored information for individual patients based on tumor stage, and the patient's age and co-morbidities, but never by marital status. Other considerations in tailoring information included education level, ethnic-based cultural interaction with medicine (American Indian), and patients' need for detail. Most radiation oncology respondents claimed that patients who were referred for consultation are preselected on the basis of older age and greater co-morbidity.

Seven of the respondents said they supplied articles, brochures, videos, or computer-based information to their patients as an adjunct to the consultation. Articles were most frequently mentioned, followed by brochures and videos. No one used computer-based patient education. Only one respondent had brochures in more than one language. (Three respondents noted that this particular question was not applicable in their practice situation). The physicians generally felt that better educated patients benefited most from these educational materials. Only two of the experts knew that patients who belong to managed care plans were given educational information by the plan. Time lost from work was not routinely discussed unless patients specifically inquired about it.

Patients' concerns. According to the expert radiation oncologists, the most important concerns their patients expressed during the initial consultation were survival, recurrence of the tumor, and sexual function. Several of the respondents noted that sexual function only seemed important to about half of their patients, and that availability of Viagra appears to mitigate most perceived and actual concerns in this area. Patients were also concerned about bowel function. Many patients had a preconception (possibly obtained from a prior urological consultation) that radiation therapy is a second choice treatment, that it is not curative, or that it has a time limit to its effectiveness. Other factors reported to be of concern to patients were recovery time, coordination of care, cost, quality of life, fear of surgery, and rectal complications.

The radiation oncologists reported discussions with patients ranging from 30 to 75 minutes (median of 50 minutes, mean of 49 minutes, a mode of 60 minutes). Most respondents felt the time spent was adequate to respond to patients' needs for information. Three of the experts identified a patient personality type who asked the same question repeatedly or lacked the cognitive ability to make a decision about any treatment modality. The experts felt that no amount of time spent in discussion would ever be adequate for these patients.

Most respondents found it "easy" to discuss treatment issues with patients, but they noted some areas of difficulty. Half of the experts noted that the most challenging communication issue was the lack of data to answer questions regarding survival. They also found it difficult to overcome patient misperceptions regarding efficacy and morbidity of radiation. In addition, two respondents said it was hard to deal with the misguided notion that surgical failures may be followed with a salvage treatment (namely radiation therapy), but that no such salvage treatment exists for radiation failures. The experts noted that it is not presently known whether radiation therapy is an effective salvage treatment for surgical failures. Furthermore, patients have difficulty accepting that surgical failure and radiation failure appear to be associated with the same ultimate outcome in terms of survival, regardless of attempts at salvage treatment. Other areas of difficulty raised by some respondents included making treatment recommendations in young patients (less than 50 years old) and the lack of long-term data for brachytherapy treatments.

Managed care. Community-based experts mentioned that managed care might affect the type of treatment offered patients because managed care was sometimes not willing to pay for implant procedures, or to recognize the increased cost involved in delivery of the technologically advanced three-dimensional conformal therapy.

Information sources available to physicians. The majority of expert radiation oncologists relied on data from multiple sources, including their own personal practice, clinic-wide experience, and the scientific literature. Both academic and community-based providers relied on scientific literature, in addition to the generally accepted peer-reviewed literature, included ASTRO consensus panel and RTOG published data. Most of the experts had tabulated data describing their own or clinic-wide experience; one physician used anecdotal experience for PSA, and another did so for treatment-related fatigue. The expert radiation oncologists were more likely to have tabulated data from personal experience or clinic-wide experience as compared to the community-based experts. Although tabulated data were more commonly available in the academic group regarding PSA, potency, and rectal bleeding, it was infrequently available with regard to recurrence rate and prostatic cancer-specific mortality.

Pre-treatment evaluation and staging. The salient feature of the pretreatment evaluation noted by all expert radiation oncologists is the conventional history and physical, paying special attention to the patient's general health, co-morbidities, and urologic system. When the experts were asked how they assessed co-morbidity, the most common answer was "by patient and family history." Other methods mentioned by several experts included review of urologic systems and Karnofsky performance status. Few obtained formal tests of potency, voiding, or continence before treatment; two respondents requested AUA symptom scores for urologic function. One respondent mentioned cystoscopy if the patient is "symptomatic."

All of the experts used measurement of PSA as part of the staging procedures. Experts also mentioned acid phosphatase, CBC, and chemistry panel (mentioned in conjunction with use of hormone ablative medications). Seven experts used CT scans as part of the work-up, and all used CT scans for treatment planning. Only one expert mentioned MRI scan with endorectal coil and/or spectrophotography. Transurethral and volumetric ultrasound were mentioned by all expert radiation oncologists for permanent seed implant. Other procedures in the work-up included multiple sextant biopsies, ProstaScint scans in postprostatectomy setting, and lymph node dissection if PSA was greater than 20.

We asked the radiation oncologists if they used tabulated estimates as part of their work-up or as an information source for their patients. Three of them used Partin tables, one used the Roach Equation, and one used his own survival curves for these purposes.

Treatment modalities and approaches. The experts we interviewed used a wide range of treatment modalities. All used external beam radiation therapy via either conventional or conformal techniques. Only one expert said that he utilized a dose escalation technique; however, three other respondents said they routinely utilize doses in the range of 7,200–7,380 cGY although they did not consider these doses consistent with dose escalation (doses of 6,600-7,000 cGY are considered conventional).

All respondents either used permanent seed implant techniques themselves or had access to these techniques by referral. Two of the radiation oncologists employed high-dose-rate interstitial implant techniques. One expert radiation oncologist had access to neutron therapy, but none had access to proton therapy other than by referral. None of the experts considered the latter two treatment modalities to be standard, and some commented that there was no evidence that these very expensive treatments were equivalent or superior to other, newer treatment modalities, such as 3-D conformal therapy or interstitial implant techniques. At the time of our interviews, none of the expert radiation oncologist had access to intensity modulated radiation therapy (IMRT technology), but some mentioned interest in this modality. None of the experts used hyperthermia; one had extensive experience with hyperthermia and prostate cancer but had abandoned the modality.

We asked the expert radiation oncologists to suggest characteristics of external beam treatment that would ensure a successful outcome for patients with localized prostate cancer. All of the respondents mentioned that machine energies of 4 MeV, or Co^{60} were associated with survival and quality of life outcomes. Machine energies considered adequate for treatment of localized prostate cancer ranged from 6 MeV to 25 MeV. It was noted that IMRT is best utilized at 6 MeV. The experts also noted that computer-generated dosimetry by FDA-approved software would allow clinicians to determine adequate radiation dose coverage for each individual patient, regardless of machine energy.

The experts agreed that four characteristics of the process of care were associated with good outcome in treatment.

1. Dose fractionation of 180 to 200 cGY per day and tumor dose of greater than or equal to 7,000 cGY;
2. Immobilization of the patient during treatment and use of multiple field techniques with treatment of all fields each day;
3. Hormone ablative therapy for high-risk patients (most experts were using hormone ablative therapy even in patients in so-called good prognostic categories);
4. Multiple-level CT planning for tumor control.

The experts thought that compulsive attention to patient management with frequent, perhaps weekly, visits produced superior outcomes. They also noted that it was beneficial to begin treatment quickly when a patient suffers from a treatment-related side effect. They thought processes – e.g., immobilizing the patient – that decrease variability in treatment setup and delivery were helpful. Other processes associated with superior outcomes included dose volume histograms for prostate and critical structures, including rectum and bladder, and customizing and modifying treatment fields with regard to the seminal vesicles to prevent excessive irradiation of rectal tissues.

Items mentioned but not consistently agreed upon included weekly port films and use of urethrograms for treatment setup. Some experts used three-dimensional CT simulation without urethrogram; they felt this technique was adequate and that the urethrogram could be anatomically misleading. No one felt MRI scans had a place in setup or management of localized prostate cancer at the present time. Multileaf collimators (MLC) and custom Cerrobend blocks were felt to be equivalent in terms of outcome of treatment.

When using permanent seed implants, experts agreed that several factors led to better outcomes: uniformity of implant placement, urethral dose sparing, supplemental seed placement in the lateral peripheral aspects of the prostate gland (8 to 12 seeds beyond that called for in the pre-plan), use of CT-based post-treatment dosimetry, and use of external beam radiation in conjunction with interstitial implant when PSA is greater than 10 or the Gleason score is greater than or equal to 7. The issue of case volume versus quality was mentioned, but there was no consensus about the answer. Some mentioned that there was a steep learning curve for brachytherapy, but the brachytherapy specialist felt that 10 cases or fewer are adequate to gain expertise.

Characteristics of treatment felt to be associated with successful outcome when utilizing HDR implant techniques included use of 3D CT treatment planning, use of dose volume histograms, rectal dose less than 70% of tumor dose, and urethral dose less than 120% of tumor dose.

Practice guidelines. Clinical pathways or practice guidelines were not used by the expert radiation oncologists. Only one community-based expert utilized a care path that was derived from the literature.

Follow-up care and measuring outcomes. Overall, the expert radiation oncologists believed that PSA evidence of recurrence, quality of life, and sexual function were the most important outcomes to measure to evaluate the success of treatment. Also mentioned were bowel function, clinical recurrence, "complications," metastasis, incontinence, and bladder function.

The experts most frequently cited PSA measurement at six-month intervals as the most important element of post-treatment follow-up. But expert opinion about what constituted adequate clinical follow-up was extremely variable, ranging from a regimen where the first follow-up visit is 4 – 6 weeks after treatment followed by visits every six months to telephone follow-up. The radiation oncologists felt it was important to have both the radiation oncologist and the urologist involved in follow-up care so that radiation-induced morbidity could be recognized early and treated. Three of the experts were uncertain about whether close follow-up makes much difference in outcome since there is no clearly defined benefit of early diagnosis and treatment of recurrence.

Summary of interviews with urology experts

Information provided to patients. All six expert urologists we interviewed said that they typically give patients newly diagnosed with localized prostate cancer a comprehensive description of the three principal management options (surgery, radiation, and watchful waiting). One stated that he usually eliminates the watchful waiting option although he encourages it in older patients. One also includes a brief discussion of the natural history of prostate cancer. Two mentioned cryotherapy although one believes it is not an appropriate recommendation for most patients.

Most patients seeking consultation from an academic urologist have already gotten over the initial shock of the diagnosis, and they come to the table fairly well-read and prepared to discuss the risks and benefits of each treatment option. Only one of the urology experts always recommends a treatment; three others insist on providing only information and leaving the decision completely up to the patient. All stressed the importance of including the spouse or family in the consultation process.

All six expert urologists used probabilistic language to describe outcomes; however, several stated that patients often do not understand information presented as percentages. The experts thought risk was better communicated with phrases such as, "one chance in ten" or, "one man in seven." They also thought it was important to provide a time frame when discussing the likelihood of impotence and incontinence. In addition, one expert underscored the importance of talking about sexual function not just as an all-or-none variable, but as a qualitative outcome with different degrees of severity, and different relevance at different ages.

Four of six urologists interviewed said that they always provide written information to newly diagnosed patients. This included articles from the scientific and lay media, brochures, monographs, newsletters, and research updates. Three recommend books published in the lay press. Two also provide patient information on a webpage. Two of the six urologists provide written information in more than one language.

The experts we interviewed said that giving patients information about alternative treatment facilities is a delicate issue for them as urologists in academic referral centers. When patients ask them about specific community urologists, the experts said they reply candidly if they know that the outside urologist is good. Indeed, most tried to refer the patient back to the primary urologist, especially when he/she was more geographically convenient than the expert. When patients expressed a strong desire to have surgery in the referral center, the six experts tended to honor that request.

When asked when they recommend radiation therapy over surgery, four of the experts said they tend to recommend it for older patients, and half advise it for patients with higher-stage tumors. Only one explicitly stated that he considered patient preference the primary factor in recommending radiation therapy, but the others mentioned a patient's predisposition as an important factor in counseling for early stage prostate cancer.

Patients' concerns. All of the experts mentioned survival as their patients' most important concern. As one urologist put it," . . . they have two main concerns . . . are they going to die of this disease, and at what price if we do something to keep them from dying." Another reported that the central concern patients have is whether they are curable. Five of six felt that these issues were easy to discuss with patients; however, one described it as difficult, primarily because few patients have had any personal experience of someone close to them dying of prostate cancer. A related issue is patient denial. In particular, once patients understand that they are potentially curable, many want to know "whether they really have it." Although survival is the most common concern, patients who are older or who have small well-differentiated tumors tend to be somewhat less concerned with survival relative to the risks of treatment.

Secondary concerns primarily include the specific potential complications of surgery, such as urinary and sexual dysfunction. Expert urologists acknowledged somewhat more difficulty talking with patients about these issues, primarily because of the paucity of reliable data. In addition, one urologist stated that the reason sexual function is more difficult to discuss is that it is harder to quantify. "There are questions about mechanical aspects as well as emotional aspects which overlay questions about sexual functioning," said one urologist. Each of the six expert urologists stated that he compiled and reported his own continence and potency statistics when talking to patients. The experts expressed frustration about the lack of valid data describing complications from other therapies.

The experts reported that all patients are interested in continence, but a large subset of patients do not have great concerns regarding potency. These men are typically older, married for many years, or already impotent, and are far less concerned about maintaining potency at the risk of compromising survival. One important consideration is not only the potential sexual dysfunction but also the degree of bother that patients experience from that dysfunction; typically these two factors are not highly correlated.

Recurrence represents another significant concern for patients. Although most realize that PSA will be used as a marker, most of the experts agreed that some men become highly focused on the PSA levels while others appeared to be much less concerned about them. One urologist joked that PSA should stand for "patient stimulated anxiety" because it often becomes a source of great stress in the post-treatment period. This is especially true with patients after radiation, since PSA can go up before it goes down. One urologist said that he tries to convince patients that "PSA is only a piece of the puzzle, not necessarily the whole puzzle and that this is still where the art rather than the science of medicine comes in."

Additional issues such as post-operative pain, blood loss, length of hospitalization, recovery time, and coordination of care are more minor patient concerns. These areas do not necessarily demand a lot of time during consultation sessions, but one urologist indicated that it is important to spend adequate time educating patients about what to expect after surgery. If patients have realistic expectations, they are more likely to be satisfied with the outcomes of surgery.

Managed care. Although expense of treatment was not mentioned as a central concern for patients on Medicare, managed care appears to have had various effects in different areas of the country. Several of the expert urologists said that they came across patients who had sought a second opinion at the academic center but whose plan would not cover the costs of the surgery out of network. This had led to situations in which patients wanted to have surgery at the academic center but could not afford to pay out-of-pocket for it. "Some will accept it, and some will make enough noise in the system that they will get it changed. Those are important issues nowadays," commented one urologist.

Five of the experts indicated that managed care had altered the way they practiced because of denied referrals, restriction of choice of providers, and limitations on available modalities. Various experts said that they did not accept HMO patients, that managed care had a bigger effect on the hospital than on the practitioners, or that managed care had not affected how patients were treated in his institution

All six experts required one visit for patients undergoing surgery, and four scheduled a second visit after the initial consultation to address patient concerns. The amount of time spent with the patient during the initial consultation ranged from 30 to 60 minutes (mode of 45 minutes). The physicians felt this was adequate time for 70% to 100% of patients, too little time for 0% to 30% of patients, and too much time for 0% to 5% of patients.

All six experts preferred to have a spouse present during the initial consultation, but most said that patients generally tend to bring a spouse with them without being told. One commented that "it depends on the dynamic of the marriage" as to whether the spouse comes along and that he did not want to insert himself into that aspect of the relationship.

Half of the urologists said the most difficult patients to counsel are men with locally advanced tumors, particularly younger men. Other challenges in counseling patients include trying to elicit patient preferences, determining what the true life expectancy is, the lack of data to answer important clinical questions, and making sure the patient understands what he has been told about the chance of cure and the risk of complications.

Information sources available to physicians. All six of the expert urologists underscored the importance of PSA as a marker of cure or recurrence following surgery, and all used their own clinical practices to generate statistics on PSA and potency. For continence and recurrence, most relied on personal clinical experience; one used facility-wide experience for these data. For cancer-specific mortality, half used their own practice experience, while others drew from the literature. None of the expert urologists used the scientific literature or other sources to provide information on specific post-operative outcomes. Each felt it was important to present his own success and complication rates to patients considering surgery.

Four of the experts used tabulated estimates of pathological stage (two of whom used the Partin tables), but two experts emphatically did not use tabulated estimates for this purpose. One stated that tabulated data seem only to frighten patients without providing clinically useful information. "They don't state anything really about the patient's chance of survival . . . when they talk about the risk of a positive margin . . . that's not really the issue." Another commented that the available tabulated estimates of pathological outcomes are so outdated as not to be clinically useful any longer.

71

All six expert urologists tailored information to the individual patient based on tumor stage or location, patient age, and co-morbidity. Two also considered marital status, life expectancy, or tumor grade. Regarding the importance of individualizing information, one urologist expressed frustration at the lack of reliable and valid methods to predict a patient's longevity. He said, "Life insurance companies seem to be able to size you up faster than anybody else, . . . but in [the assessment of patients with prostate cancer], the [co-morbidity] instruments I've seen are not all that user-friendly, and they don't seem to include . . . factors that I think would be important . . . One of the big unanswered questions, I would say, is how long is someone going to live?"

Pre-treatment evaluation and staging. Elements in the pre-operative evaluation recommended by all six urologists include a complete medical history, determination of comorbid illnesses, digital rectal examination, serum prostate specific antigen (PSA), and histological tumor grade. Four of the experts explicitly consider family history. All six recommended routine open pelvic lymphadenectomy at the time of radical prostatectomy.

Recommendations about other elements in the pre-operative evaluation varied widely. Bone scan was advised only in high-risk cases, defined variably as PSA greater than 8, 10, or 20, a Gleason score greater than 7 or 8, or bone pain. Pelvic CT scans were recommended by four of the urologists in high-risk cases, defined variably as PSA greater than 20 or 25, a Gleason score greater than 7, or in "patients at high suspicion for lymph node involvement." Endorectal MRI scans were recommended by half of the urologists for various definitions of high-risk tumors. ProstaScint scanning was used by only one urologist for patients with high Gleason scores. One urologist recommended routine complete blood counts and urinalyses; none advised routine chemistry panels. Acid phosphatase was used only rarely by two of the experts. Three urologists routinely used laparoscopic pelvic lymphadenectomy; the other three never used it.

None of the expert urologists conducted formal tests for potency or continence at baseline; however, five of them used patient self-report to document these functions. Two also used the International Prostate Symptom Score to measure urinary symptoms before treatment.

Treatment modalities and approaches. All six expert urologists employed the retropubic approach for radical prostatectomy, and one also used the perineal approach in cases of obesity. All of the surgeons routinely performed nerve sparing, though half often spared the nerves only unilaterally. One urologist routinely encouraged autologous blood storage, while the others did so only selectively at the patient's request. Only one of six was personally involved in a brachytherapy program. None routinely recommended pre-operative androgen ablation.

The characteristics of the surgery thought to be most important in determining successful outcomes included surgical volume; surgical technique, such as handling the nerves and pelvic floor muscles as little as possible and avoiding the use of electrocautery at the prostate apex; size of the prostate, and size of the patient.

Practice guidelines. Four of the six expert urologists routinely used clinical care pathways to standardize post-operative hospital care. Methods used to develop these care pathways included systematic literature review (three of six), expert judgment (two of six), and institutional data (one of six).

Follow-up care and measuring outcomes. Elements of follow-up care thought to be important for ensuring successful outcomes included counseling and management of patient expectations, PSA monitoring, and reassurance. The experts thought the most important outcomes to be measured included ongoing assessment of post-operative urinary and sexual function by patient self-report (all experts) and PSA (four experts).

Summary

The experts we interviewed had diverse approaches to diagnosing and managing early-stage localized prostate cancer and communicating with patients. However, some areas of consensus emerge. Issues involving information are summarized in Table 5.2. Key features of the structure, process, and outcomes of care, as seen by the two groups of experts, are summarized in Table 5.3. For reference, we also show the key findings on each topic from our review of the medical literature.

Table 5.2
Information given to patients and available to physicians

	Majority or all radiation oncologist experts	Majority or all urology experts
Information provided to patients		
In initial consultation, give patients information about radiation therapy, surgery, and watchful waiting	Yes	Yes
Provide information about hormone ablation therapy	Yes	No
Provide information about alternative treatment facilities	Refer to providers they know but only if asked	"delicate question"
Use probabilistic language to explain treatment outcomes	Yes	Yes
Tailor information for patients based on age, tumor stage, co-morbidity	Yes	Yes
Give patients supplementary materials for information	Yes	Yes
Find it easy to discuss treatment issues	Yes	Yes (with exception of sexual function)
Information available to physicians		
Use multiple sources of data (personal and clinical experience, scientific literature)	Yes	Yes
Use tabulated data	Yes	Yes
Find current data adequate	No	No
Baseline tests of sexual function, voiding, or continence	No	Patient self-report only

Table 5.3

Structure, process, and outcomes of care:

Judgment of experts and findings from the medical literature

	Judgment of radiation oncologists	Key findings from radiation oncology literature	Judgment of urologists	Key findings from urology literature
Structure and process of care				
Pre-treatment work-up	1. History, physical exam 2. Special attention to general and urologic health and co-morbidities	PSA	1. History 2. Co-morbidities	
Average time spent with patient	49 minutes		45 minutes	
Staging	1. PSA 2. CBC 3. Chemical panel 4. CT scans	1. PSA most important prognostic factor 2. Gleason score and clinical stage also important	1. DRE, PSA, histological tumor grade 2. Pelvic CT scans for high-risk cases 3. Endorectal MRI	1. DRE, pre-treatment PSA, bone scan, CT scan are standard, but up to 60% of patients are understaged 2. Utility of MRI or ProstaScint not yet proven
Treatment modalities and approaches				
	1. External beam radiation therapy via conventional or conformal techniques 2. Brachytherapy	1. Variables that affect outcomes are total dose, duration of treatment, number and volumes of fields used, and nature of treatment planning 2. Many questions remain re brachytherapy process and its relation to outcomes	1. Retropubic approach for radical prostatectomy 2. Nerve sparing	No randomized controlled trials have evaluated surgical treatment; only case series
Characteristics of treatment thought important for good outcomes				
	1. Dose fractionation of 180 to 200 cGY per day and tumor dose of greater than or equal to 7,000 cGY;	1. Doses below 6,000 cGY not sufficient; doses between 6,600 – 7,000 cGY adequate for low-risk patients; doses	1. Surgical volume 2. Surgical technique	1. Anatomic nerve-sparing radical retropubic prostatectomy, using a modified bladder neck

75

	2. Immobilization of the patient during treatment and use of multiple field techniques with treatment of all fields each day 3. Hormone ablative therapy for high-risk patients (most experts were using hormone ablative therapy even in patients in so-called good prognostic categories) 4. Multiple-level CT planning for tumor control	>7,000 cGY better for more advanced tumors, but have higher complication rates 2. Patient immobilization and conformal treatment effective 3. Neo-adjuvant hormone ablative therapy effective for high-risk patients; benefits for low-risk patients unknown 4. Effect of therapy on quality of life unknown		dissection and modified urethro-vesical anastomosis, shown to yield optimal results in methodologically sound, statistically valid studies 2. Little data to prove other modifications in surgical technique produce better outcomes
	Clinical pathways not used	1. Increased compliance with guidelines from Patterns of Care study 2. No proven link between use of guidelines and better outcomes	Clinical pathways used to standardize post-operative hospital care	Clinical pathways improve quality and decrease costs of surgical treatment
Outcomes to measure	1. PSA evidence of recurrence 2. Quality of life 3. Sexual function, urinary function, bowel function	1. No widely accepted way to measure side effects (bladder, bowel, and sexual function) 2. Patients exaggerate pre-treatment function 3. Best approach is prospective measurement of function via patient surveys 4. Long-term side effects should be assessed at least one year following treatment	1. PSA 2. Post-operative urinary and sexual function by patient self-report	1. PSA monitoring widely accepted but prognostic value of PSA recurrence in question 2. Doubling time of PSA better predictor of recurrence 3. Short- and long-term complications also widely used 4. Relative contribution of each outcome to patient's well-being and satisfaction unknown

Important elements of follow-up care		
Follow-up care	PSA measurement at six months	PSA
	1. DRE widely used, but findings are subjective, and predictive value of DRE is as low as 24% 2. Biopsy used, but rates of positive biopsies vary widely between centers, and relation of biopsy results to other outcomes (e.g., biochemical relapse, disease-free or overall survival) unknown 3. Some guidelines for biochemical recurrence exist, but widely accepted definition is needed	1. Appropriate follow-up undefined 2. Post-treatment PSA monitoring widely accepted, but doubling time better predictor 3. Most physicians use patient's history and physical exam to evaluate patients' post-treatment urinary tract function and quality of life. 4. More accurate way to evaluate outcomes would be prospective measurement of function via patient surveys

Table 5.3 provides a cross-tabulation of quality indicators that are either (1) judged by at least one of the respective experts to be important or (2) mentioned in the relevant literature as being important.

Chapter 6

SUMMARY OF FOCUS GROUPS WITH PATIENTS AND THEIR PARTNERS

In the last chapter, we summarized the interviews we conducted with physician experts to learn how they communicated with their patients and what their approaches were to treating prostate cancer. This chapter addresses the same issues from the patient perspective.

To gather this information, we conducted three separate focus groups: with patients who had been treated for early-stage prostate cancer with either (1) radical prostatectomy or (2) radiation therapy, and (3) with their spouses or significant others. In this chapter, we summarize what we learned from these groups.

Methods

Selecting and recruiting patients. The three focus groups were held on March 14, 1998. We began recruitment four to six weeks prior to the groups, so the patients in the focus groups were treated between January and September of 1997. Patients were eligible for the focus groups if:

1. They had been treated for localized prostate cancer by radical prostatectomy or radiation therapy;

2. Their treatment had been completed between six months and one year prior to the focus group;

3. They spoke fluent English.

We also asked patients if they were current members of a prostate cancer patient support group. Involvement in patient support groups did not exclude patients from participating. However, we wanted to balance the number of participants who were support group members (hence, more likely to be outspoken) with more timid patients in order to keep the focus groups from being dominated by any member.

We asked physician practices in the greater Los Angeles area to help us recruit patients for the focus groups. Nine practices agreed. We sent letters to the practices describing the study and asking them to identify patients who met our criteria and who might be interested in participating in the focus group. We asked the physicians to make the initial contact by discussing the study with eligible patients and gauging their interest in the study.

If patients expressed interest, RAND contacted them directly. For initial communication with patients, we worked with the individual physicians according to their preference.

Some physicians preferred to identify and speak with patients initially, then give RAND their address and phone number to proceed with further recruitment efforts. In these cases, we called the patients to introduce the project, answer any questions, and confirm interest and contact information. We then sent each interested patient a letter about the focus groups and the study in general.

Other physicians preferred not only to identify and speak with patients initially but also to contact the patients more directly for the second step as well. In these cases we prepared the recruitment letter on the referring physician's own letterhead.

Patients notified either the physician's office (who in turn notified RAND) or notified the project staff directly of their interest. We then telephoned the patient directly to confirm his interest and eligibility. In addition, we asked patients several demographic questions to ensure that we had diverse interests and backgrounds represented in our focus groups. Demographic variables included age, insurance status, ethnicity, level of education, current job or occupation (job or occupation prior to retirement where applicable), and the types of organizations at which subjects had been employees.

The focus group process

We developed a set of open-ended questions to be asked by experienced focus-group moderators. The questions were designed to identify what information was available to men newly diagnosed with prostate cancer and from what sources, and to learn what kind of potentially useful information the men felt was lacking. In addition, we wanted to find out whether patients considered the quality of providers and facilities when making their treatment decisions. The RAND Survey Group provided advice for developing the questions and interacting with patients.

We selected non-clinician moderators for each group to make participants more comfortable. Moderators were RAND staff well versed in survey methodologies and health services research, but who had no involvement with the project and were not known to the participants. An age-appropriate male led the two patient groups and a female moderated the spouse group. We designed the focus group questions so that a non-clinician moderator could identify key topics raised by patients.

After discussing the ground rules for communicating in the focus group setting, moderators asked each participant to briefly introduce him or herself. Then, the moderators opened the discussion with a question designed to take participants back to the moment they first heard the news of prostate cancer and the subsequent process of gathering information and making treatment decisions. We focused the discussion to help us understand how patients felt when they were first diagnosed and how this feeling affected their willingness or ability to gather information and make decisions.

We asked the participants what issues most influenced their treatment decisions, with whom they consulted, and generally how they proceeded. We asked about the data gathering process – what they needed to know to make their treatment decision, where they got their information, what they found helpful, whether it was too much or too little, etc. We were also interested in the role played by their physician(s), how their physicians provided information or guidance, and how comfortable they were with their physicians. We inquired about and the role of family in decision-making and support. Finally, we asked them what advice they would offer other patients or partners of patients who were facing the same decisions.

All subjects gave written informed consent to participate in the focus group and to allow audiotaping and videotaping of the sessions. Each focus group included eight to ten participants.

Overview of the focus groups

Overall, patients decisions about type of treatment appeared to reflect their personality traits and individual coping styles. In general, patients who wanted what they believed was an immediate cure chose surgery; patients who felt they could live with uncertainty chose radiation.

Patients in the surgery focus group were generally younger (range 40 to 60) and had slightly less formal education than those in the radiation group (range 60 to 80). Most of the men who chose surgery felt their decision was made quickly and easily. They wanted "certainty" and chose surgery for the feeling of cure it gave them. The general perception in this group was that surgery would "get the cancer out," and there was little appreciation of the potential for recurrence.

Men who had primary treatment with radiation took more time to make their decision. For them, sexual functioning and quality-of-life were more important than survival, a preference that may have been a function of age. These patients seemed to understand and be more comfortable with the uncertainty associated with possible side effects of treatment and cancer recurrence.

All of the men in both focus groups expressed satisfaction with their physician and felt that they had chosen the right treatment for their prostate cancer. However, they did not feel that they had been informed about the severity and duration of treatment side effects.

Surgery focus group

Gathering information and making decisions. All patients in the surgical focus group said they were extremely upset to learn that they had prostate cancer. They felt depression, anger, or fear – usually all of the above. One man described it as "a death sentence."

Most of the patients indicated that they made the decision to have surgery before doing any research. Only about one-fourth said they gathered more information before making a treatment decision. Information-gathering included speaking with friends and multiple physicians, reading books from the lay press, reviewing medical pamphlets, watching educational videos, and evaluating the experiences of others they had known who were sick.

About three-fourths of the group said selecting their treatment was a relatively quick and easy process. Interestingly, many of these same patients gathered a great deal of information after making their decision. It appears that patients who are more certain of the treatment choice appreciate information describing the disease and the treatment in more detail.

Patients also chose surgery because of age (two men in their 40s and one patient in his late 60s who was told it might not be an option for him in a few years), and the fear of perceived difficulties with radiation therapy – daily visits, an ongoing and long-term process, and ultimate uncertainty of cure.

For this group, the biggest issue affecting treatment choice was the belief that surgery was the surest approach to getting the cancer out.

"I realized that the doctor called surgery the "gold-standard." It gave me a 90% chance of cure. At my age [late 40s] for the type of [Gleason] score I had, surgery was the best."

Everyone in the surgery group spoke with at least two physicians, and some consulted with as many as eight doctors (primarily urologists and radiation oncologists) from diagnosis through treatment.

Patients obtained information from books, educational videos, and other materials from the physician. One patient referred to a 100-page packet from the doctor that included articles on all treatment choices for prostate cancer. Most had used the book by Dr. Patrick Walsh, although several were somewhat skeptical about his statistics. They commented that he did not operate on anyone over 60 and felt that this practice was too exclusive.

Two patients said that they took four to six weeks to get additional opinions, and both felt that they had enough time to do so. Everyone else said the decision was immediate – that they could not stand the uncertainty of waiting, evaluating, and deciding.

"I made my decision 5 minutes after I heard the options."
"Right away."
" Took me ½ a minute to decide."

Two other patients took time to do a lot of research, evaluated several treatment options, felt they needed extra time to make a decision, and expressed uncertainty after the diagnosis. These two men were younger, more educated, and appeared more thoughtful about the decision-making process. They expressed far less confusion about what to do and consistently commented that they did not want the decision weighing on their minds.

No patient allowed non-medical factors to affect his treatment decision. In one case, a patient was diagnosed initially at the Veterans Affairs Medical Center (VA). With the help of VA physicians, he had made the decision to have surgery but because of concerns over insurance and quality issues, he wanted to use his HMO plan for this treatment. The HMO was unwilling to pay for surgery, claiming that the patient was eligible only for radiation therapy or watchful waiting. He decided he was going to have surgery anyway, refusing to succumb to insurance obstacles. While preparing to have his surgery, the patient had to send a letter to his physician, medical center, and health plan accepting financial responsibility for any care related to his prostate cancer surgery. At the last minute the HMO said it would pay.

Role of the physician. For the patients in this focus group, the urologist who made the diagnosis of prostate cancer was their primary source of information about their treatment options for prostate cancer. Many men described their urologists as facilitators for information gathering, referring them to radiation oncologists, calling their general physicians to see if they could tolerate the surgery, and reviewing their medical records. Even when patients made their decision quickly, they felt that their doctors provided them with a great deal of information and encouraged them to take the time to evaluate their treatment decision. Two of the more educated patients said that the research they did on their own confused them somewhat.

Patients reported that their surgeons typically dichotomized outcomes, using language like "cured" or "not cured." They also indicated that physicians generally spoke about rates of recurrence and some of the side effects of treatment in qualitative terms but less often with quantitative information. Some men noted that the books their physicians recommended to them usually provided quantitative information about expected outcomes. However, the patients were frustrated that the available data were not uniform and often conflicted.

Some patients reported that their surgeons advocated radical prostatectomy over radiation therapy. One patient reported that his surgeon told him he had a 5% chance of recurrence with surgery and a 14% chance of recurrence with radiation therapy. These statistics make surgery the obvious treatment choice for this patient, even though he had also consulted with a radiation oncologist. Most patients commented that when they told their doctor (general practitioner or urologist) that they had decided to have surgery, they heard comments like, "great," "that's exactly what I would do," and "right decision."

The men in the surgery focus group did not recall much discussion about the potential risks of impotence and incontinence following surgery when they were making their treatment decision. Some said that, in retrospect, perhaps their physician had informed them about side effects of surgery but at the time they did not listen to or believe it:

"I should have listened more when doctors talked about impotence – I thought I had a 50/50 chance of a normal sex life . . . maybe I wasn't told that, but I heard it anyhow . . ."

Although side effects like impotence seemed trivial compared to survival when these men were faced with making a decision about treatment, they gained importance to many of the participants once they were actually affected by them.

Role of the patients' families. Most families were very involved in these patients' information gathering and decision-making. One man said his girlfriend was aware and involved, but he only told his mother and children about it after his surgery was over. All participants indicated that their spouse or partner typically played a major role in the information gathering, but spouses' involvement in the decision-making was more variable. Some patients said that their wives had a say in the decision; others said their wives felt "whatever you decide, I'll do."

Choice of surgeon or facility. Most patients had their surgery performed by the diagnosing urologist, usually upon referral from a primary care physician. Other considerations in selecting a surgeon included the surgeon's reputation, recommendations from other patients, and the number of surgeries performed per week. Only one participant said he considered going outside California (to the Mayo Clinic or Johns Hopkins), but because he did not want to risk a communication gap with the surgeon before or after treatment, he had his surgery locally.

Advice to other patients. Most men said that they could not tell someone in a similar situation what to do – "it has to be their own decision" – but they would advise them to see several doctors for second opinions, go to a support group, talk to others who have had surgery and radiation therapy, get the relevant data, and read and learn as much as possible. A few said they would tell other patients to "do what I did" – "get it out – see my doctor." One man said this was the advice he would give his sons.

As comfortable as these patients were, both when making the decision and now after treatment, most felt they did not know what they were getting into regarding recovery and side effects. They were "blown away" by the demeaning and uncomfortable aspects of recovery and were not prepared for it. They all still viewed the side effects of having surgery as better than dying. However, most said they would tell other patients that it is a really rough procedure and that they should be prepared for the fact that it would not be easy for three to four months.

> "... of 7 surgeries in 10 years, this was the worst."
>
> "... my doctor asked if I'd speak with someone – brought in a man going to have the same surgery next week – he was real worried – he had reason to be worried too. So afterwards I told the doctor, 'I did not tell him everything about the operation. I didn't want to frighten him.' The doctor said, 'Good.'"

Conclusions from the surgery focus group. These men felt confident about surgery because they believed the surgery would remove all the cancer, and that certainty gave them relief. Compared with the radiation therapy focus group, this group spent less time talking information and decision-making, and much more time discussing the details of staging and treatment (nodal status, pathology, etc.). All participants were satisfied with their treatment decision and certain that they had done the right thing.

> "Surgery is the gold-standard. We know we're all going to die someday, but not of prostate cancer."

The men expressed a need for accurate, current, unbiased, reputable statistics and information. They felt that no source of such information currently exists; indeed, they often felt that each new piece of information they encountered conflicted with a previous piece. One man suggested that the government or an organization such as the American Cancer Society should assist patients with gathering unbiased information. Although all participants felt that they had adequate information to make a treatment decision, most felt the information was of limited usefulness because it was not presented in lay terms. The participants emphasized that they did not want the information "dumbed down"; rather, they wanted it presented in clear language free of medical jargon. Some participants felt they did not receive enough information from their doctors and had to look elsewhere.

Radiation therapy focus group

Information gathering and decisionmaking. Patients in this group had a variety of responses to hearing they had prostate cancer. Some expressed shock and surprise, "I felt like I was kicked in the stomach." Some asked themselves, "How will I tell my family?" Others (primarily older men) said they were not surprised – many had had other illnesses or cancers and this was "just another thing" that they expected to hear about one day, although it was still hard to accept.

Age was an important factor in their decision to have radiation therapy, and in most cases, their doctors recommended radiation because of their age. One patient said his doctor told him radical prostatectomy was "a pretty rough operation" and it would not extend his life any longer than radiation therapy, "at least for someone my age." Also, perhaps because this group was somewhat older, many participants had previously had surgery for other conditions and were skeptical that surgery would provide an immediate cure.

All the participants expressed frustration that they felt pressured to make the final decision on their own. Most said it was ironic that with a diagnosis of prostate cancer they had "to figure it out," but if they had something minor like a cold, their doctor would hand them a drug and tell them what to do.

> *"Don't you think it's interesting that when you have a cold or pneumonia, the doctor says take this antibiotic or drug, but when you show up with prostate cancer they tell you here are your options, now YOU make the decision."*

Two other factors strongly influenced these men's decisions about treatment: sexual function after treatment and quality of life. All felt that quality of life was more important than quantity of life, and that radiation therapy provided a fair trade-off. Some also mentioned that information on staging was critical to decision-making. One man in the radiation therapy group had received both surgery and radiation therapy. He said when he chose to have surgery, he was thinking only about saving his life. He said he now felt that he had not considered all the important factors and would probably make a different choice.

For most of the men, non-medical factors such as insurance or hospital had no affect on their decision-making. And for most of the men, neither did the location of the radiation center. One patient said that the fact that the radiation center was five miles from his house definitely affected his treatment decision. But another commented that he lived 200 miles from the facility, but was so convinced he wanted this treatment that he made the trip for every treatment.

These patients got their information about prostate cancer and its treatment from a variety of sources including their physicians, pamphlets from their doctors, peers and family, anyone with prostate cancer, a *Fortune* magazine article written by a corporate leader (although some were skeptical of the article and his choices), the library, books, specifically Dr. Patrick Walsh's book, the Johns Hopkins "white papers," and the Internet.

However, patients commented that much of this material seemed biased. Some felt that there was not enough quantitative information. They wanted actual numbers to examine and compare. They wanted more information about staging, which some felt was critically important, as well as more data about five-year and long-term survival for each treatment. However, despite this perceived need for more detailed quantitative information, many felt that the information currently available was too technical and not written in lay terms.

> " . . . if you could take that stuff and write it in plain English so anyone could understand it, but I couldn't find it that way."
> " . . . have to dig hard to find graphs and numbers."
> " . . . there was a lot of information, but it was so extensive and not all in one place and so technical – it was hard to boil it down to help with decision-making."

Paradoxically, most patients found that they had simultaneously too much and too little information, and that they had to obtain it from too many sources. They could not always find information that they felt would be helpful. Some patients felt that the doctor did not give them enough information to make a decision, but when they had to search on their own they often felt overwhelmed. They did not like having to make the ultimate decision when there was no clear-cut answer. They particularly wanted more quantitative information about outcomes, – "real data" – but explained in clear, lay terms from a single, unbiased, readily accessible source.

Most men took three to four weeks to come to a decision. None felt he did not have enough time. Once the decision was made, everyone wanted to get started right away. They felt they had "lost enough sleep."

"I read all those books in a 3-week period. If I'd studied like that in college, I would have been a genius."

Role of the physician. Their physicians played a major role in these men's decision-making process, regardless of whether they accepted the doctor's recommendation or did their own research and made independently informed decisions. Although only two patients based their decisions solely on their physician's recommendation, all of the patients valued their doctors' opinions highly. However, most felt that they never had enough time with their physicians to get their questions answered. They felt rushed by their physicians and often did not feel comfortable asking them questions. One man said his doctor told him to read more because he asked so many questions.

" . . . felt pressured . . . you know they have a whole line of people in the waiting room."

These men seemed reluctant to be more demanding of their physicians, viewing them as authorities – "he's the doctor; he's the boss."

" . . . I brought my wife in because she's more assertive and got her questions answered. Doctors can be intimidating – especially when you feel vulnerable or rushed."

Although a few men felt they obtained sufficient information about treatment outcomes, most felt that the complications were "glossed over." Some felt their physicians spoke in terms that were too general. Many of the patients were surprised by the severity of the treatment's aftereffects. Although they were given pamphlets, few patients felt they received enough detail about side effects such as lethargy, fatigue, hot flashes, decreased libido, and shortness of breath, and enough information on the severity or duration of these symptoms. Some men acknowledged that no matter how well-informed they were, no one is ever prepared for the actual experience. Others commented that while they were told a lot about the physical side effects, they were not warned about the emotional effects of treatment and of having prostate cancer. A few said that their doctors had mentioned the emotional aspects of treatment and even had them complete a depression screening survey.

Role of the patients' families. There was general consensus that it was a good idea to involved your spouse or significant other, even among those who did not, but the level of involvement varied from couple to couple. Most partners came to the initial consultation, some came to subsequent meetings, some came during treatment. Some partners read and/or prepared questions. Although the nature of the involvement varied among couples, all of the patients said that they made their decision jointly with their partner.

All of the men felt the partner's role was critical; the decision affected them both since quality-of-life and quantity-of-life issues also affect the partner. One man said he would advise someone to bring his partner because the patient does not hear at least half of what was said at the consultation with the physician.

> *" . . . made my wife read the book – scared the hell out of her . . . told her what's coming...then we sat down and talked and looked at graphs and percentages – made the decision based on that."*
>
> *" . . . I'd tell other patients to bring your wife along to all meetings . . . because when you're emotionally involved, you don't hear . . . you need a second set of ears, that actually listens, and also [my] wife is a great disseminator of information into the family."*

Some people commented that to avoid being treated differently by friends, colleagues, and family they were pretty secretive about their illness and treatment. One person commented that "kids think you're going to live forever." He felt talking with them demystified his illness and therefore helped a lot. Some commented that there was no information available on how to deal with your family (kids) and other people.

Choice of radiation oncologist or facility. Patients spoke with their health plans representatives, physicians, spouses, friends, colleagues, peers and others who had had prostate cancer or radiation therapy to learn about prostate cancer experts in their area. They chose their physicians based on information from the Internet and on recommendations from surgeons or their HMO. One man consulted with his wife's oncologist, whom he "respected very much."

The majority of the men spoke with at least two physicians, and many consulted with as many as four. Unlike the men who chose surgery, these men had often consulted multiple radiation oncologists and were very interested in the outcomes of different radiation techniques (external beam radiation, implants, proton therapy, etc.). However, they did not focus their research or decision-making on outcomes for the same type of radiation therapy at different facilities (quality of care), but rather on the possible outcomes with each of the different radiation treatments (efficacy).

Advice for other patients. Participants said they would advise other patients to talk to their peers – "definitely speak with others who have been through it." All felt the patient perspective would be most helpful for getting the true picture. They suggested going to a prostate cancer support group to get this – in person or on-line – but they acknowledged that support groups are "not for everyone." These men said they would give any man newly diagnosed with prostate cancer all of the information they had collected to help him approach the decisions that faced him. They advocated seeking multiple medical opinions and getting "your numbers" (PSA, stage, Gleason score) so that the patient could be an active participant in the decision-making process. They also felt patients should be informed about the long-term side effects and would advise them that it takes six months to a year after treatment to feel better. Regarding the long-term effects of treatment, participants offered the following comments:

> "... be prepared for the emotional toll, especially post-treatment – later on."
>
> "... another patient perspective is most useful for actual information."
>
> "... would tell them about the long-term expectations."
>
> "... I should have been more diligent in gathering information."
>
> "... no surgeon – those butchers want to cut right away."
>
> "... support groups can be intimidating and/or depressing."

Many participants also commented that they had become more spiritual during this time and became more focused on "what is important in life."

Conclusions from the radiation therapy focus group. Participants in the radiation therapy group were older, better-educated, philosophical, more accepting of uncertainty, and more focused on the processes of gathering information and making a treatment decision. They valued quality-of-life factors over survival. Overall they were satisfied with their physician and treatment choice. However, they felt they had not been informed about the severity and duration of side effects. In addition, they would have liked to know about the emotional effects of treatment. As a group, they wanted unbiased quantitative information, from a central source, presented in a non-technical format.

The protracted course of radiation therapy provided a very supportive and helpful environment for some of these men because it gave them a chance to interact regularly with people in the treatment environment. However, one man commented, "when the treatment is over, [you] have to deal with cancer and everything that happened to you on your own. [It's] very hard emotionally."

Participants in both patient focus groups commented that they found the exercise very helpful – "we learned something from other people - hearing what the other guys had to say" – and thought it would be very helpful for doctors and other patients who had been treated to hear a recording of the conversation.

Spouse focus group

The participants in this focus group were the partners of men in one of the two patient focus groups. They were all women and, with one exception, all were married to the patient.

Information gathering and decisionmaking. These women described their first reaction to the prostate cancer diagnosis as "hit hard," "quiet terror," "I'm not going to lose him." One woman mentioned that this was the most worrisome part of the process – hearing that he had cancer. Several mentioned having nursed and lost fathers, grandfathers, or uncles through prostate cancer; because of this experience, these women were terrified about their husband's future. One woman said she was not frightened initially by her husband's diagnosis, but her fear intensified as she read and learned more about the disease.

When it came to making a treatment decision, these women unanimously felt that the decision was *his* to make. They would help, read, gather, and question as much as possible, but they all felt that ultimately he had to decide. Whether partners of a radiation therapy or a surgery patient, all seemed to feel that once they looked at all the factors, the decision process became fairly clear. Some found all of the options frightening, but once the decision was made, they felt their husbands had chosen the right treatment – whichever it was.

> " . . . *acted quickly, but looked into everything. [We] talked to as many people as possible. [My] husband was fairly young with a high PSA – because he was young, slowing down wasn't good enough. [The doctor] told him you couldn't get it all with radiation therapy. Surgery seemed the best option because you know exactly what you're up against right then and there. It's the option I was hoping he'd choose, but had to leave the final decision with him. He wanted me to make the decision for him, but I couldn't – he had to.*

Some women discovered that they were not able to offer suggestions – their husbands would not always let them into the decisionmaking process.

> " . . . *he was frightened [and told me] it's my decision because it's my body. All you can do then is be supportive and hope the doctor knows what he's talking about.*"

Some of the spouses of radiation therapy patients said that surgery had not been an option for their husband because of age, a high PSA, the tumor stage, or some combination of these factors. Others commented that they were against surgery. Most of the couples who chose surgery said the single major factor in their decision was that "surgery was a done deal – they'd get it all," or felt that surgery would "take care of it." However, several felt in retrospect that perhaps they were wrong. One woman believed "surgery meant cure." She said that made the decision easy at the time, but in reality, she and her husband were still dealing with the cancer

" . . . Initially I felt relief that the decision wasn't more difficult – it was virtually a non-decision – only one way to go – surgery. [My] husband was positive – I kept busy. I felt great and thought radical prostatectomy – cancer out – over. [That's] not true. His PSA became elevated and we may face more decisions. It's been extremely shocking because I thought this was it."

The women said that they got their information from the Internet, general physicians and medical specialists, other "veteran" patients and spouses in the waiting room of the doctor's office, the library, and books. The common complaint about books was that much of the data was outdated because the field is growing and changing so quickly.

Some women did not rely on what doctors told them and instead aggressively researched questions on their own. They felt the Internet was the best source for up-to-date information. However, they all indicated that they would have preferred to get this information from the doctor because it would have felt more personal. Others got most of their information from the doctors, feeling that doctors are the experts so patients have to trust what they say and then make a choice.

" . . . talking with veteran patients and spouses sitting in the waiting room of the doctor's office at pre-treatment and early treatment sessions. [We'd] talk about what they felt or not and what side effects they were experiencing. It was very spiritual to talk to those folks who would come in. Mostly patients in the waiting room, but sometimes spouses. It was like a support group."

None of the women felt prepared for the treatment's effect on their husbands. They wished they had known the impact and magnitude of treatment effects, what they were, and how long they would go on. These women also felt that they would have liked to know more about the disease itself – a clear sense of what was going on physiologically, and a better understanding of all the options so that they could have better evaluated and compared each one.

Role of the physicians. All the women went with their husbands to the doctor at least once. Some went to many appointments, a few to all appointments, and several attended only the initial visit. The women had mixed views about the physician as a provider of information. Some felt they received useful information from the doctor; others did not. There was tremendous variation in the amount of time they said the physicians spent with patients (a half hour on average), as well as tremendous variation in whether they felt the time spent with them or their husbands was sufficient. One woman was angered when the doctor (one she referred to as "a good one, too") told them that research, more information, and multiple options would confuse them. About half the women found nurses to be the most helpful and informative of all the people they were exposed to in the medical setting. The others said that the physicians were most helpful.

> " . . . I don't think doctors withhold things from you, they just don't remember everything."
>
> " . . . if doctors would just get down and talk with you more rather than treat it like it's a business . . ."
>
> " . . . I feel it's unrealistic to expect to get details and personal information from your doctors. They just don't seem trained or conditioned to sit down and formally have discussions with patients and families. I didn't have many problems this time – I talked to them – but from past experiences – the doctors just don't consider you to be a peer. They don't think you can understand the information or that you're prepared to hear the facts."
>
> " . . . with radiation therapy, they lose sight of you over the course of the treatment time span. That's why I attended the treatment with my husband – for the long-term upkeep."

Some women felt comfortable asking questions; some did not. Some felt they did not know what to ask. One made a list of questions for her husband to ask, but he came home without having asked them, saying that he did not want to waste the doctor's time. One woman felt that she got too much statistical information from the physician, but no explanation of the reasoning. She felt she had to learn all of the clinical information on her own – she found out how dangerously high her husband's PSA was through her own research, not through the doctor.

Everyone saw at least two doctors – on average three to four. They typically saw a urologist, radiation oncologist and general oncologist. One comment reflected the frustration with seeking multiple opinions: "you could go to ten different doctors and get ten different opinions." Most women felt that even when physicians gave them information about treatment options, it was either not in terms they could understand or was totally generic. One woman commented she had to press the physician and ask "what does that mean?"

Role of the families. These women were consistently involved with their husbands' prostate cancer treatment. They accompanied their husbands to hear about the choices, ask questions, get information, and help their husbands process the information.

> *" . . . I couldn't tell him – I was just there to help him out – be by his side"*
> *" . . . he never got answers when I wasn't there – got them when I came along . . ."*

Most of these women spoke of the tremendous support and care they received from their children, friends and family. However, several commented that the rest of their family had not been as involved as they were. Some wives observed that "kids think their parents are invincible" and in order to alleviate their own fears, their children did not take seriously what was happening to their father. No patient's children were involved in the actual information gathering or treatment decision-making.

Many of the women were afraid that they would not be prepared to care for their husbands after treatment. Spouses are expected to be supportive and optimistic caretakers. But the men often felt depressed or defeated. The women noted that coping with this situation takes a very high emotional toll on the wives. They have to remain positive and calm even though they are also very frightened.

Choice of physician or facility. Physicians or facilities were selected based on recommendations, HMO referrals, perceived physician skill, or reputation of the facility. In general, the women shared the opinion expressed in both patient focus groups: there were things they wished they had known but they were satisfied with the selection of treatment and provider.

Advice to other patients or patients' partners. If a friend, or a friend's partner were diagnosed with prostate cancer, these women would tell them to have hope, to get multiple opinions, to be informed and educate themselves, to read a lot and work with the doctor, but not to rely solely on the doctor for information. They would also share their spouse's experience with other patients and their partners.

They felt that physicians and providers of information to the prostate cancer community should explain to patients in more detail about the aftereffects of treatment and the recovery process. In particular, spouses mentioned treatment effects that they felt were never addressed, such as the effects of androgen ablation or "male menopause." They felt patients should be told to expect side effects, receive clear information about the side effects' true length and magnitude, and be informed that each man's recovery is different. They felt this kind of information would have better prepared them for much of what they and their husbands faced.

" . . . most men – even if informed of the side effects before – don't quite understand what the impact will be regarding impotence and other side effects. I think a lot of them mentally know it, but don't accept it. They don't understand how they're going to feel."

Conclusions from the spouse focus group. The spouse group was the most varied of the focus groups. They bonded over similarities, but took many different approaches to the challenge of gathering information and making a decision. But like their partners, they wished they had known certain things but remained satisfied with the treatment that was selected.

They all felt that support and education for spouses before the treatment would have been very helpful for both patients and partners, and they thought this should be available in the future to other spouses. They did not want their hands held; rather, they really wanted to be educated.

The women had many suggestions about how to give newly diagnosed patients and their families the benefit of others' experience. They liked one participant's suggestion of a class for patients and families. They also felt it would be helpful to attend a group like the focus group in which they had participated to hear about what patients and their families have already gone through. A suggestion to videotape a focus group and make it available in the doctor's office for patients and partners generated tremendous enthusiasm. The participants thought such a tape would be a reliable source of useful patient information regarding aftereffects and the variety of opinions, experiences, and outcomes. They mentioned the American Cancer Society's practice of sending breast cancer survivors to visit newly diagnosed women. They thought a similar program for prostate cancer patients might be a good idea, but worried that men might not respond as well to such a program as women do. The final suggestion was a patient/spouse hotline, staffed on a volunteer basis by previously treated patients and their families, which newly diagnosed patients and their families could call for information and advice.

Chapter 7

SELECTING CANDIDATE QUALITY INDICATORS
FOR EARLY-STAGE PROSTATE CANCER

The goal of this study is to develop the infrastructure necessary to begin evaluating quality of care provided to men with early-stage prostate cancer. In this chapter, we describe (1) the method by which we selected candidate indicators for the structure, process, and outcomes of prostate cancer care, (2) the composition of the panel of experts we convened to assess the candidate indicators, (3) the process the experts used to do their assessment, and (4) the resulting list of indicators.

Conceptual framework for organizing candidate indicators

To categorize candidate indicators into meaningful groups that can be used for research and assessment purposes, we used the terminology offered by Donabedian (Donabedian 1980) to describe the components of quality of care: *structure, process,* and *outcomes*. In addition, we included a separate category for *covariates,* measures that would be used to control for potential confounding factors when comparing quality across different facilities. Each of these constructs is described in detail below, along with specific examples illustrating their utility as reported in the scientific literature.

Structure of care. Structure of care refers to elements of the treatment facility – its inputs and organization – that may play a role in accounting for variations in treatment results. Examples of candidate structural quality indicators include: availability of certain types of medical equipment or specialized services, staff qualifications and staffing ratios (e.g., percentage of board-certified specialists, patient/staff ratios), and payer mix. Patient case-mix and volume of patients are also candidate indicators of structural quality, each being a measure of a structural input. The use of clinical pathways or guidelines can be considered a structural element of quality if a monitoring function is implemented in the facility.

The medical literature provides little empirical information with which to assess the relationship between structure and localized prostate cancer treatment outcomes. Hanks et al. (1995) studied the association between equipment types used to treat three types of cancer

(Hodgkin's disease, cervical cancer, and prostate cancer) and patient outcomes as measured by rates of disease recurrence. Facilities that used cobalt units were found to have higher stage-adjusted rates of disease recurrence for cervical and prostate cancer patients than those that used linear accelerators or betatron. The same facilities that used cobalt units were also found to have other structural indicators that could indicate lower-quality care. These facilities had lower percentages of patients staged, lower staff/patient ratios, and were more likely to have part-time therapists as compared with national averages.

The study recommends that facilities using <80 cm cobalt units should upgrade treatment equipment, treat palliative patients only, or close. However, the study does not report direct links between these measures and patient outcomes.

A potential structural measure of surgical treatment for localized prostate cancer is patient volume, where volume is defined as the number of patients treated at the facility. Preliminary findings about the relationship between volume and treatment outcomes have been identified by Lu-Yao et al. (personal communication, 1998) using Medicare claims data. They found that high-volume hospitals had more favorable surgical outcomes following radical prostatectomy (reduced mortality, complication rates, readmission rates) and shorter lengths of stay than low-volume facilities. The effect appeared linear based on analyses of hospital groups by volume quartiles. Their analyses controlled for differences in patient composition using age, race, year of surgery, and hospital teaching status. A recent publication by Ellison and colleagues also showed a positive relationship between volume and outcomes (Ellison, Heaney, and Birkmeyer 2000).

We did not have prior direct evidence either to support or refute the link between patient outcomes and a number of other structure measures. However, we asked panelists to rate the feasibility of these measures, and to provide any comments based on their own professional experience.

Process of care. Process of care refers to elements of the technical delivery of care that may be associated with variations in treatment results. Examples of domains that are included in process quality indicators include: elements of the pre-treatment work-up, primary treatment, and post-treatment follow-up and continuing care. Examples of candidate process quality indicators include: use and documentation of certain diagnostic procedures, coordination of care, and practices for monitoring patients after treatment. A number of these elements have been addressed directly in the prostate cancer treatment literature.

Pre-treatment stage, Gleason grade, and PSA assessment. Numerous studies have illustrated the prognostic usefulness of pre-treatment PSA, clinical stage, and Gleason grade in predicting post-treatment outcomes such as risk of recurrence (D'Amico et al. 1998a; Lankford et al. 1997; Pisansky et al. 1997a; 1997b). Some have found that PSA cancer volume, an estimate of cancer volume based on PSA, may improve the accuracy of outcome prediction for men who have intermediate PSA levels, from 4 to 20 ng/mL. The ratio of free to total PSA may also improve the accuracy of staging (Pannek et al. 1998). Catalona (Catalona 1996) suggests that free PSA may correlate with the potential aggressiveness of localized prostate cancer. However, Pannek et al. (1996) found that free PSA did not provide additional utility in predicting pathologic stage after controlling for Gleason score and clinical stage for early-stage prostate cancer patients.

Pelvic lymph node dissection. Rees et al. (1997) offer guidelines for when a pelvic lymph node dissection may be eliminated for some types of patients: (1) if the PSA is less than 5 ng/ml, or (2) if the Gleason score is less than or equal to 5, or (3) if the PSA is under 25 and the Gleason score is less than or equal to 7 for a patient with a negative digital rectal exam.

Assessment of co-morbidity, pre-treatment functioning, family history. In the process of conducting interviews with 14 expert urologists and radiation oncologists, we found uniform agreement about the importance of assessing patient co-morbidity during the pre-treatment work-up. However, the approaches used to assess co-morbidity varied widely. Examples of co-morbidity assessments included: Karnofsky Performance Status; documentation of patient obesity; and patient self-reported activity levels, cardiac disease, vascular disease, pulmonary disease, hypertension, diabetes, or prior surgeries. At present, there are no specific guidelines for uniformed reporting of patient co-morbidity for localized prostate cancer pre-treatment work-up.

In our interviews we found that pre-treatment urinary, bowel, and sexual function are most commonly assessed by patients' verbal reports. Some physicians reported using the American Urological Association (AUA) symptom score to assess obstruction. Formal assessment of potency, voiding symptoms, or continence is rarely performed on a routine basis.

Kupelian et al. (1997a, 1997b) found that family history of prostate cancer can be prognostic of treatment failure following radiation therapy or radical prostatectomy, even after controlling for patient age, pre-treatment PSA, Gleason sum, clinical stage, and treatment modality. Some physicians explicitly indicated that family history of prostate cancer is routinely assessed during the pre-treatment work-up. Family history of other diseases was mentioned by some physicians as a way to assess a patient's life expectancy in conjunction with the patient's age.

Pre-treatment counseling. A specific recommendation from the American Urological Association's clinical guidelines on managing localized prostate cancer is to explain to patients what the treatment options are (radical prostatectomy, radiation therapy—external beam, interstitial treatment, and expectant management).

Surgery. The use of a retropubic approach for surgery may increase the chances of nerve-sparing, and Wahle et al. (1990) found that nerve-sparing approaches do not result in increased risk of margin involvement. Blute et al. (1997) report that positive surgical margins can be a significant predictor of recurrence in stage pT2N0 prostate cancer independent of grade, PSA, and DNA ploidy. A practice protocol has been developed by the College of American Pathologists Cancer Committee for management of pathology specimens (Henson et al. 1994). We do not have evidence of whether adherence to this protocol improves patient outcomes for localized prostate cancer. About one-fourth of localized prostate cancer Medicare patients treated by radical prostatectomy undergo further cancer treatment following the surgery (Lu-Yao et al. 1996). Routine post-treatment follow-up for radical prostatectomy patients may be warranted as a result.

Radiation therapy. A substantial body of literature has developed on the use and outcomes of conformal radiation therapy. Although this method of radiation treatment is not used widely, the evidence obtained from these studies is especially useful to consider in the context of methods used for conventional external beam radiation treatment, as well as with some expectation for expanded adoption by radiation oncologists.

Hanks et al. (1995) found that conformal radiation therapy resulted in fewer Grade 2 toxicities as compared with external beam radiation. However, high-dose conformal treatment may result in increased risk of severe rectal bleeding (Hanlon et al. 1997, Teshima et al. 1997). Appropriate shielding of the rectal mucosa is recommended to reduce this risk. The prostate may have considerable movement within the body (Roeske et al. 1995). Assessment of target motion and patient immobilization (Beard et al. 1996, Soffen et al. 1991) may be recommended for radiation treatment.

Using CT-MRI image fusion, Kagawa et al. (1997) found that MRI localization of the prostate may be more accurate than CT for improving physicians' ability to locate the treatment area for 3D conformal radiation therapy treatment planning.

Outcomes of care. Outcomes refer to the results of medical treatment. They may be assessed by a clinician, patient, or, in some instances, by a proxy on behalf of the patient. Outcomes may be proximal to treatment: for example, they can include immediate complications resulting from primary treatment. They may also include intermediate markers of longer-term outcomes: for example, a serum marker may be prognostic of disease recurrence.

Kuban et al. (1998) documented the consensus guidelines developed by ASTRO for using PSA for post-treatment assessment. The recommended indicator for biochemical failure was three consecutive increases in PSA after irradiation. However, this indicator is not intended to be a surrogate for clinical progression or survival, neither is it meant by itself to indicate the need for additional treatment. In measuring surgical outcomes, a detectable PSA may be correlated with risk of recurrence, but there is no consensus on PSA outcome reporting.

The American Urological Association has endorsed the assessment of patient quality of life (Middleton et al. 1995). Litwin (1998b) and others have shown that clinicians' assessments of patient functioning may differ sharply from the patients' own assessments, with physicians underestimating rates of complications. The use of patient-reported functional status and quality of life may provide additional information about the results of treatment (Fowler et al. 1995; 1996; Litwin et al. 1995).

Covariates. We included an additional category, covariates, to describe indicators that, while not directly related to quality of care, could represent potential confounding variables or effect modifiers. Covariates are not measures of quality; rather, they represent factors that might be controlled for when comparing quality across various providers. The covariates must be tested for their effect on all of the process and outcome measures, though not necessarily on the

103

structure measures. Among the candidate covariates were tumor characteristics, such as stage, Gleason grade, and pre-treatment PSA; general health indicators, such as age and co-morbidities; and other factors, such as family history of prostate cancer and race (African-American).

Expert panel methods

We convened a panel of experts to evaluate candidate performance indicators for early-stage prostate cancer. This panel comprised 11 clinicians and researchers from the fields of urology (3 panel members), radiation oncology (3 panel members), medical oncology (3 panel members), and health services research (2 panel members). Clinical members of the panel were nominated by their professional societies for having strong expertise in localized prostate cancer treatment and research. Professional societies who provided recommendations included the American Urological Association, the American College of Radiation Oncology, the American College of Radiology, the American Society for Therapeutic Radiology and Oncology, and the American Society for Clinical Oncology. Two non-clinical members of the panel were selected for their expertise in health services and their experience in assessing prostate cancer outcomes and prostate cancer-related quality of life. Participating panel members are listed in Table 7.1.

Table 7.1
Members of the RAND expert consensus panel for the development of candidate quality indicators in localized prostate cancer

---

Health Services

David Cella, PhD

Center on Outcomes Research & Evaluation – Northwestern University

Arnold L. Potosky, PhD, MHS

Independent Consultant (Dr. Potosky's participation does not imply endorsement by the National Cancer Institute or the National Institutes of Health)

Medical Oncology

Derek Raghavan, MD

University of Southern California – Norris Cancer Center

David Reese, MD

University of California, San Francisco

William Kevin Kelly, DO

Memorial Sloan-Kettering Cancer Center

Radiation Oncology

John C. Blasko, MD

University of Washington Medical Center

Gerald E. Hanks, MD

Fox Chase Cancer Center

Deborah A. Kuban, MD

Eastern Virginia Medical School

Urology

Roy J. Correa, MD
Virginia Mason Clinic

James E. Montie, MD
University of Michigan

Horst Zincke, MD
Mayo Clinic

To assess candidate quality indicators, the panel used methods previously developed at RAND to assess appropriate care in other clinical settings (Fraser, 1994). This approach asked panel members to:

1.   Review candidate quality indicators;
2.   Provide initial ratings on the validity and feasibility of the measures as indicators of high-quality care for the treatment of localized prostate cancer;
3.   Meet collectively to discuss, re-rate, and rank these indicators; and
4.   Provide revised ratings.

Steps 1 and 2 occurred before the expert panel meeting, with panel members providing initial rankings independently. Steps 3 and 4 took place during the expert panel meeting held at RAND.

The panel's instruction materials explained that the members' role was to rate the appropriateness of candidate quality indicators to assess localized prostate cancer treatment and, where applicable, to consider alternative quality indicators for different treatment modalities. Panel members were asked not to assess the comparative efficacy of any treatment modality, because these types of recommendations would fall beyond the scope of the panel's goals.

Ratings of validity and feasibility for candidate indicators. During the initial round, panel members were asked to rate a total of 59 candidate measures, including 10 structure, 27 process, 13 outcomes, and 9 covariates using a nine-point rating scale to assess clinical validity and feasibility. In this study, a candidate quality indicator was considered *valid* if:

1. There was adequate scientific evidence or professional consensus supporting the indicator; and
2. Based on the panelists' professional experience, physicians with significantly higher rates as measured by the indicator would be considered higher-quality providers.

Ratings of 1–3 mean that the indicator would not be a valid measure for evaluating quality, ratings of 4–6 mean that the indicator would be an uncertain or equivocal measure, and ratings of 7–9 mean that the indicator would be a clearly valid measure.

In this study a candidate quality indicator was defined as *feasible* if:

1. The information necessary to assess the measure could be found in a medical record, cancer registry, or other systematically recorded data source;
2. Recorded information about the measure was likely to be reported reliably; and
3. Failure to document relevant information about the measure would itself be a marker of poor quality.

Ratings of 1–3 mean that it would not be feasible to use the indicator to evaluate quality, ratings of 4–6 mean that there would be considerable variability in the feasibility of using the measure, and ratings of 7–9 mean that it would be clearly feasible to use the measure. Table 7.2 shows an example of the rating formats.

Table 7.2
Example of pre-meeting rating form for candidate indicators

Indicator	Validity			Feasibility		
	Not valid	Equivocal	Valid	Not feasible	Varies	Feasible
Mortality	1 2 3	4 5 6	7 8 9	1 2 3	4 5 6	7 8 9

Panel members provided several additional indicators during the initial round. A total of 95 candidate measures were reviewed at the panel meeting, including 13 structure indicators, 39 process indicators, 27 outcome indicators, and 16 covariate measures.

To determine whether a candidate indicator should be included in the set of *recommended* indicators, the median rating was used to measure the central tendency for the 11 panelists, and the mean absolute deviation from the median was used to measure the dispersion of the ratings.

The final rating was based on the median score for validity and feasibility. To be included in the final set, an indicator needed a rating of 7–9 on validity and 4–9 on feasibility. If panelists disagreed strongly about an indicator, it was excluded.

Definitions of agreement and disagreement. We identified agreement and disagreement by framing their definitions as tests of hypotheses about the distribution of ratings in a hypothetical population of repeated ratings by similarly selected panelists.

For agreement, we tested the hypothesis that 80 percent of the hypothetical population of repeated ratings were within the same region (1–3, 4–6, or 7–9) as the observed median rating. If we were unable to reject that hypothesis on a binomial test at the 0.33 level, the indication was rated "with agreement." For 11 ratings, this definition of agreement required that no more than three of the ratings be outside the three-point region containing the median. For items with fewer than 11 raters – for example, if one of the raters chose to leave an item missing – then agreement required that no more than two of the ratings be outside the three-point region containing the median.

For disagreement, we tested the hypothesis that 90 percent of the hypothetical population of repeated ratings were within one of two wider regions (1–6 or 4–9). If we rejected that hypothesis on a binomial test at the 0.10 level, the indication was rated "with disagreement." For between eight and eleven raters, this definition of disagreement was satisfied when three or more ratings were in the 1–3 region and three or more were in the 7–9 region. These definitions are equivalent to those from previous studies using similar expert panel methods (Chassin et al. 1987). Table 7.3 shows the definitions of agreement and disagreement that we used.

Table 7.3
Definitions of panel agreement and disagreement

Validity	Feasibility	Disposition	
		Include	*Exclude*
1–3	1–3		√
1–3	4–6		√
1–3	7–9		√
4–6	1–3		√
4–6	4–6		√
4–6	7-9		√
7–9	1–3		√
7–9	4–6	√	
7–9	7–9	√	

Final candidate indicators

Tables 7.4 through 7.7 present the candidate quality-of-care indicators that were included and excluded by the expert panel.

Structure indicators. Of a long list of possible structure measures, panelists endorsed only a few candidate quality indicators. They included patient case-mix, provider volume, availability of counseling resources, board certification of providers, and knowledge (availability) of treating institution outcomes. The panel rejected all indicators of accreditation and clinical pathways and guidelines as potential structure indicators.

Despite the absence of published evidence to support it, the panelists thought experience (also referred to as volume or caseload) was an important indicator of quality of care. Another indicator of experience, albeit imperfect, is board certification, which the panelists also endorsed. Perhaps reflecting the penetration of the current outcomes era in medical care, panelists endorsed the availability of outcomes data specific to the treating institution. Simply quoting the literature for complications and outcomes was felt to be consistent with poorer quality care. Panelists also felt that the effect of prostate cancer on patients' mental health is so great that a provider or facility might be judged to be of higher quality if it had demonstrated availability of psychological counseling resources. Finally, panelists endorsed the availability of conformal treatment as a quality indicator for radiation therapy.

Process indictors. Process indicators included a number of pre-treatment work-up assessments including DRE, clinical stage, total PSA, and Gleason grade, and well as documentation that the physician assessed voiding, potency, family history, and co-morbidities. These panelists excluded measures of the ratio of free-to-total PSA and PSA volume as well as AUA symptom score.

Pre-treatment evaluation is critical to the accurate clinical staging of the tumor. There is general consensus in the literature and among the expert panelists that success rates of curative local therapies are enhanced when tumors are pathologically organ-confined. Although there is no absolute pre-treatment indicator of pathological stage, measures of tumor aggressiveness contribute greatly to the difficult clinical decisions that patients face.

With respect to these decisions, the expert panelists endorsed all the quality indicators related to patient counseling, including documenting the discussion of alternative treatment modalities, providing treatment outcomes based on the provider's own practice experience, and giving patients the opportunity to consult with other specialists. Each of these clearly improves the decision-making process.

For surgery, the only specific process indicator endorsed was intraoperative blood loss. The consensus is that this measure, although imperfect, provides at least a rough proxy for the surgeon's skills. Nonetheless, it is important to control for covariates, such as clinical tumor stage, which can affect the technical difficulty of the procedure. Decision rules regarding when pelvic lymph node dissection might be avoidable were not considered by the panel to be useful indicators of quality of care. Neither were other measures, such as surgical approach, use of nerve-sparing method, and operating room time.

Adherence to the College of American Pathologists guidelines for managing pathology specimens was endorsed as a potential indicator of institutional quality. Although we did not include a pathologist on our panel, members were acutely aware of the importance of uniform handling of specimens and reporting of histologic findings.

For radiation, expert panelists endorsed the use of CT scans during planning for standard and conformal external beam treatment. CT scans, and *not* MRI scans, were felt to contribute critical information to the accurate pre-treatment determination of exactly where and how to target the radiation dose. Patient immobilization and rectal mucosa protection during treatment were also endorsed for both external beam and conformal treatment, although assessment of target motion was not endorsed. A final quality indicator endorsed by the panelists was adherence to standard dose recommendations, specific to either external beam or conformal treatment.

For both surgery and radiation, adequate follow-up was endorsed as a potential indicator of high quality, as evidenced by at least two visits by the treating physician during the first year after treatment.

Outcome indicators. Panel members endorsed a number of clinical and patient-reported outcomes as candidate quality indicators. These included biochemical failure using PSA assessment, although endorsed methods differed by treatment modality. After surgery, PSA should become undetectable; after radiation it should drop to very low levels and remain there. Recognizing the importance of patient self-assessment, panelists endorsed patient reports of urinary, sexual, and bowel functioning following treatment and did not endorse physician assessments of patient functioning. Again, emphasizing the importance of patient-centered outcomes, panelists endorsed indicators of patients' satisfaction with their treatment choice, continence, and potency (and for surgery, length of hospital stay).

Fundamental to using outcome measures is including covariates to control for various aspects of case mix. For example, although the panelists endorsed inclusion of pre-treatment PSA and Gleason score in determining whether to proceed with curative therapy, the actual values must be adjusted for when examining outcome measures. The higher the PSA and Gleason score, the more likely the patient is to have non-organ – confined disease, and hence the more likely he is to experience biochemical failure or shorter survival. If a provider takes on more of the challenging cases, then these factors must be considered when judging measures of the provider's quality of care. Likewise, patients who are impotent before treatment will certainly be impotent afterward, and any assessment of provider quality must take this into account. To that end, the panel also endorsed acute surgical complication rates and the need to treat specific complications (e.g., bowel and bladder dysfunction) as valid and feasible candidate outcome measures.

Panelists endorsed various measures of survival, such as 10-year overall survival and 5-, 10-, and 15-year disease-free survival. However, although these outcomes are easy to measure, they are problematic in prostate cancer because the disease has a long natural history, but treatment approaches are evolving rapidly. By the time long-term survival data are collected and analyzed, they may be irrelevant because they represent the outcomes of treatments that have been substantially revised or are no longer in use. Biochemical recurrence rate is a more useful proxy, although it must be carefully controlled for case mix. Five-year overall survival was excluded by the panelists as too short to be meaningful in the context of the long survival of most patients.

Panelists excluded measures of clinical local control, positive surgical margins, assessment of perineural invasion, and patient-reported satisfaction with doctor.

Covariates. The expert panel endorsed all candidate covariates except one as being important measures to control when comparing outcomes across institutions. The single exclusion was race (African American) because panel members believed that the literature did not clearly show that differences in outcomes by race could not be attributable to other clinical factors such as stage at diagnosis. Certain covariates are more appropriate for some candidate quality indicators than for others. Several candidate quality indicators do not need to be adjusted for any of the covariates.

Summary

Table 7.8 contains a final proposed list of candidate quality indicators, each of which is flagged with its relevant covariates. The list was developed by synthesizing the results of the expert panel in the context of the literature reviews, the interviews with experts, and the focus groups. Related and redundant indicators have been combined.

The list of candidate quality indicators provides the foundation for several potential next steps. We describe these in the next chapter.

Table 7.4 Quality-of-care measures included and excluded by the panel: STRUCTURE

	Include	Exclude
S1	Volume (number) of patients treated	
S2		Provider use and documentation of adherence to clinical guidelines
S3		Provider use and documentation of adherence to clinical pathways
S4		Joint Committee on the Accreditation of Healthcare Organizations (JCAHO) accreditation
S5		American College of Radiology (ACR) accreditation (XRT only)
S6		American College of Radiation Oncology (ACRO) accreditation (XRT only)
S7		Access to National Cancer Institute (NCI) or cooperative group trials (for surgery and XRT)
S8		Availability of multidisciplinary clinic for prostate cancer patients
S9	Availability of conformal radiation therapy treatment (radiation oncology facilities)	
S10	Availability of psychological counseling resources	
S11		Risk assessment program for relatives of patients
S12	Board certification of urologists and radiation oncologists	
S13	Knowledge of treating institution outcomes	

Table 7.5 Quality-of-care measures included and excluded by the panel: PROCESS

	Include	Exclude
P1	Pre-treatment clinical staging with digital rectal exam (DRE), total PSA, Gleason grade	
P2		Free/total PSA
P3		PSA volume
P4	Documented assessment of voiding	
P5	Documented assessment of potency	
P6		AUA symptom score assessment (obstruction)
P7	Documented assessment of co-morbidity	
P8	Assessment of family history of prostate cancer	
P9		Pelvic lymph node dissection in patients with (PSA < 5 ng/ml and Gleason score ≤ 5)
P10		Pelvic lymph node dissection in patients with (PSA < 25, Gleason < 7, and negative DRE)
P11	Documentation that alternative treatment modalities (radical prostatectomy, radiation therapy – external beam, interstitial treatment, and expectant management) were presented to patient	
P12	Documentation that complications from treatment, based on the practitioner's or facility's own experience, were presented to patient	
P13	Documentation that patient was offered the opportunity to consult with a urologist or medical oncologist (if provider is radiation oncologist), or with a radiation oncologist or medical oncologist (if provider is urologist)	
P14		Use of retropubic surgical approach, unless contraindicated

P15	Evidence of institutional adherence to practice protocol of the College of American Pathologists Cancer Committee for management of pathology specimens	

Table 7.5 – Continued

P16	Use of CT in conventional (external beam) radiation therapy treatment planning	
P17		Use of Magnetic Resonance Imaging (MRI) in conventional (external beam) radiation therapy treatment planning
P18		Assessment of target motion in conventional (external beam) radiation therapy treatment planning
P19	Immobilization of patient during conventional (external beam) radiation treatment	
P20	Use of CT in conformal radiation therapy treatment planning	
P21		Use of MRI in conformal radiation therapy treatment planning
P22		Assessment of target motion in conformal radiation treatment planning
P23	Immobilization of patient during conformal radiation treatment	
P24	Appropriate protection of rectal mucosa in high-dose conformal treatment	
P25		Routine use of post-treatment (XRT) biopsy to evaluate outcome
P26	At least 2 visits for follow-up by treating physician during the first year post-treatment	
P27	Documentation or evidence of communication with patient's primary care physician or provision of continuing care	
P28	Operative blood loss	
P29		Operating room time
P30		Percentage of positive lymph nodes
P31	Use of clinical and pathological Tumor-Nodes-Metastasis (TNM) staging by the treating physicians	

P32		Use of nerve-sparing method
P33		Use of ICRU for reporting dose
P34	Delivering recommended doses (68 – 72 Gy isocenter [ICRU]) for conventional external beam radiation therapy	

Table 7.5 – Continued

P35	Delivering escalated doses (70–80 Gy ICRU) with conformal radiation therapy	
P36	High energy linear accelerator (≥10 MV)	
P37		Documented second opinion with urologist or radiation oncologist
P38		Presence of independent written information with signature of patient
P39	Documentation of pre-treatment urinary, sexual, and bowel functioning	

Table 7.6 Quality-of-care measures included and excluded by the panel: OUTCOMES

	Include	Exclude
O1	Primary treatment failure indicated by 3 consecutive rising PSA values after primary treatment by radiation therapy	
O2	Primary treatment failure indicated by any confirmed detectable PSA value after primary treatment by radical prostatectomy	
O3	Clinical detection of post-treatment recurrence with biopsy confirmation	
O4		Physician assessment of urinary, sexual, and bowel functioning following primary treatment by radiation therapy or radical prostatectomy
O5	Hospitalization for cystitis, proctitis, hematuria, rectal bleeding following primary treatment by radiation therapy	
O6	Surgical treatment for cystitis, proctitis, hematuria, rectal bleeding following primary treatment by radiation therapy	
O7	Medical treatment for cystitis, proctitis, hematuria, rectal bleeding following primary treatment by radiation therapy	
O8	Hospitalization for bladder neck contracture/urethral stricture following radical prostatectomy or radiation therapy	
O9	Surgical treatment for bladder neck contracture/urethral stricture following radical prostatectomy or radiation therapy	
O10	Medical treatment for bladder neck contracture/urethral stricture following radical prostatectomy or radiation therapy	
O11	Patient assessment of urinary, sexual, and bowel functioning following primary treatment by radiation therapy or radical prostatectomy, using a reliable, validated survey instrument	
O12		Clinical local control following primary treatment by radiation therapy or radical prostatectomy
O13	10-year clinical and/or biochemical *disease-free* survival following primary treatment by radiation therapy or radical prostatectomy (see also 10, 11, 15, 16, 22)	
O14	5-year clinical and/or biochemical *disease-free* survival following primary treatment by radiation therapy or radical prostatectomy	

Table 7.6 – Continued

O15		5-year case mix adjusted *overall* survival following primary treatment by radiation therapy or radical prostatectomy
O16		Positive surgical margins adjusted for pathological technique, stage, grade, PSA, neoadjuvant hormone therapy
017	Patient satisfaction with treatment choice	
O18		Clinical finding of no post-treatment local recurrence with negative biopsy
O19	10-year overall survival	
O20	15-year disease free survival	
O21	Patient satisfaction with continence	
O22	Patient satisfaction with potency	
O23		Perineural invasion on pathology
O24	Acute surgical complication rate (death, cardiovascular complications, deep vein thrombosis, pulmonary embolus, blood loss necessitating transfusions, etc.)	
O25	Hospital length of stay (surgery)	
O26	15-year overall survival	
O27		Satisfaction with doctor

Table 7.7 Quality-of-care measures included and excluded by the panel: COVARIATES

	Include	Exclude
C1	Patient age	
C2	Patient life expectancy	
C3	Pre-treatment total PSA	
C4	Clinical stage	
C5	Gleason grade	
C6	Family history of prostate cancer	
C7	History of other cancer	
C8		Patient race (African American)
C9	Co-morbidity indicators	
C10	Use of neoadjuvant hormone therapy (surgery)	
C11	Use of neoadjuvant hormone therapy (XRT)	
C12	Use of temporary (e.g., 6 months) adjuvant hormonal treatment	
C13	Use of adjuvant hormonal treatment	
C14	Insurance plan coverage	
C15	Educational attainment	
C16	Patient income	

Table 7.8 Short list of candidate quality indicators with relevant covariates

	Indicator	Covariates
STRUCTURE		
1	Volume (number) of patients treated	Age, life expectancy, pre-treatment PSA, clinical stage, Gleason grade, history of other cancer, co-morbidity indicators, insurance, education, income
2	Availability of conformal therapy (radiation oncology facilities)	
3	Availability of psychological counseling resources	
4	Knowledge of treating institution outcomes	
PROCESS		
5	Pre-treatment assessment with DRE, PSA, and Gleason grade	
6	Documentation of pre-treatment urinary, sexual, and bowel function	
7	Assessment of family history of prostate cancer	
8	Documentation that the patient was presented with alternative treatment modalities; the opportunity to consult with a provider of an alternative treatment modality; and the risk of treatment complications in the experience of the practitioner or facility	
9	Evidence of institutional adherence to practice protocol of College of American Pathologists Cancer Committee for management of pathology specimens	
10	For conventional external beam radiation therapy: use of CT during treatment planning; use of patient immobilization during treatment; delivering recommended doses (68–72 Gy isocenter [ICRU]	
11	For conformal external beam radiation therapy: use of CT during treatment planning; use of patient immobilization during treatment; appropriate protection of rectal mucosa during high-dose conformal treatment; delivering escalated doses (70–80 Gy ICRU)	

Table 7.8 – Continued

12	For radiation therapy: use of high energy linear accelerator (≥10 MV)	
13	At least 2 follow-up visits by treating physician during the first year post-treatment	
14	Documentation or evidence of communication with patient's primary care physician or provision of continuing care	
15	Operative blood loss	Pre-treatment PSA, clinical stage, Gleason grade, use of neoadjuvant hormone therapy
16	Use of clinical and pathological TNM staging by treating physicians	
OUTCOME		
17	Primary treatment failure indicated by 3 consecutive rising PSA values after radiation therapy or any confirmed detectable PSA value after radical prostatectomy	Pre-treatment PSA, clinical stage, Gleason grade, use of neoadjuvant or adjuvant hormone therapy, insurance, education, income
18	Following primary treatment by radiation therapy: hospitalization, medical, or surgical treatment for cystitis, proctitis, hematuria, or rectal bleeding	Age, pre-treatment PSA, clinical stage, Gleason grade, history of other cancer, co-morbidity indicators, use of neoadjuvant or adjuvant hormone therapy, insurance, education, income
19	Following primary treatment by radiation therapy or radical prostatectomy: hospitalization, medical or surgical treatment for bladder neck contracture/urethral stricture	Age, pre-treatment PSA, clinical stage, Gleason grade, history of other cancer, co-morbidity indicators, use of neoadjuvant or adjuvant hormone therapy, insurance, education, income
20	Acute surgical complication rate (death, cardiovascular complications, deep vein thrombosis, pulmonary embolus, blood loss necessitating transfusions, etc.)	Age, pre-treatment PSA, clinical stage, Gleason grade, history of other cancer, co-morbidity indicators, use of neoadjuvant or adjuvant hormone therapy, insurance, education, income
21	Patient assessment of urinary, sexual, and bowel functioning following primary treatment by radiation therapy or radical prostatectomy, using a reliable, validated survey instrument	Age, pre-treatment PSA, clinical stage, Gleason grade, family history of prostate cancer, history of other cancer, co-morbidity indicators, use of neoadjuvant or adjuvant hormone therapy, insurance, education, income

Table 7.8 – Continued

22	Patient satisfaction with treatment choice, continence, and potency	Age, pre-treatment PSA, clinical stage, Gleason grade, family history of prostate cancer, history of other cancer, comorbidity indicators, use of neoadjuvant or adjuvant hormone therapy, insurance, education, income

Chapter 8

RECOMMENDATIONS FOR A RESEARCH AGENDA

Each year, more than 100,000 men face the decision about where and how to be treated for localized prostate cancer. Although a number of information sources are available about treatment options, there is no comprehensive source that provides guidance about the quality of care and resulting outcomes across treatment facilities in the United States. We need valid measures for assessing quality of care for prostate cancer, and we need to understand how variations in quality of care affect treatment outcomes.

But prostate cancer provides a particular challenge for quality-of-care assessment:

- We have methods for early detection, but we do not yet have definitive information about the efficacy of early detection.

- We have a number of treatment modalities for early-stage disease, but we do not yet have definitive information about the efficacy of early treatment.

- Primary treatment itself can have complications that may be relatively short term and manageable, but for many patients, treatment of prostate cancer can result in long-term problems such as urinary incontinence, bowel dysfunction, or impotence.

An additional challenge that lies ahead in the process of developing and testing quality indicators and introducing them for widespread adoption will be provider resistance. Physicians are often reluctant to accept that not everyone is above average, and as a result some may have a strong negative reaction to the implication that choice of provider affects survival and quality of life. These issues have been discussed in the literature by authors such as Epstein (1995) and will no doubt provide a significant challenge to moving this work from the research stage to widespread application.

Based on a synthesis of the medical literature, the opinions of physicians working in this field, the views of patients and their families, and the judgment of an expert panel, we make the following recommendations for further research so that we can understand and measure variations in quality of care provided to men with early-stage prostate cancer.

1. **Pilot test the candidate quality indicators to look for real variation across providers.**

   The next step in finalizing the list of quality indicators for early-stage prostate cancer is to conduct pilot tests to determine whether there is measurable variation across providers. Identifying variation is requisite to the continued development and validation of the list of candidate quality indicators. A limited pilot test will determine the likelihood of success in a larger field test of the indicators' reliability and validity. It will also provide evidence for the feasibility of actually measuring these indicators.

2. **Field test the candidate quality indicators in a national sample of institutions to empirically test their validity and demonstrate their feasibility**

   The set of quality indicators endorsed by the RAND expert panel represents measures of structure and process of care for early-stage prostate cancer that may be important to producing good outcomes. But because of the paucity of strong evidence from randomized controlled trials in early-stage prostate cancer, the links between structure, process, and outcomes that are essential for good quality indicators are not yet clearly established. Therefore, these links and the quality indicators' validity must be established empirically. This validation would require collecting and analyzing data about approximately 60–100 patients at each of 30 urology and 30 radiation oncology facilities. This sample size would provide adequate power (80% or better) to test for significant associations between processes and outcomes of care for the candidate quality indicators.

3. **Identify what aspects of structure and process of care are important to producing excellent outcomes in early-stage prostate cancer.**

   Establishing the validity of the candidate quality indicators is necessary but not sufficient for improving care for prostate cancer. We also need to determine the links between structure and process of care and patient outcomes.

126

Establishing such links will require additional research. Because prostate cancer typically has a very long natural history, survival outcomes of greater than 5 to 10 years may not be practical for assessing quality of care. And given the rapid rate technological and pharmacological innovation in prostate cancer treatment, 5- to 10-year outcomes represent treatment techniques, patient selection criteria, and clinical stratification approaches that are likely to be dated or obsolete at the time of the reporting. Hence, there is an urgent need to develop structure and process indicators that can serve as accurate surrogates for survival. Such measures will make it possible to measure quality of care within a time frame that benefits current patients who are attempting to determine the quality of care of potential providers.

4. **Determine which patient characteristics among those endorsed by the expert panel must be adjusted for when comparing institutions so that factors beyond the providers' control will not confound quality measurement.**

Many factors that affect outcomes are outside the providers' control. The RAND Prostate Cancer Outcomes and Patient Choice Expert Panel endorsed a number of patient characteristics that may be important to measure and adjust for in quality assessment. Although many of these patient characteristics have important clinical implications, their necessity and significance in case-mix adjustment need to be established.

5. **Develop a program for men newly diagnosed with early-stage prostate cancer to help them interpret scientific data and use information about treatment outcomes in their treatment.**

Men newly diagnosed with prostate cancer lack information about the expected outcomes of treatment options. Although data about the frequency and severity of side effects after the different treatments exist, the men in our focus groups reported difficulty in obtaining such information from their physicians. Prostate cancer patients need a program that reviews the current medical evidence about available treatments and delivers this information in ways that are consistent with what is known about patient decisionmaking. There was virtual unanimity within the focus groups on the observation

127

that patients had not been adequately informed about the potential side effects of treatment. Hence, an important next step will be to work to improve the way that treating physicians talk with newly diagnosed patients about side effects.

6. **Develop a national, population-based cohort to track quality-of-life outcomes, determine which quality-of-life components are both measurable and meaningful to patients over time, and determine whether these factors are associated with structure and process indicators.**

   Although the focus groups clearly define survival as the most critical factor in selecting treatment, they also expressed substantial interest in quality-of-life factors. In addition to the effects of treatment-related morbidities such as incontinence, bowel dysfunction, and impotence on quality of life, we need to explore how the cancer diagnosis and treatment affect the emotional and social well-being of the patient, his partner, and his family. Such studies should be designed to elucidate and quantify the relative incidence and importance of potentially significant treatment side effects and to relate this information to the quality of care. Results of such research will improve patients' ability to select a provider once a mode of therapy has been chosen.

References

Abdel-Nabi, H., G. L. Wright, J. V. Gulfo, D. P. Petrylak, C. E. Neal, J. E. Texter, F. P. Begun, I. Tyson, A. Heal, E. Mitchell, and et al. 1992. Monoclonal antibodies and radioimmunoconjugates in the diagnosis and treatment of prostate cancer [published erratum appears in *Semin Urol* 1992 May;10(2):138]. *Semin Urol* 10, no. 1: 45-54.

Aharony, L. and S. Strasser. 1993. Patient satisfaction: what we know about and what we still need to explore. *Med Care Rev* 50, no. 1: 49-79.

Albertsen, P. C., D. G. Fryback, B. E. Storer, T. F. Kolon, and J. Fine. 1995. Long-term survival among men with conservatively treated localized prostate cancer. *Jama* 274, no. 8: 626-31.

Albertsen, P. C., J. A. Hanley, and M. Murphy-Setzko. 1999. Statistical considerations when assessing outcomes following treatment for prostate cancer. *J Urol* 162, no. 2: 439-44.

Amdur, R. J., J. T. Parsons, L. T. Fitzgerald, and R. R. Million. 1990. The effect of overall treatment time on local control in patients with adenocarcinoma of the prostate treated with radiation therapy. *Int J Radiat Oncol Biol Phys* 19, no. 6: 1377-82.

Anonymous. 1997. Immediate versus deferred treatment for advanced prostatic cancer: initial results of the Medical Research Council Trial. The Medical Research Council Prostate Cancer Working Party Investigators Group. *Br J Urol* 79, no. 2: 235-46.

Anscher, M. S. and L. R. Prosnitz. 1991. Transurethral resection of prostate prior to definitive irradiation for prostate cancer. Lack of correlation with treatment outcome. *Urology* 38, no. 3: 206-11.

Arcangeli, G., A. Micheli, L. Verna, B. Saracino, G. Giovinazzo, L. D'Angelo, V. Pansadoro, and C. N. Sternberg. 1995. Prognostic impact of transurethral resection on patients irradiated for localized prostate cancer. *Radiother Oncol* 35, no. 2: 123-8.

Asbell, S. O., J. M. Krall, M. V. Pilepich, H. Baerwald, W. T. Sause, G. E. Hanks, and C. A. Perez. 1988. Elective pelvic irradiation in stage A2, B carcinoma of the prostate: analysis of RTOG 77-06. *Int J Radiat Oncol Biol Phys* 15, no. 6: 1307-16.

Asbell, S. O., K. L. Martz, M. V. Pilepich, H. H. Baerwald, W. T. Sause, R. L. Doggett, and C. A. Perez. 1989. Impact of surgical staging in evaluating the radiotherapeutic outcome in RTOG phase III study for A2 and B prostate carcinoma. *Int J Radiat Oncol Biol Phys* 17, no. 5: 945-51.

ASTRO. 1997. Consensus statement: guidelines for PSA following radiation therapy. American Society for Therapeutic Radiology and Oncology Consensus Panel. *Int J Radiat Oncol Biol Phys* 37, no. 5: 1035-41.

Austin, J. P. and K. Convery. 1993. Age-race interaction in prostatic adenocarcinoma treated with external beam irradiation. *Am J Clin Oncol* 16, no. 2: 140-5.

Bauer, H. W. and N. T. Schmeller. 1984. Clinical assessment of solid phase immunoadsorbent assay of human prostatic acid phosphatase. *Urology* 23, no. 3: 247-51.

Beard, C. J., P. Kijewski, M. Bussiere, R. Gelman, D. Gladstone, K. Shaffer, M. Plunkett, P. Castello, and C. N. Coleman. 1996. Analysis of prostate and seminal vesicle motion: implications for treatment planning. *Int J Radiat Oncol Biol Phys* 34, no. 2: 451-8.

Beard, C. J., K. J. Propert, P. P. Rieker, J. A. Clark, I. Kaplan, P. W. Kantoff, and J. A. Talcott. 1997. Complications after treatment with external-beam irradiation in early- stage prostate cancer patients: a prospective multiinstitutional outcomes study. *J Clin Oncol* 15, no. 1: 223-9.

Bell, D. G. 1993. A simple technique to facilitate vesicourethral anastomosis following radical prostatectomy. *Br J Urol* 72, no. 1: 124-5.

Berlin, J. W., P. Ramchandani, M. P. Banner, H. M. Pollack, C. F. Nodine, and A. J. Wein. 1994. Voiding cystourethrography after radical prostatectomy: normal findings and correlation between contrast extravasation and anastomotic strictures. *AJR Am J Roentgenol* 162, no. 1: 87-91.

Beyer, D. C. and J. B. Priestley, Jr. 1997. Biochemical disease-free survival following 125I prostate implantation. *Int J Radiat Oncol Biol Phys* 37, no. 3: 559-63.

Bigg, S. W., L. R. Kavoussi, and W. J. Catalona. 1990. Role of nerve-sparing radical prostatectomy for clinical stage B2 prostate cancer. *J Urol* 144, no. 6: 1420-4.

Blackwell, K. L., D. G. Bostwick, R. P. Myers, H. Zincke, and J. E. Oesterling. 1994. Combining prostate specific antigen with cancer and gland volume to predict more reliably pathological stage: the influence of prostate specific antigen cancer density. *J Urol* 151, no. 6: 1565-70.

Blute, M. L., D. G. Bostwick, E. J. Bergstralh, J. M. Slezak, S. K. Martin, C. L. Amling, and H. Zincke. 1997. Anatomic site-specific positive margins in organ-confined prostate cancer and its impact on outcome after radical prostatectomy. *Urology* 50, no. 5: 733-9.

Boeckmann, W. and G. Jakse. 1995. Management of rectal injury during perineal prostatectomy. *Urol Int* 55, no. 3: 147-9.

Bolla, M., X. Artignan, E. Chirpaz, J. Balosso, and J. L. Descotes. 1998. Current studies of combined radiotherapy-hormone therapy in localized and locally advanced prostatic cancers. *Cancer Radiother* 2, no. 6: 783-6.

Bolla, M., D. Gonzalez, P. Warde, J. B. Dubois, R. O. Mirimanoff, G. Storme, J. Bernier, A. Kuten, C. Sternberg, T. Gil, L. Collette, and M. Pierart. 1997. Improved survival in patients with locally advanced prostate cancer treated with radiotherapy and goserelin. *N Engl J Med* 337, no. 5: 295-300.

Bostwick, D. G. 1994. Gleason grading of prostatic needle biopsies. Correlation with grade in 316 matched prostatectomies. *Am J Surg Pathol* 18, no. 8: 796-803.

Brandeis, J. M., M. S. Litwin, C. M. Burnison, and R. E. Reiter. 2000. Quality of life outcomes after brachytherapy for early stage prostate cancer. *J Urol* 163, no. 3: 851-7.

Brook, R. H., C. J. Kamberg, K. N. Lohr, G. A. Goldberg, E. B. Keeler, and J. P. Newhouse. 1990. Quality of ambulatory care. Epidemiology and comparison by insurance status and income. *Med Care* 28, no. 5: 392-433.

Catalona, W. J. 1990. Patient selection for, results of, and impact on tumor resection of potency-sparing radical prostatectomy. *Urol Clin North Am* 17, no. 4: 819-26.

Catalona, W. J. 1996. Clinical utility of measurements of free and total prostate-specific antigen (PSA): a review. *Prostate Suppl* 7: 64-9.

Cella, D. F. 1995. Methods and problems in measuring quality of life. *Support Care Cancer* 3, no. 1: 11-22.

Cella, D. F. and A. E. Bonomi. 1995. Measuring quality of life: 1995 update. *Oncology (Huntingt)* 9, no. 11 Suppl: 47-60.

Chassin, M. R., J. Kosecoff, R. E. Park, C. M. Winslow, K. L. Kahn, N. J. Merrick, J. Keesey, A. Fink, D. H. Solomon, and R. H. Brook. 1987. Does inappropriate use explain geographic variations in the use of health care services? A study of three procedures [see comments]. *Jama* 258, no. 18: 2533-7.

Cleary, P. D. and B. J. McNeil. 1988. Patient satisfaction as an indicator of quality care. *Inquiry* 25, no. 1: 25-36.

Critz, F. A., A. K. Levinson, W. H. Williams, and D. A. Holladay. 1996. Prostate-specific antigen nadir: the optimum level after irradiation for prostate cancer. *J Clin Oncol* 14, no. 11: 2893-900.

Crook, J. M., E. Choan, G. A. Perry, S. Robertson, and B. A. Esche. 1998. Serum prostate-specific antigen profile following radiotherapy for prostate cancer: implications for patterns of failure and definition of cure. *Urology* 51, no. 4: 566-72.

D'Amico, A. V., R. Whittington, I. Kaplan, C. Beard, D. Schultz, S. B. Malkowicz, A. Wein, J. E. Tomaszewski, and C. N. Coleman. 1998a. Calculated prostate carcinoma volume: The optimal predictor of 3-year prostate specific antigen (PSA) failure free survival after surgery or radiation therapy of patients with pretreatment PSA levels of 4-20 nanograms per milliliter. *Cancer* 82, no. 2: 334-41.

D'Amico, A. V., R. Whittington, S. B. Malkowicz, K. Loughlin, D. Schultz, M. Schnall, C. M. Tempany, J. E. Tomaszewski, A. Renshaw, and A. Wein. 1996. An analysis of the time course of postoperative prostate-specific antigen failure in patients with positive surgical margins: implications on the use of adjuvant therapy. *Urology* 47, no. 4: 538-47.

D'Amico, A. V., R. Whittington, S. B. Malkowicz, M. Schnall, J. Tomaszewski, D. Schultz, G. Kao, K. VanArsdalen, and A. Wein. 1994. A multivariable analysis of clinical factors predicting for pathological features associated with local failure after radical prostatectomy for prostate cancer. *Int J Radiat Oncol Biol Phys* 30, no. 2: 293-302.

D'Amico, A. V., R. Whittington, S. B. Malkowicz, D. Schultz, K. Blank, G. A. Broderick, J. E. Tomaszewski, A. A. Renshaw, I. Kaplan, C. J. Beard, and A. Wein. 1998b. Biochemical outcome after radical prostatectomy, external beam radiation therapy, or interstitial radiation therapy for clinically localized prostate cancer [see comments]. *Jama* 280, no. 11: 969-74.

D'Amico, A. V., R. Whittington, S. B. Malkowicz, D. Schultz, M. Schnall, J. E. Tomaszewski, and A. Wein. 1995. A multivariate analysis of clinical and pathological factors that predict for prostate specific antigen failure after radical prostatectomy for prostate cancer. *J Urol* 154, no. 1: 131-8.

D'Amico, A. V., R. Whittington, D. Schultz, S. B. Malkowicz, J. E. Tomaszewski, and A. Wein. 1997. Outcome based staging for clinically localized adenocarcinoma of the prostate. *J Urol* 158, no. 4: 1422-6.

Davies, A. R. and J. E. Ware, Jr. 1988. Involving consumers in quality of care assessment. *Health Aff (Millwood)* 7, no. 1: 33-48.

Davis, B. E. and W. R. Fair. 1994. Technique for the management of Santorini's deep venous plexus during radical retropubic prostatectomy. *J Surg Oncol* 55, no. 1: 24-5.

deKernion, J.B., A. Belldegrun, and J. Naitoh. 1998. Radical prostatectomy for localized prostate cancer: indications, techniques and results. In A. Belldegrun, R.S. Kirby, and T. Oliver, eds. *New perspectives in the treatment of prostate cancer*: 195-204. London: Isis Medical Media.

Desch, C. E., L. Penberthy, C. J. Newschaffer, B. E. Hillner, M. Whittemore, D. McClish, T. J. Smith, and S. M. Retchin. 1996. Factors that determine the treatment for local and regional prostate cancer. *Med Care* 34, no. 2: 152-62.

Diamond, J. J., A. D. Steinfeld, and G. E. Hanks. 1991. The relationship between facility structure and outcome in cancer of the prostate and uterine cervix. *Int J Radiat Oncol Biol Phys* 21, no. 4: 1085-7.

Donabedian, A. 1980. *Explorations in quality assessment and monitoring I: the definition of quality and approaches to its assessment.* Ann Arbor, MI: Health Administration Press.

Douglas, L., M. Cadogan, and R. Wan. 1997. Easy visualization of the membranous urethral stump in radical prostatectomy. *J Urol* 157, no. 2: 576-7.

Douglas, T. H., T. O. Morgan, D. G. McLeod, J. W. Moul, G. P. Murphy, R. Barren, 3rd, I. A. Sesterhenn, and F. K. Mostofi. 1997. Comparison of serum prostate specific membrane antigen, prostate specific antigen, and free prostate specific antigen levels in radical prostatectomy patients. *Cancer* 80, no. 1: 107-14.

Duchesne, G. M. and L. J. Peters. 1999. What is the alpha/beta ratio for prostate cancer? Rationale for hypofractionated high-dose-rate brachytherapy [editorial]. *Int J Radiat Oncol Biol Phys* 44, no. 4: 747-8.

Eastham, J. A., M. W. Kattan, E. Rogers, J. R. Goad, M. Ohori, T. B. Boone, and P. T. Scardino. 1996. Risk factors for urinary incontinence after radical prostatectomy. *J Urol* 156, no. 5: 1707-13.

Egawa, S., T. M. Wheeler, D. R. Greene, and P. T. Scardino. 1992. Detection of residual prostate cancer after radiotherapy by sonographically guided needle biopsy. *Urology* 39, no. 4: 358-63.

Ellison, L. M., J. A. Heaney, and J. D. Birkmeyer. 2000. The effect of hospital volume on mortality and resource use after radical prostatectomy. *J Urol* 163, no. 3: 867-9.

Ennis, R. D., S. D. Flynn, D. B. Fischer, and R. E. Peschel. 1994. Preoperative serum prostate-specific antigen and Gleason grade as predictors of pathologic stage in clinically organ confined prostate cancer: implications for the choice of primary treatment. *Int J Radiat Oncol Biol Phys* 30, no. 2: 317-22.

Epstein, A. 1995. Performance reports on quality--prototypes, problems, and prospects. *N Engl J Med* 333, no. 1: 57-61.

Epstein, J. I., A. W. Partin, J. Sauvageot, and P. C. Walsh. 1996. Prediction of progression following radical prostatectomy. A multivariate analysis of 721 men with long-term follow-up. *Am J Surg Pathol* 20, no. 3: 286-92.

Eskew, L. A., R. D. Woodruff, R. L. Bare, and D. L. McCullough. 1998. Prostate cancer diagnosed by the 5 region biopsy method is significant disease. *J Urol* 160, no. 3 Pt 1: 794-6.

Ferguson, J. K. and J. E. Oesterling. 1994. Patient evaluation if prostate-specific antigen becomes elevated following radical prostatectomy or radiation therapy. *Urol Clin North Am* 21, no. 4: 677-85.

Forman, J. D., R. Kumar, G. Haas, J. Montie, A. T. Porter, and C. F. Mesina. 1995. Neoadjuvant hormonal downsizing of localized carcinoma of the prostate: effects on the volume of normal tissue irradiation [see comments]. *Cancer Invest* 13, no. 1: 8-15.

Forman, J. D., T. Oppenheim, H. Liu, J. Montie, P. W. McLaughlin, and A. T. Porter. 1993. Frequency of residual neoplasm in the prostate following three- dimensional conformal radiotherapy. *Prostate* 23, no. 3: 235-43.

Foti, A. G., J. F. Cooper, H. Herschman, and R. R. Malvaez. 1977. Detection of prostatic cancer by solid-phase radioimmunoassay of serum prostatic acid phosphatase. *N Engl J Med* 297, no. 25: 1357-61.

Fowler, F. J., Jr., M. J. Barry, G. Lu-Yao, J. Wasson, A. Roman, and J. Wennberg. 1995. Effect of radical prostatectomy for prostate cancer on patient quality of life: results from a Medicare survey. *Urology* 45, no. 6: 1007-13; discussion 1013-5.

Fowler, F. J., Jr., M. J. Barry, G. Lu-Yao, J. H. Wasson, and L. Bin. 1996. Outcomes of external-beam radiation therapy for prostate cancer: a study of Medicare beneficiaries in three surveillance, epidemiology, and end results areas. *J Clin Oncol* 14, no. 8: 2258-65.

Frank, E., O. P. Sood, M. Torjman, S. G. Mulholland, and L. G. Gomella. 1998. Postoperative epidural analgesia following radical retropubic prostatectomy: outcome assessment. *J Surg Oncol* 67, no. 2: 117-20.

Fraser, G. M., D. Pilpel, J. Kosecoff, and R. H. Brook. 1994. Effect of panel composition on appropriateness ratings. *Int J Qual Health Care* 6, no. 3: 251-55.

Fuks, Z., S. A. Leibel, K. E. Wallner, C. B. Begg, W. R. Fair, L. L. Anderson, B. S. Hilaris, and W. F. Whitmore. 1991. The effect of local control on metastatic dissemination in carcinoma of the prostate: long-term results in patients treated with 125I implantation. *Int J Radiat Oncol Biol Phys* 21, no. 3: 537-47.

Fukunaga-Johnson, N., H. M. Sandler, P. W. McLaughlin, M. S. Strawderman, K. H. Grijalva, K. E. Kish, and A. S. Lichter. 1997. Results of 3D conformal radiotherapy in the treatment of localized prostate cancer. *Int J Radiat Oncol Biol Phys* 38, no. 2: 311-7.

Ganz, P. A., C. A. Schag, J. J. Lee, and M. S. Sim. 1992. The CARES: a generic measure of health-related quality of life for patients with cancer. *Qual Life Res* 1, no. 1: 19-29.

Gao, X., A. T. Porter, D. J. Grignon, J. E. Pontes, and K. V. Honn. 1997. Diagnostic and prognostic markers for human prostate cancer. *Prostate* 31, no. 4: 264-81.

Geara, F. B., G. K. Zagars, and A. Pollack. 1994. Influence of initial presentation on treatment outcome of clinically localized prostate cancer treated by definitive radiation therapy. *Int J Radiat Oncol Biol Phys* 30, no. 2: 331-7.

Gervasi, L. A., J. Mata, J. D. Easley, J. H. Wilbanks, C. Seale-Hawkins, C. E. Carlton, Jr., and P. T. Scardino. 1989. Prognostic significance of lymph nodal metastases in prostate cancer. *J Urol* 142, no. 2 Pt 1: 332-6.

Glick, A. J., C. B. Philput, A. el Mahdi, L. Ladaga, and P. F. Schellhammer. 1990. Are three substages of clinical B prostate carcinoma useful in predicting disease-free survival? *Urology* 36, no. 6: 483-7.

Goh, M., C. G. Kleer, P. Kielczewski, K. J. Wojno, K. Kim, and J. E. Oesterling. 1997. Autologous blood donation prior to anatomical radical retropubic prostatectomy: is it necessary? *Urology* 49, no. 4: 569-73; discussion 574.

Gomez, C. A., M. S. Soloway, F. Civantos, and T. Hachiya. 1993. Bladder neck preservation and its impact on positive surgical margins during radical prostatectomy. *Urology* 42, no. 6: 689-93; discussion 693-4.

Goodnough, L. M., J. E. Grishaber, J. D. Birkmeyer, T. G. Monk, and W. J. Catalona. 1994a. Efficacy and cost-effectiveness of autologous blood predeposit in patients undergoing radical prostatectomy procedures. *Urology* 44, no. 2: 226-31.

Goodnough, L. T., J. E. Grishaber, T. G. Monk, and W. J. Catalona. 1994b. Acute preoperative hemodilution in patients undergoing radical prostatectomy: a case study analysis of efficacy [see comments]. *Anesth Analg* 78, no. 5: 932-7.

Grumbach, K., G. M. Anderson, H. S. Luft, L. L. Roos, and R. Brook. 1995. Regionalization of cardiac surgery in the United States and Canada. Geographic access, choice, and outcomes [see comments]. *Jama* 274, no. 16: 1282-8.

Hanash, K. A. 1992. Balloon pull-out or push-in technique for vesicourethral anastomosis after radical prostatectomy or enterocystoplasty. *Urology* 40, no. 3: 243-4.

Hanks, G. E. 1992. Post treatment biopsies of the prostate: a stalking horse for improving local control [editorial; comment]. *Int J Radiat Oncol Biol Phys* 24, no. 3: 571-2.

Hanks, G. E., S. Asbell, J. M. Krall, C. A. Perez, S. Doggett, P. Rubin, W. Sause, and M. V. Pilepich. 1991. Outcome for lymph node dissection negative T-1b, T-2 (A-2,B) prostate cancer treated with external beam radiation therapy in RTOG 77-06. *Int J Radiat Oncol Biol Phys* 21, no. 4: 1099-103.

Hanks, G. E., A. Hanlon, J. B. Owen, and T. E. Schultheiss. 1994a. Patterns of radiation treatment of elderly patients with prostate cancer. *Cancer* 74, no. 7 Suppl: 2174-7.

Hanks, G. E., A. L. Hanlon, G. Hudes, W. R. Lee, W. Suasin, and T. E. Schultheiss. 1996a. Patterns-of-failure analysis of patients with high pretreatment prostate-specific antigen levels treated by radiation therapy: the need for improved systemic and locoregional treatment. *J Clin Oncol* 14, no. 4: 1093-7.

Hanks, G. E., J. M. Krall, A. L. Hanlon, S. O. Asbell, M. V. Pilepich, and J. B. Owen. 1994b. Patterns of care and RTOG studies in prostate cancer: long-term survival, hazard rate observations, and possibilities of cure. *Int J Radiat Oncol Biol Phys* 28, no. 1: 39-45.

Hanks, G. E., J. M. Krall, K. L. Martz, J. J. Diamond, and S. Kramer. 1988. The outcome of treatment of 313 patients with T-1 (UICC) prostate cancer treated with external beam irradiation. *Int J Radiat Oncol Biol Phys* 14, no. 2: 243-8.

Hanks, G. E., W. R. Lee, A. L. Hanlon, M. Hunt, E. Kaplan, B. E. Epstein, B. Movsas, and T. E. Schultheiss. 1996b. Conformal technique dose escalation for prostate cancer: biochemical evidence of improved cancer control with higher doses in patients with pretreatment prostate-specific antigen > or = 10 NG/ML. *Int J Radiat Oncol Biol Phys* 35, no. 5: 861-8.

Hanks, G. E., S. A. Leibel, J. M. Krall, and S. Kramer. 1985. Patterns of care studies: dose-response observations for local control of adenocarcinoma of the prostate. *Int J Radiat Oncol Biol Phys* 11, no. 1: 153-7.

Hanks, G. E., K. L. Martz, and J. J. Diamond. 1988. The effect of dose on local control of prostate cancer. *Int J Radiat Oncol Biol Phys* 15, no. 6: 1299-305.

Hanks, G. E., T. E. Schultheiss, M. A. Hunt, and B. Epstein. 1995. Factors influencing incidence of acute grade 2 morbidity in conformal and standard radiation treatment of prostate cancer. *Int J Radiat Oncol Biol Phys* 31, no. 1: 25-9.

Hanlon, A. L., T. E. Schultheiss, M. A. Hunt, B. Movsas, R. S. Peter, and G. E. Hanks. 1997. Chronic rectal bleeding after high-dose conformal treatment of prostate cancer warrants modification of existing morbidity scales. *Int J Radiat Oncol Biol Phys* 38, no. 1: 59-63.

Hannan, E. L., M. Racz, T. J. Ryan, B. D. McCallister, L. W. Johnson, D. T. Arani, A. D. Guerci, J. Sosa, and E. J. Topol. 1997. Coronary angioplasty volume-outcome relationships for hospitals and cardiologists. *Jama* 277, no. 11: 892-8.

Hayward, R. A., L. F. McMahon, Jr., and A. M. Bernard. 1993. Evaluating the care of general medicine inpatients: how good is implicit review? *Ann Intern Med* 118, no. 7: 550-6.

Henson, D. E., R. V. Hutter, and G. Farrow. 1994. Practice protocol for the examination of specimens removed from patients with carcinoma of the prostate gland. A publication of the Cancer Committee, College of American Pathologists. Task Force on the Examination of Specimens Removed From Patients With Prostate Cancer. *Arch Pathol Lab Med* 118, no. 8: 779-83.

Hoppe, R. T., A. L. Hanlon, G. E. Hanks, and J. B. Owen. 1994. Progress in the treatment of Hodgkin's disease in the United States, 1973 versus 1983. The Patterns of Care Study. *Cancer* 74, no. 12: 3198-203.

Hrebinko, R. L., and W. F. O'Donnell. 1993. Control of the deep dorsal venous complex in radical retropubic prostatectomy. *J Urol* 149, no. 4: 799-800; discussion 800-1.

Huggins, C. and C.V. Hodges. 1941. Studies on prostatic cancer: the effects of castration, of estrogen and of androgen injection on serum phosphatases in metastatic carcinoma of the prostate. *Cancer Research* 1: 293.

Iezzoni, L. I. 1996. An introduction to risk adjustment. *Am J Med Qual* 11, no. 1: S8-11.

Iezzoni, L. I., A. S. Ash, M. Shwartz, J. Daley, J. S. Hughes, and Y. D. Mackiernan. 1996. Judging hospitals by severity-adjusted mortality rates: the influence of the severity-adjustment method. *Am J Public Health* 86, no. 10: 1379-87.

Israeli, R. S., M. Grob, and W. R. Fair. 1997. Prostate-specific membrane antigen and other prostatic tumor markers on the horizon. *Urol Clin North Am* 24, no. 2: 439-50.

Israeli, R. S., C. T. Powell, J. G. Corr, W. R. Fair, and W. D. Heston. 1994. Expression of the prostate-specific membrane antigen. *Cancer Res* 54, no. 7: 1807-11.

Johnstone, P. A., C. R. Powell, R. Riffenburgh, K. J. Bethel, and C. J. Kane. 1998. The fate of 10-year clinically recurrence-free survivors after definitive radiotherapy for T1-3N0M0 prostate cancer. *Radiat Oncol Investig* 6, no. 2: 103-8.

Jonler, M., E. M. Messing, P. R. Rhodes, and R. C. Bruskewitz. 1994. Sequelae of radical prostatectomy. *Br J Urol* 74, no. 3: 352-8.

Kabalin, J. N., K. K. Hodge, J. E. McNeal, F. S. Freiha, and T. A. Stamey. 1989. Identification of residual cancer in the prostate following radiation therapy: role of transrectal ultrasound guided biopsy and prostate specific antigen. *J Urol* 142, no. 2 Pt 1: 326-31.

Kagawa, K., W. R. Lee, T. E. Schultheiss, M. A. Hunt, A. H. Shaer, and G. E. Hanks. 1997. Initial clinical assessment of CT-MRI image fusion software in localization of the prostate for 3D conformal radiation therapy. *Int J Radiat Oncol Biol Phys* 38, no. 2: 319-25.

Kaplan, I. D., R. S. Cox, and M. A. Bagshaw. 1994. Radiotherapy for prostatic cancer: patient selection and the impact of local control. *Urology* 43, no. 5: 634-9.

Kaplan, I. D., B. R. Prestidge, M. A. Bagshaw, and R. S. Cox. 1992. The importance of local control in the treatment of prostatic cancer. *J Urol* 147, no. 3 Pt 2: 917-21.

Katz, A. E., G. M. de Vries, M. D. Begg, A. J. Raffo, C. Cama, K. O'Toole, R. Buttyan, M. C. Benson, and C. A. Olsson. 1995. Enhanced reverse transcriptase-polymerase chain reaction for prostate specific antigen as an indicator of true pathologic stage in patients with prostate cancer. *Cancer* 75, no. 7: 1642-8.

Kavadi, V. S., G. K. Zagars, and A. Pollack. 1994. Serum prostate-specific antigen after radiation therapy for clinically localized prostate cancer: prognostic implications. *Int J Radiat Oncol Biol Phys* 30, no. 2: 279-87.

Kitahata, M. M., T. D. Koepsell, R. A. Deyo, C. L. Maxwell, W. T. Dodge, and E. H. Wagner. 1996. Physicians' experience with the acquired immunodeficiency syndrome as a factor in patients' survival. *N Engl J Med* 334, no. 11: 701-6.

Klein, E. A. 1993. Modified apical dissection for early continence after radical prostatectomy. *Prostate* 22, no. 3: 217-23.

Klein, E. A., J. A. Grass, D. A. Calabrese, R. A. Kay, W. Sargeant, and J. F. O'Hara. 1996. Maintaining quality of care and patient satisfaction with radical prostatectomy in the era of cost containment. *Urology* 48, no. 2: 269-76.

Koch, M. O. and J. A. Smith, Jr. 1995. Clinical outcomes associated with the implementation of a cost- efficient programme for radical retropubic prostatectomy. *Br J Urol* 76, no. 1: 28-33.

Komaki, R., T. J. Brickner, A. L. Hanlon, J. B. Owen, and G. E. Hanks. 1995. Long-term results of treatment of cervical carcinoma in the United States in 1973, 1978, and 1983: Patterns of Care Study (PCS). *Int J Radiat Oncol Biol Phys* 31, no. 4: 973-82.

Kuban, D. A., A. M. el-Mahdi, and P. F. Schellhammer. 1993. Prognostic significance of post-irradiation prostate biopsies. *Oncology (Huntingt)* 7, no. 2: 29-38; discussion 40, 43-4, 47.

Kuban, D. A., A. M. el-Mahdi, and P. F. Schellhammer. 1998. PSA for outcome prediction and posttreatment evaluation following radiation for prostate cancer: do we know how to use it? *Semin Radiat Oncol* 8, no. 2: 72-80.

Kupelian, P., J. Katcher, H. Levin, C. Zippe, and E. Klein. 1996. Correlation of clinical and pathologic factors with rising prostate- specific antigen profiles after radical prostatectomy alone for clinically localized prostate cancer. *Urology* 48, no. 2: 249-60.

Kupelian, P. A., E. A. Klein, J. S. Witte, V. A. Kupelian, and J. H. Suh. 1997a. Familial prostate cancer: a different disease? *J Urol* 158, no. 6: 2197-201.

Kupelian, P. A., V. A. Kupelian, J. S. Witte, R. Macklis, and E. A. Klein. 1997b. Family history of prostate cancer in patients with localized prostate cancer: an independent predictor of treatment outcome. *J Clin Oncol* 15, no. 4: 1478-80.

Lai, P. P., C. A. Perez, and M. A. Lockett. 1992. Prognostic significance of pelvic recurrence and distant metastasis in prostate carcinoma following definitive radiotherapy. *Int J Radiat Oncol Biol Phys* 24, no. 3: 423-30.

Lai, P. P., M. V. Pilepich, J. M. Krall, S. O. Asbell, G. E. Hanks, C. A. Perez, P. Rubin, W. T. Sause, and J. D. Cox. 1991. The effect of overall treatment time on the outcome of definitive radiotherapy for localized prostate carcinoma: the Radiation Therapy Oncology Group 75-06 and 77-06 experience [see comments]. *Int J Radiat Oncol Biol Phys* 21, no. 4: 925-33.

Landis, S. H., T. Murray, S. Bolden, and P. A. Wingo. 1999. Cancer statistics, 1999. *CA Cancer J Clin* 49, no. 1: 8-31, 1.

Lange, P. H., C. J. Ercole, D. J. Lightner, E. E. Fraley, and R. Vessella. 1989. The value of serum prostate specific antigen determinations before and after radical prostatectomy. *J Urol* 141, no. 4: 873-9.

Lankford, S. P., A. Pollack, and G. K. Zagars. 1997. Prostate-specific antigen cancer volume: a significant prognostic factor in prostate cancer patients at intermediate risk of failing radiotherapy. *Int J Radiat Oncol Biol Phys* 38, no. 2: 327-33.

Lassen, P. M. and W. S. Kearse, Jr. 1995. Rectal injuries during radical perineal prostatectomy. *Urology* 45, no. 2: 266-9.

Lee, C. T. and J. E. Oesterling. 1997. Using prostate-specific antigen to eliminate the staging radionuclide bone scan. *Urol Clin North Am* 24, no. 2: 389-94.

Lee, R. J. and W. T. Sause. 1994. Surgically staged patients with prostatic carcinoma treated with definitive radiotherapy: fifteen-year results. *Urology* 43, no. 5: 640-4.

Lee, W. R., G. E. Hanks, and A. Hanlon. 1997. Increasing prostate-specific antigen profile following definitive radiation therapy for localized prostate cancer: clinical observations. *J Clin Oncol* 15, no. 1: 230-8.

Lee, W. R., R. P. McQuellon, L. D. Case, A. F. deGuzman, and D. L. McCullough. 1999. Early quality of life assessment in men treated with permanent source interstitial brachytherapy for clinically localized prostate cancer. *J Urol* 162, no. 2: 403-6.

Leibel, S. A., G. E. Hanks, and S. Kramer. 1984. Patterns of care outcome studies: results of the national practice in adenocarcinoma of the prostate. *Int J Radiat Oncol Biol Phys* 10, no. 3: 401-9.

Leibel, S. A., G. J. Kutcher, M. J. Zelefsky, C. M. Burman, R. Mohan, C. C. Ling, and Z. Fuks. 1996. 3-D conformal radiotherapy for carcinoma of the prostate. Clinical experience at the Memorial Sloan-Kettering Cancer Center. *Front Radiat Ther Oncol* 29: 229-37.

Lerner, S. E., M. L. Blute, E. J. Bergstralh, D. G. Bostwick, J. T. Eickholt, and H. Zincke. 1996. Analysis of risk factors for progression in patients with pathologically confined prostate cancers after radical retropubic prostatectomy [see comments]. *J Urol* 156, no. 1: 137-43.

Lerner, S. E., J. Fleischmann, H. C. Taub, J. W. Chamberlin, N. Z. Kahan, and A. Melman. 1994. Combined laparoscopic pelvic lymph node dissection and modified belt radical perineal prostatectomy for localized prostatic adenocarcinoma. *Urology* 43, no. 4: 493-8.

Lerner, S. P., C. Seale-Hawkins, C. E. Carlton, Jr., and P. T. Scardino. 1991. The risk of dying of prostate cancer in patients with clinically localized disease. *J Urol* 146, no. 4: 1040-5.

Levy, D. A., and M. I. Resnick. 1997. Staging of prostate cancer. In *Principles and Practice of Genitourinary Oncology*, ed. D. Raghavan, H. I. Scher, S. A. Leibel, and P. Lange: 480-481. Philadelphia: Lippincott Raven Publishers.

Licht, M. R., E. A. Klein, L. Tuason, and H. Levin. 1994. Impact of bladder neck preservation during radical prostatectomy on continence and cancer control. *Urology* 44, no. 6: 883-7.

Litwin, M. S., R. D. Hays, A. Fink, P. A. Ganz, B. Leake, and R. H. Brook. 1998a. The UCLA Prostate Cancer Index: development, reliability, and validity of a health-related quality of life measure. *Med Care* 36, no. 7: 1002-12.

Litwin, M. S., R. D. Hays, A. Fink, P. A. Ganz, B. Leake, G. E. Leach, and R. H. Brook. 1995. Quality-of-life outcomes in men treated for localized prostate cancer. *Jama* 273, no. 2: 129-35.

Litwin, M. S., D. P. Lubeck, J. M. Henning, and P. R. Carroll. 1998b. Differences in urologist and patient assessments of health related quality of life in men with prostate cancer: results of the CaPSURE database. *J Urol* 159, no. 6: 1988-92.

Litwin, M. S. and K. A. McGuigan. 1999. Accuracy of recall in health-related quality-of-life assessment among men treated for prostate cancer. *J Clin Oncol* 17, no. 9: 2882-8.

Litwin, M. S., A. I. Shpall, and F. Dorey. 1997. Patient satisfaction with short stays for radical prostatectomy. *Urology* 49, no. 6: 898-905; discussion 905-6.

Litwin, M. S., R. B. Smith, A. Thind, N. Reccius, M. Blanco-Yarosh, and J. B. deKernion. 1996. Cost-efficient radical prostatectomy with a clinical care path. *J Urol* 155, no. 3: 989-93.

Lowe, F. C. and S. J. Trauzzi. 1993. Prostatic acid phosphatase in 1993. Its limited clinical utility. *Urol Clin North Am* 20, no. 4: 589-95.

Luft, H. S., D. W. Garnick, D. H. Mark, D. J. Peltzman, C. S. Phibbs, E. Lichtenberg, and S. J. McPhee. 1990. Does quality influence choice of hospital? *Jama* 263, no. 21: 2899-906.

Lu-Yao, G. L., A. L. Potosky, P. C. Albertsen, J. H. Wasson, M. J. Barry, and J. E. Wennberg. 1996. Follow-up prostate cancer treatments after radical prostatectomy: a population-based study. *J Natl Cancer Inst* 88, no. 3-4: 166-73.

Maggio, M. I., R. A. Costabile, and J. P. Foley. 1992. Endoscopically controlled placement of urethrovesical anastomotic sutures after radical retropubic prostatectomy. *J Urol* 147, no. 3 Pt 2: 903-4.

Malkowicz, S. B. 1996. Serum prostate-specific antigen elevation in the post-radical prostatectomy patient. *Urol Clin North Am* 23, no. 4: 665-75.

Mazur, D. J. and D. H. Hickam. 1996. Patient preferences for management of localized prostate cancer. *West J Med* 165, no. 1-2: 26-30.

Mazur, D. J. and J. F. Merz. 1995. Older patients' willingness to trade off urologic adverse outcomes for a better chance at five-year survival in the clinical setting of prostate cancer [see comments]. *J Am Geriatr Soc* 43, no. 9: 979-84.

Mazur, D. J. and J. F. Merz. 1996. How older patients' treatment preferences are influenced by disclosures about therapeutic uncertainty: surgery versus expectant management for localized prostate cancer. *J Am Geriatr Soc* 44, no. 8: 934-7.

McGowan, D. G. and J. Hanson. 1985. The national Canadian study of carcinoma of the prostate treated by external beam radiation (1970-1978): I. A medical audit. *J Can Assoc Radiol* 36, no. 3: 216-22.

McNeil, C. 1996. PSA levels after radiotherapy: how low must they go? *J Natl Cancer Inst* 88, no. 12: 791-2.

Menon, M. and S. Vaidyanathan. 1995. The University of Massachusetts technique of radical retropubic prostatectomy. *Eur J Surg Oncol* 21, no. 1: 66-8.

Messing, E. M., J. Manola, M. Sarosdy, G. Wilding, E. D. Crawford, and D. Trump. 1999. Immediate hormonal therapy compared with observation after radical prostatectomy and pelvic lymphadenectomy in men with node-positive prostate cancer [see comments]. *N Engl J Med* 341, no. 24: 1781-8.

Mettlin, C. J., G. P. Murphy, J. Sylvester, R. F. McKee, M. Morrow, and D. P. Winchester. 1997. Results of hospital cancer registry surveys by the American College of Surgeons: outcomes of prostate cancer treatment by radical prostatectomy. *Cancer* 80, no. 9: 1875-81.

Middleton, R. G., I. M. Thompson, M. S. Austenfeld, W. H. Cooner, R. J. Correa, R. P. Gibbons, H. C. Miller, J. E. Oesterling, M. I. Resnick, S. R. Smalley, et al. 1995. Prostate Cancer Clinical Guidelines Panel Summary report on the management of clinically localized prostate cancer. The American Urological Association. *J Urol* 154, no. 6: 2144-8.

Movsas, B., A. L. Hanlon, T. Teshima, and G. E. Hanks. 1997. Analyzing predictive models following definitive radiotherapy for prostate carcinoma. *Cancer* 80, no. 6: 1093-102.

Naitoh, J., F. Dorey, and J. B. deKernion. 1997. Predicting pathological stage of localized prostate cancer. *Jama* 278, no. 12: 980-1; discussion 981-2.

Narayan, P., V. Gajendran, S. P. Taylor, A. Tewari, J. C. Presti, Jr., R. Leidich, R. Lo, K. Palmer, K. Shinohara, and J. T. Spaulding. 1995. The role of transrectal ultrasound-guided biopsy-based staging, preoperative serum prostate-specific antigen, and biopsy Gleason score in prediction of final pathologic diagnosis in prostate cancer. *Urology* 46, no. 2:

205-12.

O'Dowd, G. J., R. W. Veltri, R. Orozco, M. C. Miller, and J. E. Oesterling. 1997. Update on the appropriate staging evaluation for newly diagnosed prostate cancer [published erratum appears in *J Urol* 1997 Dec;158(6):2253]. *J Urol* 158, no. 3 Pt 1: 687-98.

Oesterling, J. E. 1993. Using PSA to eliminate the staging radionuclide bone scan. Significant economic implications. *Urol Clin North Am* 20, no. 4: 705-11.

Oesterling, J. E., C. B. Brendler, J. I. Epstein, A. W. Kimball, Jr., and P. C. Walsh. 1987. Correlation of clinical stage, serum prostatic acid phosphatase and preoperative Gleason grade with final pathological stage in 275 patients with clinically localized adenocarcinoma of the prostate. *J Urol* 138, no. 1: 92-8.

Pannek, J., H. G. Rittenhouse, D. W. Chan, J. I. Epstein, P. C. Walsh, and A. W. Partin. 1998. The use of percent free prostate specific antigen for staging clinically localized prostate cancer. *J Urol* 159, no. 4: 1238-42.

Pannek, J., E. N. Subong, K. A. Jones, P. L. Marschke, J. I. Epstein, D. W. Chan, H. B. Carter, A. A. Luderer, and A. W. Partin. 1996. The role of free/total prostate-specific antigen ratio in the prediction of final pathologic stage for men with clinically localized prostate cancer. *Urology* 48, no. 6A Suppl: 51-4.

Partin, A. W., M. W. Kattan, E. N. Subong, P. C. Walsh, K. J. Wojno, J. E. Oesterling, P. T. Scardino, and J. D. Pearson. 1997. Combination of prostate-specific antigen, clinical stage, and Gleason score to predict pathological stage of localized prostate cancer. A multi-institutional update [see comments] [published erratum appears in *JAMA* 1997 Jul 9;278(2):118]. *JAMA* 277, no. 18: 1445-51.

Partin, A. W., J. D. Pearson, P. K. Landis, H. B. Carter, C. R. Pound, J. Q. Clemens, J. I. Epstein, and P. C. Walsh. 1994. Evaluation of serum prostate-specific antigen velocity after radical prostatectomy to distinguish local recurrence from distant metastases. *Urology* 43, no. 5: 649-59.

Paulson, D. F., J. W. Moul, and P. J. Walther. 1990. Radical prostatectomy for clinical stage T1-2N0M0 prostatic adenocarcinoma: long-term results. *J Urol* 144, no. 5: 1180-4.

Perez, C. A., D. Garcia, J. R. Simpson, F. Zivnuska, and M. A. Lockett. 1989. Factors influencing outcome of definitive radiotherapy for localized carcinoma of the prostate. *Radiother Oncol* 16, no. 1: 1-21.

Perez, C. A., H. K. Lee, A. Georgiou, and M. A. Lockett. 1994. Technical factors affecting morbidity in definitive irradiation for localized carcinoma of the prostate. *Int J Radiat Oncol Biol Phys* 28, no. 4: 811-9.

Perez, C. A., H. K. Lee, A. Georgiou, M. D. Logsdon, P. P. Lai, and M. A. Lockett. 1993. Technical and tumor-related factors affecting outcome of definitive irradiation for localized carcinoma of the prostate [see comments]. *Int J Radiat Oncol Biol Phys* 26, no. 4: 581-91.

Perez, C. A., M. V. Pilepich, D. Garcia, J. R. Simpson, F. Zivnuska, and M. A. Hederman. 1988. Definitive radiation therapy in carcinoma of the prostate localized to the pelvis: experience at the Mallinckrodt Institute of Radiology. *NCI Monogr* 7: 85-94.

Petroski, R. A., J. B. Thrasher, and K. L. Hansberry. 1996. New use of Foley catheter for precise vesicourethral anastomosis during radical retropubic prostatectomy. *J Urol* 155, no. 4: 1376-7.

Pilepich, M. V. 1988. Radiation Therapy Oncology Group studies in carcinoma of the prostate.

NCI Monogr 7: 61-5.

Pilepich, M. V., R. Caplan, R. W. Byhardt, C. A. Lawton, M. J. Gallagher, J. B. Mesic, G. E. Hanks, C. T. Coughlin, A. Porter, W. U. Shipley, and D. Grignon. 1997. Phase III trial of androgen suppression using goserelin in unfavorable- prognosis carcinoma of the prostate treated with definitive radiotherapy: report of Radiation Therapy Oncology Group Protocol 85-31. *J Clin Oncol* 15, no. 3: 1013-21.

Pilepich, M. V., J. M. Krall, M. al-Sarraf, M. J. John, R. L. Doggett, W. T. Sause, C. A. Lawton, R. A. Abrams, M. Rotman, P. Rubin, and et al. 1995. Androgen deprivation with radiation therapy compared with radiation therapy alone for locally advanced prostatic carcinoma: a randomized comparative trial of the Radiation Therapy Oncology Group [see comments]. *Urology* 45, no. 4: 616-23.

Pilepich, M. V., J. M. Krall, R. J. Johnson, W. T. Sause, C. A. Perez, M. Zinninger, and K. Martz. 1986. Extended field (periaortic) irradiation in carcinoma of the prostate-- analysis of RTOG 75-06. *Int J Radiat Oncol Biol Phys* 12, no. 3: 345-51.

Pisansky, T. M., M. J. Kahn, and D. G. Bostwick. 1997a. An enhanced prognostic system for clinically localized carcinoma of the prostate [published erratum appears in *Cancer* 1997 Jul 15;80(2):350]. *Cancer* 79, no. 11: 2154-61.

Pisansky, T. M., M. J. Kahn, G. M. Rasp, S. S. Cha, M. G. Haddock, and D. G. Bostwick. 1997b. A multiple prognostic index predictive of disease outcome after irradiation for clinically localized prostate carcinoma. *Cancer* 79, no. 2: 337-44.

Pollack, A., G. K. Zagars, A. K. el-Naggar, and N. H. Terry. 1994. Relationship of tumor DNA-ploidy to serum prostate-specific antigen doubling time after radiotherapy for prostate cancer. *Urology* 44, no. 5: 711-8.

Pontes, J. E., Z. Wajsman, R. P. Huben, R. M. Wolf, and L. S. Englander. 1985. Prognostic factors in localized prostatic carcinoma. *J Urol* 134, no. 6: 1137-9.

Potosky, A. L., B. A. Miller, P. C. Albertsen, and B. S. Kramer. 1995. The role of increasing detection in the rising incidence of prostate cancer. *Jama* 273, no. 7: 548-52.

Pound, C. R., A. W. Partin, M. A. Eisenberger, D. W. Chan, J. D. Pearson, and P. C. Walsh. 1999a. Natural history of progression after PSA elevation following radical prostatectomy. *JAMA* 281, no. 17: 1591-7.

Pound, C. R., A. W. Partin, M. A. Eisenberger, D. W. Chan, J. D. Pearson, and P. C. Walsh. 1999b. Natural history of progression after PSA elevation following radical prostatectomy [see comments]. *Jama* 281, no. 17: 1591-7.

Prestidge, B. R., I. Kaplan, R. S. Cox, and M. A. Bagshaw. 1992. The clinical significance of a positive post-irradiation prostatic biopsy without metastases. *Int J Radiat Oncol Biol Phys* 24, no. 3: 403-8.

Quinlan, D. M., J. I. Epstein, B. S. Carter, and P. C. Walsh. 1991. Sexual function following radical prostatectomy: influence of preservation of neurovascular bundles. *J Urol* 145, no. 5: 998-1002.

Ragde, H., J. C. Blasko, P. D. Grimm, G. M. Kenny, J. E. Sylvester, D. C. Hoak, K. Landin, and W. Cavanagh. 1997. Interstitial iodine-125 radiation without adjuvant therapy in the treatment of clinically localized prostate carcinoma [see comments]. *Cancer* 80, no. 3: 442-53.

Ragde, H., A. A. Elgamal, P. B. Snow, J. Brandt, A. A. Bartolucci, B. S. Nadir, and L. J. Korb. 1998. Ten-year disease free survival after transperineal sonography-guided iodine-125 brachytherapy with or without 45-gray external beam irradiation in the treatment of patients with clinically localized, low to high Gleason grade prostate carcinoma [see comments]. *Cancer* 83, no. 5: 989-1001.

Rees, M. A., M. I. Resnick, and J. E. Oesterling. 1997. Use of prostate-specific antigen, Gleason score, and digital rectal examination in staging patients with newly diagnosed prostate cancer. *Urol Clin North Am* 24, no. 2: 379-88.

Ritter, M. A., E. M. Messing, T. G. Shanahan, S. Potts, R. J. Chappell, and T. J. Kinsella. 1992. Prostate-specific antigen as a predictor of radiotherapy response and patterns of failure in localized prostate cancer [see comments]. *J Clin Oncol* 10, no. 8: 1208-17.

Roach, M., 3rd, D. M. Chinn, J. Holland, and M. Clarke. 1996. A pilot survey of sexual function and quality of life following 3D conformal radiotherapy for clinically localized prostate cancer. *Int J Radiat Oncol Biol Phys* 35, no. 5: 869-74.

Roach, M. 3rd, J. Krall, J. W. Keller, C. A. Perez, W. T. Sause, R. L. Doggett, M. Rotman, H. Russ, M. V. Pilepich, S. O. Asbell, et al. 1992. The prognostic significance of race and survival from prostate cancer based on patients irradiated on Radiation Therapy Oncology Group protocols (1976-1985). *Int J Radiat Oncol Biol Phys* 24, no. 3: 441-9.

Roeske, J. C., J. D. Forman, C. F. Mesina, T. He, C. A. Pelizzari, E. Fontenla, S. Vijayakumar, and G. T. Chen. 1995. Evaluation of changes in the size and location of the prostate, seminal vesicles, bladder, and rectum during a course of external beam radiation therapy. *Int J Radiat Oncol Biol Phys* 33, no. 5: 1321-9.

Rosen, E., J. R. Cassady, J. Connolly, and J. T. Chaffey. 1985. Radiotherapy for prostate carcinoma: the JCRT experience (1968-1978). II. Factors related to tumor control and complications. *Int J Radiat Oncol Biol Phys* 11, no. 4: 723-30.

Russell, K. J., C. Dunatov, M. D. Hafermann, J. T. Griffeth, L. Polissar, J. Pelton, S. B. Cole, E. W. Taylor, L. W. Wiens, W. J. Koh, and et al. 1991. Prostate specific antigen in the management of patients with localized adenocarcinoma of the prostate treated with primary radiation therapy. *J Urol* 146, no. 4: 1046-52.

Sandler, H. M., D. L. McShan, and A. S. Lichter. 1992. Potential improvement in the results of irradiation for prostate carcinoma using improved dose distribution. *Int J Radiat Oncol Biol Phys* 22, no. 2: 361-7.

Schag, C. A. and R. L. Heinrich. 1990. Development of a comprehensive quality of life measurement tool: CARES. *Oncology (Huntingt)* 4, no. 5: 135-8;discussion 147.

Schellhammer, P. F., A. M. el-Mahdi, D. A. Kuban, and G. L. Wright, Jr. 1997. Prostate-specific antigen after radiation therapy. Prognosis by pretreatment level and post-treatment nadir. *Urol Clin North Am* 24, no. 2: 407-14.

Schellhammer, P. F., A. M. el-Mahdi, G. L. Wright, Jr., P. Kolm, and R. Ragle. 1993. Prostate-specific antigen to determine progression-free survival after radiation therapy for localized carcinoma of prostate. *Urology* 42, no. 1: 13-20.

Schipper, H., J. Clinch, A. McMurray, and M. Levitt. 1984. Measuring the quality of life of cancer patients: the Functional Living Index-Cancer: development and validation. *J Clin Oncol* 2, no. 5: 472-83.

Schneider, S. B., V. G. Schweitzer, R. G. Parker, and P. W. Bycott. 1996. The prognostic value of PSA levels in radiation therapy of patients with carcinoma of the prostate: the UCLA experience 1988-1992. *Am J Clin Oncol* 19, no. 1: 65-72.

Seltzer, M., J. Naitoh, T. Cangiano, R. Reiter, P. Rosen, J. B. deKernion, A. Belldegrun, and C.

Hoh. In press. A prospective comparison of CT scan, positron emmission tomography, and Prostascint scanning for patients who have biochemical relapse following definitive therapy for prostate cancer. *J Urol.*

Seltzer, M. A., Z. Barbaric, A. Belldegrun, J. Naitoh, F. Dorey, M. E. Phelps, S. S. Gambhir, and C. K. Hoh. 1999. Comparison of helical computerized tomography, positron emission tomography and monoclonal antibody scans for evaluation of lymph node metastases in patients with prostate specific antigen relapse after treatment for localized prostate cancer. *J Urol* 162, no. 4: 1322-8.

Shipley, W. U., H. D. Thames, H. M. Sandler, G. E. Hanks, A. L. Zietman, C. A. Perez, D. A. Kuban, S. L. Hancock, and C. D. Smith. 1999. Radiation therapy for clinically localized prostate cancer: a multi- institutional pooled analysis. *JAMA* 281, no. 17: 1598-604.

Shir, Y., S. N. Raja, S. M. Frank, and C. B. Brendler. 1995. Intraoperative blood loss during radical retropubic prostatectomy: epidural versus general anesthesia. *Urology* 45, no. 6: 993-9.

Shrader-Bogen, C. L., J. L. Kjellberg, C. P. McPherson, and C. L. Murray. 1997. Quality of life and treatment outcomes: prostate carcinoma patients' perspectives after prostatectomy or radiation therapy. *Cancer* 79, no. 10: 1977-86.

Singer, P. A., E. S. Tasch, C. Stocking, S. Rubin, M. Siegler, and R. Weichselbaum. 1991. Sex or survival: trade-offs between quality and quantity of life. *J Clin Oncol* 9, no. 2: 328-34.

Smith, D. S. and W. J. Catalona. 1995. Interexaminer variability of digital rectal examination in detecting prostate cancer. *Urology* 45, no. 1: 70-4.

Soffen, E. M., G. E. Hanks, M. A. Hunt, and B. E. Epstein. 1992. Conformal static field radiation therapy treatment of early prostate cancer versus non-conformal techniques: a reduction in acute morbidity. *Int J Radiat Oncol Biol Phys* 24, no. 3: 485-8.

Soffen, E. M., G. E. Hanks, C. C. Hwang, and J. C. Chu. 1991. Conformal static field therapy for low volume low grade prostate cancer with rigid immobilization. *Int J Radiat Oncol Biol Phys* 20, no. 1: 141-6.

Soh, S., M. W. Kattan, S. Berkman, T. M. Wheeler, and P. T. Scardino. 1997. Has there been a recent shift in the pathological features and prognosis of patients treated with radical prostatectomy? [see comments]. *J Urol* 157, no. 6: 2212-8.

Stamey, T. A. 1995. Some concerns about prostate cancer location, Gleason grade, and postradiation doubling times [editorial; comment]. *Int J Radiat Oncol Biol Phys* 33, no. 4: 967-8; discussion 972.

Stamey, T. A., N. Yang, A. R. Hay, J. E. McNeal, F. S. Freiha, and E. Redwine. 1987. Prostate-specific antigen as a serum marker for adenocarcinoma of the prostate. *N Engl J Med* 317, no. 15: 909-16.

Stanford, J. L., Z. Feng, A. S. Hamilton, F. D. Gilliland, R. A. Stephenson, J. W. Eley, P. C. Albertsen, L. C. Harlan, and A. L. Potosky. 2000. Urinary and sexual function after radical prostatectomy for clinically localized prostate cancer: the Prostate Cancer Outcomes Study. *Jama* 283, no. 3: 354-60.

Stein, A., J. B. deKernion, R. B. Smith, F. Dorey, and H. Patel. 1992. Prostate specific antigen levels after radical prostatectomy in patients with organ confined and locally extensive prostate cancer. *J Urol* 147, no. 3 Pt 2: 942-6.

Stock, R. G., N. N. Stone, J. K. DeWyngaert, P. Lavagnini, and P. D. Unger. 1996. Prostate specific antigen findings and biopsy results following interactive ultrasound guided transperineal brachytherapy for early stage prostate carcinoma. *Cancer* 77, no. 11: 2386-92.

Stone, N. N. and R. G. Stock. 1999. Prostate brachytherapy: treatment strategies. *J Urol* 162, no. 2: 421-6.

Suit, H. D., J. Becht, J. Leong, M. Stracher, W. C. Wood, L. Verhey, and M. Goitein. 1988. Potential for improvement in radiation therapy. *Int J Radiat Oncol Biol Phys* 14, no. 4: 777-86.

Sylvester, J., J. C. Blasko, P. Grimm, and H. Ragde. 1997. Interstitial implantation techniques in prostate cancer. *J Surg Oncol* 66, no. 1: 65-75.

Talcott, J. A., P. Rieker, J. A. Clark, K. J. Propert, J. C. Weeks, C. J. Beard, K. I. Wishnow, I. Kaplan, K. R. Loughlin, J. P. Richie, and P. W. Kantoff. 1998. Patient-reported symptoms after primary therapy for early prostate cancer: results of a prospective cohort study. *J Clin Oncol* 16, no. 1: 275-83.

Tefilli, M. V., E. L. Gheiler, R. Tiguert, W. Sakr, D. J. Grignon, M. Banerjee, J. E. Pontes, and D. P. Wood, Jr. 1999. Should Gleason score 7 prostate cancer be considered a unique grade category? *Urology* 53, no. 2: 372-7.

Ten Haken, R. K., C. Perez-Tamayo, R. J. Tesser, D. L. McShan, B. A. Fraass, and A. S. Lichter. 1989. Boost treatment of the prostate using shaped, fixed fields. *Int J Radiat Oncol Biol Phys* 16, no. 1: 193-200.

Teshima, T., G. E. Hanks, A. L. Hanlon, R. S. Peter, and T. E. Schultheiss. 1997. Rectal bleeding after conformal 3D treatment of prostate cancer: time to occurrence, response to treatment and duration of morbidity. *Int J Radiat Oncol Biol Phys* 39, no. 1: 77-83.

Troyer, J. K., M. L. Beckett, and G. L. Wright, Jr. 1997. Location of prostate-specific membrane antigen in the LNCaP prostate carcinoma cell line. *Prostate* 30, no. 4: 232-42.

Wahle, S., M. Reznicek, B. Fallon, C. Platz, and R. Williams. 1990. Incidence of surgical margin involvement in various forms of radical prostatectomy. *Urology* 36, no. 1: 23-6.

Wasserman, T. H., and A. McDonald. 1995. Quality of life: the patient's endpoint [editorial; comment]. *Int J Radiat Oncol Biol Phys* 33, no. 4: 965-6.

Weyrich, T. P., S. J. Kandzari, and P. R. Jain. 1993. Iodine 125 seed implants for prostatic carcinoma. Five- and ten-year follow-up. *Urology* 41, no. 2: 122-6.

Wilson, J. W., A. Morales, and A. W. Bruce. 1983. The prognostic significance of histological grading and pathological staging in carcinoma of the prostate. *J Urol* 130, no. 3: 481-3.

Winter, H. I., P. R. Bretton, and H. W. Herr. 1991. Preoperative prostate-specific antigen in predicting pathologic stage and grade after radical prostatectomy. *Urology* 38, no. 3: 202-5.

Witherspoon, L. R. 1997. Early detection of cancer relapse after prostatectomy using very sensitive prostate-specific antigen measurements. *Br J Urol* 79 Suppl 1: 82-6.

Yang, R. M., J. Naitoh, M. Murphy, H. J. Wang, J. Phillipson, J. B. deKernion, M. Loda, and R. E. Reiter. 1998. Low p27 expression predicts poor disease-free survival in patients with prostate cancer. *J Urol* 159, no. 3: 941-5.

Yu, H., E. P. Diamandis, A. F. Prestigiacomo, and T. A. Stamey. 1995. Ultrasensitive assay of prostate-specific antigen used for early detection of prostate cancer relapse and estimation of tumor-doubling time after radical prostatectomy. *Clin Chem* 41, no. 3: 430-4.

Zagars, G. K. 1993. Serum PSA as a tumor marker for patients undergoing definitive radiation therapy. *Urol Clin North Am* 20, no. 4: 737-47.

Zagars, G. K., A. G. Ayala, A. C. von Eschenbach, and A. Pollack. 1995a. The prognostic importance of Gleason grade in prostatic adenocarcinoma: a long-term follow-up study of 648 patients treated with radiation therapy [see comments]. *Int J Radiat Oncol Biol Phys* 31, no. 2: 237-45.

Zagars, G. K., V. S. Kavadi, A. Pollack, A. C. von Eschenbach, and M. E. Sands. 1995b. The source of pretreatment serum prostate-specific antigen in clinically localized prostate cancer--T, N, or M? *Int J Radiat Oncol Biol Phys* 32, no. 1: 21-32.

Zagars, G. K. and A. Pollack. 1995. Radiation therapy for T1 and T2 prostate cancer: prostate-specific antigen and disease outcome. *Urology* 45, no. 3: 476-83.

Zagars, G. K., A. Pollack, V. S. Kavadi, and A. C. von Eschenbach. 1995c. Prostate-specific antigen and radiation therapy for clinically localized prostate cancer. *Int J Radiat Oncol Biol Phys* 32, no. 2: 293-306.

Zagars, G. K., A. C. von Eschenbach, D. E. Johnson, and M. J. Oswald. 1988. The role of radiation therapy in stages A2 and B adenocarcinoma of the prostate. *Int J Radiat Oncol Biol Phys* 14, no. 4: 701-9.

Zelefsky, M. J., K. E. Wallner, C. C. Ling, A. Raben, T. Hollister, T. Wolfe, A. Grann, P. Gaudin, Z. Fuks, and S. A. Leibel. 1999. Comparison of the 5-year outcome and morbidity of three-dimensional conformal radiotherapy versus transperineal permanent iodine-125 implantation for early-stage prostatic cancer. *J Clin Oncol* 17, no. 2: 517-22.

Zietman, A. L., J. J. Coen, K. C. Dallow, and W. U. Shipley. 1995. The treatment of prostate cancer by conventional radiation therapy: an analysis of long-term outcome. *Int J Radiat Oncol Biol Phys* 32, no. 2: 287-92.

Zietman, A. L., R. A. Edelstein, J. J. Coen, R. K. Babayan, and R. J. Krane. 1994. Radical prostatectomy for adenocarcinoma of the prostate: the influence of preoperative and pathologic findings on biochemical disease-free outcome. *Urology* 43, no. 6: 828-33.

Zietman, A. L., M. K. Tibbs, K. C. Dallow, C. T. Smith, A. F. Althausen, R. A. Zlotecki, and W. U. Shipley. 1996. Use of PSA nadir to predict subsequent biochemical outcome following external beam radiation therapy for T1-2 adenocarcinoma of the prostate. *Radiother Oncol* 40, no. 2: 159-62.

Allen et al. Local Tumor Recurrence Following RP. Urology, 1992	
Treatment modality	RP
Site	University of TN, Memphis, TN
Study design	Case report on one patient with local tumor recurrence after initial nerve sparing surgery failed to adequately operate on the cancer. Second surgery done to "salvage"

Anscher et al. Multivariate analysis of factors predicting local relapse after RP - possible indications for postoperatic radiotherapy. Int J Radiation Oncology Biol. Phys, 1991	
Treatment modality	Radical surgery; radiotherapy; adjuvant XRT for patients at risk for recurrence
Site	Duke University Medical Center, Durham, NC
Study design	Observational study of 273 patients who underwent radical surgery for newly diagnosed adenocarcinoma and who received no adjuvant radiotherapy, were reviewed for local recurrence
Sample Size	273
Accrual dates	1970-1983
Patient stage	Retrospectively staged at pre-op evaluation using medical records. Post-op, patients were retrospectively assigned a WJ patholog stage using pathol reports.
Patient age	Mean = 64.
Duration of follow-up	5, 10, 15 years
Other Patient characteristics	Provided
Other Eligibility Criteria	Patients receiving adjuvant post-operative irradiation were excluded from analysis
Univar/Multiv Analyses (Covariates)	Multivar analysis to measure influence on the development of local recurrence and distant metastases using age, hormone theraphy, histologic grade, clin stage, histologic involvement of seminal vesicles, and elevated acid phosphatase
Outcome Definitions	Local recurrence. Probability of local return as a function of risk factors. Predictors of local relapse – Development of distant metastases followed closely on the heels of local recurrence.
Method of Survival Analysis	5,10,15 year. Variables combined in stepwise fashion to determine combination most powerful in distinguishing between groups. Chi sq method to determine significance of group differencess. Actuarial method use to calculate curves of local control
Survival Curves	Provided
Other outcomes/Results	Patients with poorly differentiated tumors, PSMs, or elevated preoperative acid phosphatase are at high risk for local relapse after RP

Berlin et al. Voiding cystourethrograhy after RP: Normal findings and correlation between contrast and extravasation and anastomotic strictures. AJR, 1994	
Treatment modality	RP
Site	Univ of Pennsylvania, Philadelphia, PA
Study design	Retrospective study to evaluate the relationship of extravasation of urine and surgical technique to the formation of an anastomotic stricture and to assess the radiographic appearance of the vesicourethral anastomosis after retropubic RP.
Sample Size	142
Accrual dates	1987-1991
Patient stage	Clinically staged A or B
Patient age	Not Available
Duration of follow-up	Voiding cystourethograms at 3 weeks after RP
Other Patient characteristics	Reviewed patient medical record to determine any other post-op complications
Other Eligibility Criteria	At least 12 months of follow-up
Univar/Multiv Analyses (Covariates)	No mention. Used z-test of independent proportions to see if the difference between the 2 proportions was statistically significant.
Outcome Definitions	Presence of anastomotic stricture. Confirmed by dynamic retrograde urethrography, cystoscopy, or both.
Other outcomes/Results	As long as catheters are left in place until anastomotic healing is complete, extravasation of contrast material does not influence subsequent formation of anastomotic strictures. Vest procedure is significant risk factor for stricture formation.

Bigg et al. Role of ns RP for clinical stage B2 Prostate Cancer. J Urology, 1990.	
Treatment modality	RP - unilateral and bilateral ns
Site	Washington Univ School of Medicine, St. Louis, MO
Study design	Asks does ns RP compromise the adequacy of tumor excision & specifically deals with the appropriateness of performing ns RP in patients with clin stage B2 disease because of the extraordinarily high incid. of extracapsular tumor extension and positive surgical margins at this stage
Sample Size	77
Accrual dates	1st 77 consec. preop potent clin stage B2 PC patients (in series) since surg team adopted ns technique in 1984
Patient stage	Clinical stage B2
Patient age	Mean = 65 (Range 48-76year)
Duration of follow-up	Every 3 - 6 months for 12 months
Univar/Multiv Analyses (Covariates)	See Table 4 +disc of analysis of preop staging to predict extracapsular tumor on pg. 1422
Outcome Definitions	Tumor excision was primary goal, potency was secondary. Pts followed with DRE and PSA every 3-6 months. PSA considered undetectable if <=0.6ng/ml. Pts considered potent if had erection sufficient for vaginal penetration and sexual intercourse.
Method of Survival Analysis	Provided
Survival Curves	Provided
Impotence	Potency preserved in 66% of bilateral ns and 37% of unilateral ns
Other outcomes/Results	Complete tumor excision in 36% of bilateral and 27% of unilateral. Patients with poorly diff tumors and/or bulky disease had higher incidence of extracapsular extension.

Blackwell et al. Combining PSA with CA and gland volume to predict more reliably pathological stage: the influence of PSA CA density. Urology, 1994	
Treatment modality	ns RP + pelvic lymphadectomy
Site	Mayo Clinic, Rochester, MN
Study design	Study to evaluate the correlation of serum PSA level with variety of prognostic factors + to determine predictive value of preop PSA level in determining tumor burden + path stage in effort to control for pros volume and ca. volume. PSA's eval'd 3 diff ways
Sample Size	320 consec pts with appropriate staging operated on by 1 of 3 Mayo Clinic surgeons
Accrual dates	1991-1992
Patient stage	T1c through T2b
Patient age	Mean = 64.8 (Range = 45-78)
Other Eligibility Criteria	No clinical evidence of metastases preop. Preop serum PSA determined within 120 days of surgery.
Univar/Multiv Analyses (Covariates)	Spearman rank corr coeff. Mult regr + stepwise regr used to study relation between preop serum PSA +mult path factors. Independent vars in regression include serum PSA, pathologic PSA density, PSA-CA density.
Statistical Estimates Related to Survival Analyses	BiVar anal shows strongest corr of serum PSA level with CA vol, % poorly differentiated CA, PSMs, and path stage. Multivariable analysis showed CA vol was major contrib to serum PSA level. PSA-CA density showed sig corr with path stage + % poorly diff CA.
Other outcomes/Results	Serum PSA strongly corr with CA vol, tumor grade, + path stage. These variables seemed to have indpt predictive value for serum PSA.

Braslis et al. Quality of Life 12 months after RP. Br J Urol, 1995	
Treatment modality	RP
Site	University of Miami School of Med, Miami, FL
Study design	Recruited patients to evaluate the impact of RP on QOL in pts 12 months after surgery
Sample Size	79
Patient age	Mean = 63 (Range = 43-76)
Duration of follow-up	Group 1: evaluatons 12+ months post RP. Group 2: evaluations 1 month prior to RP.
Other Patient characteristics	Provided
Univar/Multiv Analyses (Covariates)	Group comparisons made using 1 way ANOVA. Correl coeffs derived using Pearson correl analysis.
Outcome Definitions	QOL Measures: FLIC, POMS, bladder, bowel, sex function inventory.
Incontinence	12 month followup shows sig change in continence. Min voiding + bowel dysf reported
Impotence	12 month follow-up shows sig change in sex function. Patients were most disatisfied with postoperative sexual function.
Other outcomes/Results	Satisfaction with choice. 12 month followup shows sig change in hardship scores. Tension scores improved. RP has minimal overall impact upon patient QOL.

Brendler et al. The Role of RP in the Tx of Prostate Cancer - Ca-A Cancer J for Clinicians, 1992	
Treatment modality	ns RP
Site	Johns Hopkins University, Baltimore, MD
Study design	Article is mostly a series report - surgery done and results reported. Outcomes mentioned, but not truly measured or validated. Mostly discussion ns RP.
Sample Size	600 consecutive pts undergoing RP
Accrual dates	1982-1988
Patient stage	Those with clinically localized (A+B) classified by pathological stage into (1) Organ confined, (2) Specimen confined,and (3) Not confined
Duration of follow-up	5 years. (Mention need for 10 +15 year to confirm findings)
Outcome Definitions	Main outcomes of interest: cancer control; sexual function; urinary continence.
Method of Survival Analysis	Provided
Survival Curves	5 year actuarial status based on pathologic stage
Incontinence	Complete urin control achieved in 92%. Stress incont present in 8%. 98% dry or 1 pad/day. None totally incontinent. At 3 mo: 47% dry; at 6mo: 75% dry; at 9 months: 82% dry; at 12 months: 89% dry; at 2 years: 92% dry. Age was only factor to influence long term continence.
Impotence	Sig correlation between age + recovery of sexual function. Greater potency associated with stage A, rather than B. Influence of ns on surgical margins.
Other outcomes/Results	Structure--outcomes link - new technque improved other outcomes. 9 patients had positive margins in area of preserved neurovasc bundle. Followed separately for 2-5 years post-op and showed no local recurrence of disease.

Catalona, WJ. Patient selection for results of , and impact on tumor resection of potency – sparing RP. Urologic Clinics of N. America, 1990	
Treatment modality	RP
Site	Washington Univ Schoiol of Medicine, St Louis, MO
Study design	Retrospectively examined their own series of nsRP's to determ how often both goals (pot sparing + complete tumor excision) were achieved simultaneously. Looked at outcomes separately and together for simultaneous achievement of both goals. Looked at by number of pts at each stage.
Sample Size	250 consecutive patients treated with RP
Patient stage	Clin stage A or B. Used various staging techniques
Patient age	Range approx <50 to 74
Duration of follow-up	6 month minimum follow-up
Outcome Definitions	Completeness of tumor excision determined by tumor volume + histologic tumor grade
Method of Survival Analysis	Link disease free survival + pathologic stage
Impotence	Retention of potency unclear. Appeared to be function of age, pathol stage, +# neurovasc bundles preserved. Patient age most highly significant. See disc on pp. 821,823,824, 825. And see Table 2. For disc of simul achievement (both o/c) see Tables 3+4 and pg.825
Other outcomes/Results	Results suggest standards for potency sparing RP should be more restrictive than those for standard RP.

Chodak et al., Results of conservative management of clinically localized prostate cancer, NEJM, 1994	
Treatment modality	Observation and delayed hormone therapy
Site	6: 1 Israel, 1 Scotland, 2 in US, 2 in Sweden. After adjustment for stage, patients with grade 1 tumors from each cohort had ns differences in disease-specific survival. The same was found for grade 2, but not 3. All cohorts analyzed together.
Study design	Pooled analysis of case records from 6 nonrandomized studies.
Sample Size	828
Accrual dates	Medline articles published from January 1985 through July 1992
Patient stage	T0a, T01, A1 or focal; T0b, T0d, A2, or diffuse; T1 or B1; T2, B2, or B3
Patient age	mean= 69.6 +/- 7.8, median= 69, range 37-93
Duration of follow-up	mean= 79.5 months +/- 49.9, median=78 months
Univar/Multiv Analyses (Covariates)	Grades 1-3, 4 staging systems were used: TNM ('74 and '78), Jewett-Whitmore, and Chisholm (comparable stages were identified except for stages A1, focal, T01, and T0a).
Outcome Definitions	Disease-specific survival: survival among only those patients who did not die of causes other than prostate CA.
Method of Survival Analysis	Kaplan-Meier with log-rank or Mantel-Haenszel test.
Survival Curves	5-y and 10-y disease-specific and metastasis-free survival by grade (all stages), by grade 1 or 2 and age <61 or >=61, by grade 1 or 2 and stage. ~820 (gives number censored by grade and year). Figures 1 & 2 out to 15 years.
Statistical Estimates Related to Survival Analyses	98% (95% CI 96-99) for 5-year disease-specific, grade 1, all stages. 87% (95% CI 81-91) for 10-year, grade 1, all stages. 93% (95% CI 90-95) for 5-year metastasis-free, grade 1, all stages. 81% (95% CI 75-86) for 10-year, grade 1, all stages.

Coetzee et al., Postoperative PSA as a prognostic indicator in patients w/margin-positive prostate CA, undergoing adjuvant radiotherapy after radical prostatectomy, Urology, 1996

Treatment modality	Adjuvant radiotherapy within 6 months of radical prostatectomy
Site	Duke University Medical Center, NC
Study design	Evaluated 45 patients with margin positive disease who were pN0 at radical prostatectomy. Divided into 2 groups, initially undetectable PSA but later elevated, and persistently elevated.
Sample Size	45; Undetetectable PSA = 30; Elevated PSA = 15
Accrual dates	Unknown
Patient stage	T1-2 M0 and pN0
Patient age	Undet. PSA mean =68.4, range= 57.8-78.9; Elev. PSA mean =67.4, range=51-82
Duration of follow-up	mean since XRT=33 mos
Outcome Definitions	Using post-op PSA levels, patients divided into 2 groups: those who initially attained undet. PSA levels but later had progressive PSA elev, and those in who the PSA level never reached undetectable levels.
Method of Survival Analysis	Kaplan-Meier method.
Survival Curves	Time to PSA failure by post-op PSA level out to 13 years.
Statistical Estimates Related to Survival Analyses	Undet. PSA: Mean time to failure (elev. PSA) = 2.1 y; Median=3.31 year; range=4 mo-4.8 y. Elev. PSA: Mean time to failure (progr. incr. in PSA) = 0.95 y; Median=0.92 y; Range=4 mo-2.02 y

Coleman et al. Rate of relapse following tx for localized PC: a critical analysis of retrospective reports. Int J Rad Oncol Biol Phys, 1994

Treatment modality	ns RP; XRT
Site	Clinical reports from major surgery + rad onc institutions (8 sites)
Study design	Meta-analysis/ critical analysis of retrospective reports
Sample Size	4446
Patient stage	A+B.
Duration of follow-up	Papers selected had minimum follow-up of 5 years. to est rate of failure in 5 year intervals. Calc's actuarial % of patients who were dis free at 0,5,10,15,+20 years post surgery.
Method of Survival Analysis	Hazard function calculation to estimate + compare rate of relapse for different tx
Survival Curves	See disc on pg. 304 .
Statistical Estimates Related to Survival Analyses	Patients risk free for relapse through length of series. Recurr rates by stage were similar for patients with RT or surg. Lesions >12cm3 pose greater risk of extra-protastatic disease.
Other outcomes/Results	Tx outcomes for pts may be more dependent on inherent tumor biology than particular type of tx. Analysis indicates for tumors larger than stage A1, pts continue to be at risk for relapse.

Connolly et al. Local recurrence after RP: characteristics in size, location, + rel to PSA + surgical margins. Urology, 1996.

Treatment modality	ns RP
Study design	Series/observational study. Local recurrence detected by DRE/TRUS biopsies. Use of TRUS to define sonographic appearance of local RP incl loc, size, +rel to serum PSA.
Sample Size	114
Accrual dates	1988-1993
Patient stage	T1- T3
Other Eligibility Criteria	patients with elevated PSA + negative bone scan
Outcome Definitions	define songraphic characteristics of local cancer recurrence post RP
Statistical Estimates Related to Survival Analyses	Examination of RP specimens in patients with local recurrence showed +surgical margins in 66% + organ confined disease in 20%. TRUS is useful adjunct to PSA + DRE in detection of local recurrence post RP.

Cookson et al. Pathological staging + biochemical recurrence a/f neoadjuvant androgen deprivation therapy in combination with RP in clinically localized prostate CA: results of a Phase II study. British J Urol, 1997.	
Treatment modality	RP; neoadjuvant androgen depravation therapy (ADT)
Site	Memorial Sloan Kettering CA Center, New York
Study design	prospective case control study comparing patients with combo therapy (neoadjuvant hormone therapy followed by RP) or just RP for pathological staging + biochemical progression free recurrence.
Sample Size	147 total. Group1= 69 with ADT. Group2= 72 without ADT.
Accrual dates	July 1991 to Dec 1992
Patient stage	Table 3 outlines clinical + pathological staging for both groups. Also see table 1.
Patient age	mean = 62 (Range: 45-72)
Duration of follow-up	All patients followed @ 3 month intervals 1st 2 years + 6 month intervals thereafter Total followup = 35 mo
Other Patient characteristics	Clinical characteristics of patients in group 1 +2
Univar/Multiv Analyses (Covariates)	Chi square analysis of pathological stages between groups. Preop PSA level + pathological stage comparison (for Group 1) evaluated using Fisher's exact test.
Outcome Definitions	Pathological staging + biochemical progression free recurrence.
Method of Survival Analysis	Kaplan Meier used to determ biochem recurrence. Differences between curves evaluated using log rank test.
Survival Curves	Provided
Statistical Estimates Related to Survival Analyses	No significant difference for patients with pT2 disease between biochemical failure between 2 groups in 35 months follow-up. In patients with postive margins, biochemical failure rate was significantly higher in ADT group.
Other outcomes/Results	Study showed significant difference in rate of organ + specimen confined tumors in patients with T1/T2 PC tx with combo therapy over patients tx only with surgery.

D'Amico et al. An analysis of the time course of Postop PSA failure in patients with positive surgical margins: Implications on the use of adjuvant therapy. Urology, 1996.	
Treatment modality	RP + adjuvant therapy
Site	Hospital of Univ Penn, Philadelphia, PA ; Brigham & Women's Hospital, Boston, MA
Study design	Series /observational study intended to provide rationale for Phase III trials
Sample Size	143 of 554 consecutive PC patients undergoing RP
Accrual dates	1989- 994
Patient stage	T3A + T3B .
Duration of follow-up	1 months post surg; every 3 months for 2 years; every 6 months thereafter 36 months total follow-up for disease free survival PSM patients.
Other Eligibility Criteria	positive margin patients with pelvic lymph nodes, seminal vesicle invasion, or prostatectomy Gl sum >= 8 were excluded
Univar/Multiv Analyses (Covariates)	Cox regr multivar anal used to determine significance of independent clinical + pathol predictors of early+ delayed postop PSA failure.Cox regr + multvar anal +1 univar anal were perf'd to test for o/c PSA failure within 12 months postop in positive margin pts
Outcome Definitions	impact of adjuvant therapy on survival in POSITIVE MARGIN CA patients
Method of Survival Analysis	Kaplan-Meier method used to calc actuarial PSA failure in patients with close, focally positive, and diffusely PSMs. Test comparisons evaluated using log-rank test.
Survival Curves	Provided
Statistical Estimates Related to Survival Analyses	Gleason sum 7 + preop PSA > 20ng/ml + erMRI showing extensive disease were sig predictors of early postop PSA failure. Gleason sum <=6 + preop PSA <=20ng/ml + erMRI showing limited disease predict delayed PSA failure. Kaplan Meier subgroup anal presented
Other outcomes/Results	Results support the hypothesis that early PSA failure in a pt with positive margins is associated with distant disease as site of primary failure

D'Amico et al. Combined modality of prostate carcinoma + its utility in predicting pathologic stage + postop PSA failure. Urology, 1997	
Site	Hospital of Univ Penn, Philadelphia, PA
Study design	Series/observational study to predict factors that can optimize preop staging for clinically localized prostate cancer patients.
Sample Size	480
Accrual dates	1989 - 1995
Patient stage	T1 - T2
Duration of follow-up	1 month post surgery; every 3 months for 2 years; every 6 months thereafter
Other Patient characteristics	Provided
Univar/Multiv Analyses (Covariates)	logistic + cox regression multivariable analyses performed to evaluate ability of clin stage, PSA, biopsy Gleason sum, % + biopsies, erMRI results to predict for path established ECE, SVI, + time to postop PSA failure.
Outcome Definitions	Combined modality staging is useful, through multivar analysis, all predictors that have independent prognostic sig for a given outcome for determining probability of that outcome
Method of Survival Analysis	Kaplan-Meier method used. Comparisons made using the log-rank test.
Survival Curves	Actuarial calculations provided
Statistical Estimates Related to Survival Analyses	Provided
Other outcomes/Results	Combined modality staging in select patients can predict pathol stage + postop failure. Found that PSA, biopsy Gleason sum, + clinical stage all contributed independent information in predicting outcome

D'Amico et al. A Multivariable Analysis of clinical factors predicting for pathological features associated with local failure a/f RP for Prostate CA. Int J Rad Onc Biol Phys, 1994	
Treatment modality	RP
Site	Hospital of Univ Penn, Philadelphia, PA
Study design	Retrospective review of pathological findings in Prostate CA patients who had RP
Sample Size	235
Accrual dates	1990 - 1993
Patient stage	Provided
Univar/Multiv Analyses (Covariates)	Multivariate anal used to determ predictive value of pretx clin indicators on path features assoc with local failure post RP. Multivar anal used preop serum PSA, clin stage, GI, with + wtihout erMRI to id high risk patients + determ o/c of +surg margins.
Other outcomes/Results	Use of er surface coil mag res scan in conjunction with serum PSA + GI sum improves clin acc of predicting those patients at high risk for clinically extra protastatic disease.

151

D'Amico et al. A Multivariate Analysis of clinical + pathological factors that predict for PSA failure after RP for Prostate Cancer. J Urol, 1995

Treatment modality	RP
Study design	Series/observational study.
Sample Size	347
Accrual dates	1989 - 1993
Other Patient characteristics	Provided
Univar/Multiv Analyses (Covariates)	Cox regression multivariate analysis to determine clinical + pathological indicators predictive of PSA failure. Use to test outcome of PSA failure over time. See table 3.
Survival Curves	Provided
Statistical Estimates Related to Survival Analyses	2 year actuarial PSA failure rates were 84% vs 23% in patients with & without SVI on MRI and 58% vs 21% in those with without ECE. In patients with ECE and no SVI or poorly diff tumors. 2 year actuarial PSA failure rates were 50% (pos margin), 28% (neg margin with ECE), and 9% (neg margin with focal microscopic ECE).
Other outcomes/Results	er MRI showing SVI or ECE when PSA level is <20 ng/ml + path GI sum is 5-7, or PSA level is >10 and < 20 and pathbiol GI is 2 - 4 is predictive of PSA failure.

D'Amico et al. Outcome based staging for clinical localized adenocarcinoma of the prostate. J Urol, 1997

Treatment modality	ns RP
Site	Hospital of Univ Penn, Philadelphia, PA
Study design	Series/observational study evaluating patients for clinical features predictive of time to PSA failure after RP.
Sample Size	688
Accrual dates	1989-1996
Patient stage	Clinical T1 and T2.
Duration of follow-up	Median followup 30 months. Every 3 months for 1st 2 years, then every 6 months
Other Patient characteristics	Provided
Other Eligibility Criteria	No neoadjuvant hormonal therapy preop or postop prior to PSA failure
Univar/Multiv Analyses (Covariates)	Cox multivar regr anal. Eval'd calc'd Pr CA col + its abil to predict time to PSA failure in conjunc with PSA, biopsy, GI score, + clin stage. Step down regr methods used to build parsimonious stat models for the assoc of the clin sig prognostic factors + time to PSA failure.
Outcome Definitions	PSA failure = 2 consec non-0 PSAs obtained postop after an undetectable PSA. Freedom from PSA failure after RP. Calculated PCA vol = quotient of CA-specific PSA + serum PSA per cm3 of PC of a given score. Other definitions provided
Method of Survival Analysis	Kaplan Meier and log rank tests
Survival Curves	Provided
Statistical Estimates Related to Survival Analyses	Pathologic organ confined disease noted in 69% of all clinically confined patients.
Other outcomes/Results	Calculated PC volume + PSA may provide clinically useful info re: outcomes after RP. Process - Outcome link : Correlated CA vol with likelihood of failure of surgery to cure cancer.

Dillioglugil et al. Hazard rates for progression after RP for clinically localized prostate cancer. Urology, 1997

Treatment modality	RP
Site	Baylor College of Medicine; Houston, TX
Study design	series/observational
Sample Size	611
Accrual dates	1983 - 1995
Patient stage	Clinically localized cT1 - 2, NX, MO
Patient age	mean = 62. Range = 40-79
Duration of follow-up	5,10 years
Other Eligibility Criteria	no other documented progression
Outcome Definitions	Progression-free survival (PFS) to show pattern of tx failure over time + to assess efficacy of definitive therapy. PSA based look at disease free survival - over on average 30 months.
Method of Survival Analysis	Calculated PFSfor PC recurrence after RP.
Statistical Estimates Related to Survival Analyses	PFS 78% at 5 years and 76% at 10 yrs. Highest Hazard Rate (0.09) observed in the year immediately post RP and dropped by year 7. No patient recurred after year 6. The more ominous the prognostic factors, the higher the initial Hazard Rate.
Other outcomes/Results	PSA progression after RP occurred early (77% in 1st 2 years), often due to understaging. Late recurrence rare for patients evaluated with PSA

Douglas L et al. Easy Visualization of the membranous urethral stump in RP. J Urol, 1997

Treatment modality	RP
Site	Dept of Surgery; University Hospital of the West Indies; Mona, Kingston, JAMAICA
Study design	series/observational. This paper studies efficacy of using 20 Foley catheters with 5 ml balloon inflated 10 ml in bulbous urethra to elevate urethral stump during surgery
Sample Size	50
Incontinence	Decreased leakage of urine & no anastomotic stricture. No urethral trauma or incontinence attributable to technique.
Other outcomes/Results	No complications attributed to technique

Douglas T, et al. Comparison of serum prostate specific membrane antigen, PSA, + free PSA levels in RP patients. Cancer, 1997

Treatment modality	RP
Site	Walter Reed Army Medical Center, Washington, DC
Study design	series/observational study to evaluate various PSA-related serum markers in men undergoing RP.
Sample Size	63
Accrual dates	1994 - 1996
Patient stage	Clin loc T1c, T2
Other Patient characteristics	Provided
Other Eligibility Criteria	no preop hormonal therapy; voluntary participation; written informed consent
Univar/Multiv Analyses (Covariates)	serum values for markers were compared with path stage, surg margin status, Gl sum, prostate size, tumor size, + WHO tumor grade. Markers also compared against demog info + pt age + race. ROC anal comparing sensitivity & specificity to pos and neg margins and SVI
Survival Curves	Areas under curve for PSA + Free PSA were 0.7318 & 0.7432, respectively.
Statistical Estimates Related to Survival Analyses	Weak correlation between serum PSA + PSM, higher Gl sum, + WHO grade. ROC demonstrated PSA + FPSA predictive ability for SVI. Total PSA best marker. High PSA & Free PSA associated with locally advanced disease

Drago et al. RP 1972 - 1987 single institutional experience: comparison of stnd RP and nerve-sparing techniques. Urology, 1990

Treatment modality	RP + ns RP
Site	Ohio State University
Study design	combined retrospective + prospective evaluation of 1 institution's experience with RP. series/observ study comparing 66 standdard RP patients with 44 ns RP patients. Latter study (ns) prospective evaluation available with regard to pre & postoperative staging, erectile function, bloof loss + replacement, PSA data, clinical & pathological stage
Sample Size	104 (60 standard RP from 1972-85) (44 ns RP from 1986-1987)
Accrual dates	1972-87
Patient stage	Clinically organ confined PC.
Patient age	<50 to 74
Survival Curves	Group1= ½ (30patients) had organ confined disease
Statistical Estimates Related to Survival Analyses	Standard = 51% identified with organ confined disease. ns = 75% identified with organ confined disease.
Incontinence	All patients exp some urinary incontinence 3-6 weeks post surg. Only 1 patient in Group2 (2%) was incontinent postop at 6 months. 4 patients in group 2 developed postop bladder neck contracture
Impotence	Group1 = > 90% impotent. 2 variables play role in potency - age + pathologic stage. Ns resulted in increased reservation of erectile function in 70% preoperatively potent pts
Other outcomes/Results	ns resulted in decreased blood loss + more accurate assessment of clinical staging prior to surgery through use of TRUS

Epstein JI et al. Prediction of progression following RP. A multivariate analysis of men with long-term follow up. Am J of Surgical Pathology, 1996

Treatment modality	RP
Site	Johns Hopkins University, Baltimore, MD
Study design	series/observational study to determine whether with longer follow-up + large number of pts progression could be more accurately predicted by combining GI score, surgical margin status, + capsular penetration to give doctors + patients more accurate prognostic info post RP.
Sample Size	617
Accrual dates	1982 - 1990
Patient stage	T1 - T2 and T2 - T4
Duration of follow-up	mean=6.5 years. For no progression patients every 3 months for 1 year; every 6 months for next 2 years; annual thereafter. All followups include physical examination, PSA + some include DRE + bone scan.
Other Eligibility Criteria	no pre or post op XRT or hormone therapy until progression. No lymph node metastases or SVI.
Univar/Multiv Analyses (Covariates)	Multivar analysis: GI score (p<0.0001), surg marg (p=0.004),+ cap pen(p=0.007) were all indepedent. Predictors of progr cox proportional hazard anal used to assess multiple variables to determine indpt prognostic indicators of dis progression.
Outcome Definitions	Tumor progression = increasing PSA (>.2 ng/ml); evidence of local recurrence; or radiological evidence of distant metastases.
Method of Survival Analysis	Kaplan-Meier method used for estimation. Wilcoxan-Gehan test to test diffs between K-M curves.
Survival Curves	Actuarial curves within study allow docs to more accurately determine risk of progression following RP based on GI score, ECE, + surgica margin status – especially for mid-range GI which are more difficult to prognosticate
Statistical Estimates Related to Survival Analyses	Tumors with GI 2-4 often curved with 10 year progression-free risk of 96%. 10 year actuarial progression-free risk for men with GI score 8-9 was 35%.

Elias et al. Adjuvant Radiation Therapy after RP for carcinoma of the prostate. Am J Clin Oncol, 1997	
Treatment modality	RP with adjuvant XRT
Site	UCLA Medical Center, Los Angeles, CA
Study design	Retrospective observational study comparing disease progression in men who had only prostatectomy vs men who had prostatectomy and adjuvant XRT
Sample Size	110 total. 79=RP only. 31=RP with adjuvant XRT
Accrual dates	1965 - 1989. (58 tx between 1965-80 + 52 patients tx between 1980-89)
Patient age	mean= 64 years
Duration of follow-up	All followed for at least 5 years. 64 patients followed for >10years post tx.
Other Patient characteristics	Provided
Other Eligibility Criteria	Patients with pathology specimens showing capsular invasion without capsular penetration were excluded from study. Patients receiving XRT after documented local recurrence not included in adjuvant therapy group.
Univar/Multiv Analyses (Covariates)	Cox regression model used to compare disease progression while controlling for difference between 2 tx groups
Outcome Definitions	Patients felt to be at risk for recurrence based on pathologic finding of stage C dis. Clin endpts/clin ev of local tumor regrowth of metas. Local recurrence def as an enlarging mass palpable in site of resection. Endpoints are clinical because PSA was only available after 1987.
Method of Survival Analysis	Kaplan-Meier method used.
Survival Curves	Actuarial plots provided
Statistical Estimates Related to Survival Analyses	Differences in clinical stages not statistically significant. Status of pelvic LN: differences not statistically significant. Cox regression model showed advantage of recurrence free surv in combination pts. 20 combination pts fared better in all categories than the 45 with RP only. Differences in freedom from local recurrence were statistically significant (p=0.0095)

Ennis et al. Preoperative serum PSA + Gleason Grade as Predictors of Pathologic Stage in Clinically Organ Confined Prostate Cancer: Implications for the Choice of Primary Treatment. Int J Radiation Oncology Biol Phys, 1994	
Treatment modality	RP; XRT; pelvic lymphadectomy
Site	Yale New Haven Hospital; New Haven, CT
Study design	Retrospective study to determine if preop PSA + Gl grade predict pathologic stage among patients with clinically organ confined prostate cancer.
Sample Size	63
Accrual dates	1990 - 1991
Patient stage	2 stage A; 10 stage B (T2); 37 stage B1 (T2a); 13 stage B2 (T2a-c); 1 stage C.
Other Patient characteristics	Provided
Method of Survival Analysis	Summay of literature on rate of pathologic upstaging vs PSA and vs histologic grade .
Statistical Estimates Related to Survival Analyses	Table shows relation between clin stage + path stage. TABLE 3 shows incidence of pathologic features vs PSA. Table also shows incidence of pathologic features vs PSA for intermediate grade (Gl 5-7) tumors. Study finds preop serum PSA highly predictive of pathologic stage.
Other outcomes/Results	XRT is localized tx of choice for patients with seminal vesicle involvement + capsular margins because outcomes post RP are poor.

155

Forman et al. Definitive Radiotherapy following prostatectomy: Results and complications, Int J Rad Oncol Biol Phys, 1986

Treatment modality	XRT after prostatectomy
Site	Johns Hopkins University, Baltimore, MD
Study design	Retrospective analysis of 34 patients with localized carcinoma of the prostate who had been treated with prostatectomy (radical or simple) and postop XRT
Sample Size	34
Accrual dates	1975-1984
Patient age	age at tx=67.3; range=55-78
Duration of follow-up	median=4 years; range=1-4; 1 month posttx, quarterly for 3 years, twice yearly for 2 years, and yearly thereafter
Other Patient characteristics	Grade I-III, lymph node pos/neg/unk, 3 groups: 1 (RP with extracapsular extension, 2 (SP with extracapsular extension), 3 (palpable local recur after RP) See Table 1 (p 186)
Outcome Definitions	Survival calculated from the date of first radiation tx. Patients scored as relapsed if palpable local recurrence detected on rectal exam or metastatic dx found on physical exam or radiographic studies. Comparisons using Gehan's gen. Wilcoxan 2-sided test.
Method of Survival Analysis	Kaplan-Meier actuarial method.
Survival Curves	Actuarial survival for 3 groups out 8 years with table of patients at risk Disease-free survival for 3 groups out 8 years with table of patients at risk.
Statistical Estimates Related to Survival Analyses	5-year actuarial survival and disease-free survival for all patients were 82 and 72%, respectively. Survival significantly worse for ots irradiated for recurrence.
Incontinence	% affected overall and by group. 5 patients (15%) had urinary stress incontinence (3 of 5 incontinent prior to XRT). 2 patients (6%) had urinary outlet obstruction.
Impotence	17 ot 19 pts (89%) who had radical prostatectomy were impotent before and after XRT. 2 of 6 pts who were potent following simple prostatectomy became impotent after XRT.
Other outcomes/Results	Tx-related complications. % of total and by group who had edema, urinary incontinence, urinary obstruction, proctitis. Complication by tx modality (surg only vs XRT only).

Fowler et al., Outcomes of external-beam radiation therapy for prostate cancer: A study of Medicare beneficiaries in 3 surveillance, epidemiology, and end results areas, JCO, 1996

Treatment modality	High-energy XRT compared to RP
Site	3 SEER sites (XRT); 5% sample of Medicare (radical prostatectomy)
Study design	Sample of 799 eligible XRT patients drawn from 3 SEER regions (GA, CT, MI). 5% sample of all Medicare beneficiaries used to identify men who had undergone RP during a 3-y period plus Massachusetts sample. Survey in Appendix A.
Sample Size	621 XRT, 373 surgery
Accrual dates	Diagnosis 1989-1991 (XRT), Claim 1988-1990 (surgery)
Patient stage	Not specifically reported: "local or regional prostate CA"
Patient age	At tx: 37% 70-74 y XRT; 41% 70-74 surgery
Other Eligibility Criteria	All patients with XRT eligible except those with confirmed distant metastases
Univar/Multiv Analyses (Covariates)	"The analysis was primarily descriptive, as our goal was to estimate the prob that patients would find themselves in various outcome states, and how problemative they felt those states to be."
Outcome Definitions	Survey in this study modeled closely after the survey used for RP pts in other work. Patients were asked to describe current status with regard to sexual function, continence, and bowel function. Questions reproduced in Appendix A of article.
Incontinence	Self-report of dripping, leaking urine in past month by tx
Impotence	Self-report of sexual functioning in past month by tx
Other outcomes/Results	Self-report of bowel problems, follow-up tx, perceived CA status, worry, etc

Fowler FJ et al. Effect of Radical Prostatectomy for Prostate Cancer on Patient QOL. Results from a Medicare Survey. Urology, 1995

Treatment modality	RP
Site	National sample of Medicare patients – HCFA Claims file on 5% representative sample and Massachusetts Medicare patients.
Study design	QOL survey of national sample of Medicare patients who underwent RP (mail, phone, + in-person interviews) to assess patients responses to RP + its effects on their lives.
Sample Size	744 survey respondents + 328 MA pts = 1072 total respondents. (92% resp rate)
Accrual dates	1988 - 1990
Patient age	All >=65 47% >70 years. 29% >75 years
Duration of follow-up	2 and 4 years post surgery
Other Patient characteristics	84% married. Education: 27% less than high school, 39% some college, 20% college graduates.
Univar/Multiv Analyses (Covariates)	For analyses with variables in ordered categories, used chi sq test to assess sig of associations. For contin variable analyses, standard analyses of variance + t-tests were used to assess associations + significance of diffs between groups
Outcome Definitions	1)extent to which sexual + urinary dysfunction were "problems" 2)QOL=mental health index (MHI5) and general health index (GHI) 3)patient satisfaction reports - feelings about results and if patients would select tx option again
Incontinence	Incontinence had more sig effect on patients than impotence. Incontinence had sig adverse effects on QOL measures + self reported satisfac. Table shows post-surg continence status.
Impotence	Table shows ratings of concern about sexual functioning by reported sexual function. Table shows results of surgery + if would choose again as compared to sexual + urinary functioning.
Other outcomes/Results	Table shows general QOL data (including incontinence+impotence). High post surgical QOL measurements, high satisfaction with results (81%). 89% would choose RP again. Table shows opinions about surg results + pt choice, Generally very postive. Only sig demog variable was educ: higher education = more positive about surgery

Gee WF et al. Practice Patterns in the Diagnosis and Management of Prostate Cancer in the US. J Urol, 1995

Site	AUA - Health Policy Survey and Research Committee
Study design	AUA sponsored Gallop org to administer survey of urologists' practice patterns used in the staging and treatment of prostate cancer . 1994 survey also asked about dx and management of PC.
Sample Size	514
Patient stage	Table shows diagnostic tests routinely ordered in staging a newly diagnosed PC patient (PSA <10)
Other outcomes/Results	95% respondents recommended RP for men < 70 years with confirmed clinically localized prostate cancer. Tables show recommended pt tx and management by age.

Gomez CA et al. Bladder neck preservation and its impact on positive surgical margins during RP. Urology, 1993

Treatment modality	RP (8 of which were ns)
Site	Univ of Miami School of Med, Miami, FL
Study design	Study assessing the efficacy of modified bladder neck dissection during RP in effort to improve continence + diminishi anastomotic stricture without compromising CA removal
Sample Size	50
Accrual dates	1991 - 1992
Patient stage	Standard preop staging .
Patient age	mean= 66 years (Range= 54-76)
Duration of follow-up	minimum 6 month follow-up
Survival Curves	Figures show relationships between margin status and mean GI score, serum PSA, and mean tumor volume.
Statistical Estimates Related to Survival Analyses	There was a tumor at inked margin in 18 patients (36%), but only in 3 cases (6%) was tumor at bladder neck margin. Bladder neck was never the only positive margin.
Incontinence	Good continence rate can be achieved. All patients fully continent during routine activities at 6 month follow-up
Other outcomes/Results	Technique can be performed without compromising surgical margins. GI score >=7 and serum PSA > 10 are correlated with a greater chance of tumor at inked margin.

Goodnough LT et al. Acute Preoperative Hemodilution in Patients Undergoing RP: A case study analysis. Anesth Analg, 1994

Study design	Not applicable - case study analysis of efficacy. Retrospective case study analysis of preop hemodilution technique in large surgery program to estimate degree of efficacy as practiced routinely + to better define role as blood conservation strategy
Sample Size	16
Accrual dates	3 years
Patient age	mean= 60 years. Range= 50-75
Duration of follow-up	
Other Patient characteristics	Clinical characteristics of patients undergoing acute preop hemodilution
Outcome Definitions	efficacy of technique and blood conservation
Other outcomes/Results	Preoperative hemodilution as a single blood conservation intervention, contributes onl modestly to blood conservation.

Gould DL + Borer J. Applies stapling technique in radical retropublic prostatectomy: efficient, effective, + efficacious. J Urol, 1996

Treatment modality	RP
Study design	observational study analyzing applicability + efficacy of endovascular GIA stapler to effect ligation and division of dorsal vein complex and lateral prostatic pedicles in Group 1 vs using stapler only for lateral prostatic pedicles or not at all in Group 2
Sample Size	Group 1 = 21. Group 2 = 7
Duration of follow-up	Surgery done within 9 months of writing results
Outcome Definitions	Ease/efficacy
Statistical Estimates Related to Survival Analyses	30% had positive surgical margins
Incontinence	17 achieved urinary continence (at time article was written)
Impotence	6 patients potent (at time article was written)
Other outcomes/Results	Mean operating time = 2 hours, a decrease of 40 minutes Mean blood loss= 400cc - a decrease from the norm. Signs of improved anastomosis. Technique makes procedure easier + more approachable for less experienced surgeons.

Harlan et al. Geographic, age, and racial variation in the treatment of local/regional carcinoma of the prostate. J of Clinical Oncology, 1995	
Treatment modality	RP; XRT; WW
Study design	series/observational study that examines variation in use of RP and XRT by geographic area, age , + race. Used NCI's SEER database data for analysis.
Sample Size	67,693 (53,024 with local disease 14,669 with regional disease)
Accrual dates	1984 - 1991
Patient stage	Provided
Patient age	>=50 years.
Other Patient characteristics	Tables outline distribution of patients by stage and race, and by region respectively
Univar/Multiv Analyses (Covariates)	"chi square test of association used to calculate p values. P values used to calculate differences in tx between years or races by creating contingency tables of tx by year or race." Used Cochran-Mantel-Haenszel test for diffs in age- adjusted tx.
Outcome Definitions	Outcome studied was tx choice. Clear trend towards "more aggressive" tx (surgery).
Other outcomes/Results	Among men with localized disease, proportion >=50 receiving RP during 1984-1991 increased from 11% to32.3%. Figure 1. Tx choice varied by geographic region. Choice of XRT was more uniform across region. Increase in RP not linked to age. Proportion of blacks with RP was lower lower than whites. Rates increased for but had lower age-adjusted rates than whites for all years of study. WW as tx option seen more in blacks than whites in all ages and all years.

Hrebinko RL and O'Donnell WF. Urologists at Work: Control of the deep dorsal venous complex in radical retropublic prostatectomy. J Urol, 1993	
Treatment modality	RP
Site	Univ of Pittsburgh; Pittsburgh, PA
Study design	study describes technique/method to control deep dorsal venous complex + then evaluates patients with technique for decrease in blood loss, OR time, complications, postop hospitalization, + transfusion requrement.
Sample Size	28
Accrual dates	1991 - 1992
Patient age	Mean= 68.7 years
Duration of follow-up	3 months post surgery
Univar/Multiv Analyses (Covariates)	Wilcoxon 2 sample rank sum test
Incontinence	2 of 28 patients reported urinary incontinence (full or minimal stress incont [1pad/day]) 3 months a/f removal of Foley catheter.1 was incontinent pre-surgery; 1 gained control more slowly.
Impotence	Not solicited
Other outcomes/Results	Mean blood loss= 982ml which is a significant decrease. No significant postoperative bleeding. Could be due to increase experience with RP. Not just technique.

Huland et al. Systematic biopsies and DRE to identify the nerve sparing side for radical prostatectomy without risk of positive margin in patients with clinical stage T2, no prostatic carcinoma. Urology, 1994	
Treatment modality	ns RP
Site	Univ Clinic Eppendorf; Hamburg, GERMANY
Study design	"series/observational study of patients to see whether DRE or use of 6 systematic biopsies could identify side where nerve sparing could be used without risk of positive margin"
Sample Size	73
Patient stage	clinical stage T2a-c
Patient age	mean= 63.1 years (Range= 45-72)
Other outcomes/Results	"unilateral contralateral ns can be done safely in patients with t2a + t2b lesions without risk of positive margins when 3 biopsies on contralateral side are negative."

Isaacs JT. Commentary: Molecular markers for prostate cancer metastasis. Developing diagnostic methods for predicting the aggressiveness of prostate cancer. Am J of Pathology, 1997

Site	Johns Hopkins University; Baltimore, MD
Study design	commentary reviewing series of proteins that may be useful in predicting the clinical aggressiveness of newly diagnosed prostate cancer.

Jonler et al. Sequelae of radical prostatectomy. Br J Urol, 1994

Treatment modality	nsRP; adjuvant tx (16% of patients had adjuv ther post surgery)
Site	Division of Urology; University of Wisconsin Hospital + Clinics; Madison, WI
Study design	series/observational study of patients tx with surgery > 1 year prev, to evaluate the sequelae of RP using a survey validated instrument (Fowler). Also used 2 non-validated questions to assess effects of post-surgical radiotherapy.
Sample Size	93 sent questnr. 86 compl + respd. 92% response rate.
Accrual dates	1990 - 1992
Patient stage	T1-2. 51% organ confined (T2). 3% positive nodes (N1). Table provides staging + PSA at time of surgery
Patient age	At time of surgery:mean= 64 years. Range= 49-75 At time of follow-up: mean= 66years
Duration of follow-up	12-48 months (mean= 22.5 months)
Other Patient characteristics	Patient demographics provided
Univar/Multiv Analyses (Covariates)	Fisher's exact test (2 tail) and significance level of 0.05 used for stat analysis
Outcome Definitions	Satisfaction with tx and tx choice, as well as standard QOL (incont/impot) measures
Statistical Estimates Related to Survival Analyses	16% (14 of 86) patients had adjuvant tx (RT and/or orchidectomy) after RP. OF those patients, 31% (4 of 13) had tx >1 year. post surgery for suspected or proven local recurrence.
Incontinence	47% used pad + 59% leaked urine daily. 30% > few drops/day. 34% found incontinence bothersome. Pts receiving adjuvant XRT reported unchanged continence
Impotence	84% reported potency pre-surgery. Post surg 9% full potency and 38% partial. 51% reported substantial prob with reduced or absent potency. Pts receiving adjuvant XRT reported unchanged potency
Other outcomes/Results	Survey showed adverse sequelae of RP to be high, yet patients generally satisfied with tx decision. In all, 24% reported some persisting degree of "physical unpleasantness" which they believe was secondary to the PC or effects of its tx. But, 74% were satisfied with surg +88% said would undergo it again.

Kaplan and Bagshaw. Serum prostate-specific antigen after post-prostatectomy radiotherapy. Urology, 1992.

Treatment modality	XRT after RP
Site	Stanford University Hospital, Stanford, CA
Study design	Reporting on the 39 post-prostatectomy patients who were later treated with XRT
Sample Size	39
Accrual dates	1985 - 1991
Patient age	mean at time of XRT=65; range=46-78
Duration of follow-up	Time between surgery and XRT range=6 weeks-7 years. In 20 patients XRT begun within 6 monthss, in 19 XRT after >6months. Exams every 3-4 months after XRT
Other Patient characteristics	Define 3 risk groups based on PSA level and changes in PSA
Other Eligibility Criteria	Table provides # of patients who had detectable or undetectable PSA, neg DRE, local tumor recurrence, pos margins, pos seminal vesicles, pos nodes, and Gleason. Table describes dose to pelvis and prostatic fossa.
Outcome Definitions	"Outcomes" ltd to changes in PSA level over time. Table IV reviews the incidence of surgical upstaging in the literature. Table V reviews the results of post-radical prostatectomy radiotherapy , including % local tumor control and DFS (year varies).
Other outcomes/Results	PSA trend after post-prostatectomy XRT for low risk, 3 indeterminate risk patients, 4 high-risk patients

Keisch ME et al. Preliminary Report of 10 patients treated with radiotherapy after radical prostatectomy for isolated elevation of serum PSA levels. Int J Rad Oncol Biol Phys, 1990

Treatment modality	RP and (post-surg) XRT
Site	Mallinckrodt Institute of Radiology; Washington Univ Medical Center; St. Louis, MO
Study design	series/ observational study of patients treated with RT 3 - 43 months post RP
Sample Size	10
Accrual dates	1987 - 1990
Patient stage	Post-surg/ Pre RT: 8 had stage C; 5 had >=1 pos margins; 10 had neg staging lymphadenectomy
Patient age	mean= 63.5 years Range= 45-72
Duration of follow-up	3 to 43 months
Statistical Estimates Related to Survival Analyses	Post irradiation, 8 patients had decreases in isolated PSA levels (indicative of response to local disease). Data suggest post-RP PSA levels useful in detecting subclinical local recurrence or persistence.

Kerr LA and Zincke H. Radical retropubic prostatectomy for prostate cancer in the elderly and the young: complications and prognosis. Eur Urol, 1994

Treatment modality	RP
Site	Mayo Clinic, Rochester, MN
Study design	Review of Mayo's experience with young and elderly patients who have undergone bilateral pelvic lymphadectomy and RP for PC. 2 cohorts - "young" and "older"
Sample Size	242
Accrual dates	1966 - 1988
Patient stage	Stage pT1-pT3; NO-N2. Grade 1-4.
Patient age	191 patients= <= 55 years "young" 51 patients >= 75 years "older"
Duration of follow-up	5 (older's only follow-up), 10 + 15 years.
Univar/Multiv Analyses (Covariates)	Karnofsky scores show strong correlation admission performance status and survival in the elderly.
Survival Curves	Disease free survival + overall survival evaluated at 5 (older), 10, + 15 years
Statistical Estimates Related to Survival Analyses	Elderly had >path stage. 71% elderly vs 45% younger had state >pt3, p<0.001; And higher grade lesions - 4% elderly vs 21%, p<0.001. No elderly patients died within 1st 5 yrs post-surgery. Correlate pt age to disease control, tumor stage, complications, + survival.
Incontinence	Significant urinary incontinence (>=3 pads/day) occurred in 16% of elderly compared with 3% of younger patients. (p=0.001) at 1 year. Found Increased risk in elderly independent of stage.
Other outcomes/Results	Table shows various complications experienced 1 month after RP.

Klein EA. Modified apical dissection for early continence after radical prostatectomy. The Prostate, 1993.

Treatment modality	ns RP
Site	Cleveland Clinic Foundation. Cleveland, OH
Study design	Prospective evaluation of urinary continence in (83) consecutive patints undergoing RP using modified apical urethral dissection technique. Patients kept daily continence diary of # times voided, # pads, and subjective scale of incontinence
Sample Size	83
Patient stage	Localized
Patient age	mean= 64. Range= 42-77.
Duration of follow-up	mean = 17 months Follow-up range= 4 to 31 months
Univar/Multiv Analyses (Covariates)	statistical analysis= Fisher's exact test. Wilcoxon rank sum test. Least squares linear regression analysis.
Outcome Definitions	complete continence= urinary control without need for protective pads. Stress incontinence= urinary leakage with any activity that results in increased intra-abdominal pressure. Total continence= absence of urinary control while upright.
Incontinence	Total cont in 88%. (17% week 1, 53% week 6, 81% 3 months, rest 4 months); stress incont in 11%; total incont in 1%. Median time to continence= 5 weeks post surgery (range, 1-16 wks). Median age of continent pts sig lower than incont pts. Patient age was only predictor of continence

Klein EA et al. Maintaining quality of care and patient satisfaction with radical prostatectomy in the era of cost-containment. Urology, 1996.

Treatment modality	RP
Study design	study to determine effect of shortened hospital stay a/f RRP on costs, adverse surgical o/c, and pt satisfaction. Assessed satisfaction with LOS, analgesic regimen, + surgical outcome in random subset of 150 patients by anonymous questionnaire - went to ppl with surg between 1/94 and 6/95. looked at effects of preop counseling, periop care, and analgesic management on LOS.
Sample Size	374
Accrual dates	1989 - 1995. Questionnaire administered to pts wtih surg between 1/94 and 6/95 only.
Patient stage	clinically localized cT1 - 2a
Patient age	mean= 60 years.
Other Patient characteristics	Provided
Univar/Multiv Analyses (Covariates)	LOS/age analyzed using 1 way ANOVA using Knuskal - Wallis test. Chi sq test for trend data. Diferences between groups analyzed by Mann-Whitney test. Cost calculations. Diffs between satisfaction response analyzed by Fisher's exact test.
Outcome Definitions	satisfaction - QOL instrument / Likert + VAS scales + 2 add global satsfac questions from prev used Medicare survey. Costs= mean cost/ case + cost/ hospital day. Adverse surgical o/c/ Patient satisfaction= 30 day complication, hospital readmission, and mortality rates
Other outcomes/Results	Decreased LOS= p<0.0001. LOS + adverse outcomes. Care was shorter, more intense. Decreased LOS resulted in 43% decrease in cost per case, but increase in mean cost per day by 22-35%. Overall patient satisfaction high = 83.5% for LOS, 89.2% for pain control post-surg. Acute complications, 30 day readmission, 30 day mortality rates remained constant.

Kupelian et al. Correlation of clinical + pathological factors with rising PSA profiles after radical prostatectomy alone for clinically localized prostate cancer. Urology, 1996.	
Treatment modality	RP (1/2 nsRP)
Site	Cleveland Clinic Foundation. Cleveland, OH
Study design	Retrospective review of charts for 337 RP cases to identify factors affecting PSA level elvation after RP (only) in patients with clinical stage T1-T2 prostate cancer.
Sample Size	337
Accrual dates	1987 - 1993
Patient stage	clinically localized T1-T2; GI 2-10. Table shows case distribution
Patient age	mean= 63. Range= 43-77
Duration of follow-up	5+7 years. Median follow-up= 36 months (3 years.)
Other Patient characteristics	Pts with clinical stage T3, without pre-op GI or PSA, with synchronous bladder CA who received adjuvant or neoadjuvant therapy were excluded from study.
Univar/Multiv Analyses (Covariates)	Cox multivar regr time-to-failure analysis. Pre-tx PSA most potent clin predictor of relapse. Relapse-free suirvival predicted by preop PSA, GI score, ECE, + surg margins. Analysis endpoints were: biochemical and clinical repalse-free survival and overall survival. Failure endpoint was detectable PSA levels post-surgery
Outcome Definitions	relapse= either clinically detectable recurrence or detectable/rising PSA levels. biochemical failure = rise in PSA levels.
Method of Survival Analysis	Kaplan-Meier method + log rank statistic used.
Survival Curves	3 and 5 year RFS = 74% and 61%.
Statistical Estimates Related to Survival Analyses	Correlate preop PSA to disease control. Survival rates were 96% + 94% at 5 and 7 years respectively. Figures 1a-c. 34 patients (10%) had detectable PSA immediately post-surg - 28 of whom had PSM.

Leandri et al. Radical retropubic prostatectomy - morbidity and quality of life. Experience with 620 consecutive cases. J Urol, 1992.	
Treatment modality	RP + nsRP
Site	Department of Urology; St. Jean Languedoc-Cerou; Cedex, FRANCE
Study design	series/ observational study describing investigators' experiences and complications with RRP in 620 consecutive cases.
Sample Size	620 (167 had ns)
Accrual dates	1983 - Dec
Patient stage	pre-clinical: A-C. post-clinical: A-D.
Patient age	mean= 68 range= 46-84
Duration of follow-up	6 months
Statistical Estimates Related to Survival Analyses	In 60% of patients (371) disease was upstaged. Total of 93 patients had microscopic involv w/PLN. Downstaging occurred in 2% of patients.
Incontinence	No patient was totally incontinent. 90% had complete control within 6 months 95% had normal continence within 1 year. The remaining 5% had stress incontinence.
Impotence	Performed nerve preserving in patients who were potent preop. Sent questionnaire to these patients + partners. 30% achieved full potency; 38% partially potent at 6 mo. At 1 year, 56% were completely potent + 15% were partially potent.
Other outcomes/Results	Mean OR time decreased from 3 hr with 1st 100 pts to 1.5 hour in last 220 pts. Average blood loss decreased over time span. 6.9%(43 patients) had early complications, including 2 cases(0.3%) anastomotic urinary leakage. 1.3% had late complications. 1 death

Lerner SE. Analysis of risk factors for progression in patients with pathologically confined prostate cancers after radical retropubic prostatectomy. J Urol, 1996

Treatment modality	RP + bilateral pelvic lymphadectomy
Site	Mayo Clinic; Rochester, MN
Study design	series/ observational study attempting to identify patients at greatest risk for future clinical failure despite favorable pathological outcome.
Sample Size	904
Accrual dates	1987 - Dec
Patient stage	pT1, T2a-c. Table shows clinical + pathological variables of patients.
Patient age	mean= 66 years (Range= 33-80)
Duration of follow-up	quarterly for 1st year; biannual for 2nd year.; annually thereafter to 5 years.
Other Eligibility Criteria	no patients received adjuvant therapy
Univar/Multiv Analyses (Covariates)	multivar analysis of PSA, clin stage, path grade + stage, + DNA ploidy to determine rel value in predicting tx failure. Cox proportional hazards model for multivar analysis. Use prognostic scoring system fr regr coeffs from cox multivar model to classify patients further accord to risk of progression. Pt age, GI score, + serumPSA were initially analyzed as continuous factors in the multivar anal.
Outcome Definitions	Disease progression= elevated PSA, local recurrence, or distant metastases
Method of Survival Analysis	Kaplan Meier method. Log rank test for univariate survival comparisons.
Survival Curves	Survival estimates for a) preop PSA, b)clin stage, c)path grade, d) DNA ploidy. Figure 2 Survical estimates according to pathologic stage.
Statistical Estimates Related to Survival Analyses	Overall + CA specif survival for all at 5 years= 96 + 99.5% respectively. Disease recurred locally in 29 patients. Systematic progression seen in 15. Projected 5 year surv free of local recurrence, systematic progression + overall progression rates were 98,95,+78% respectively Preop PSA, clin stage, grade, +DNA ploidy highly significant (p<=0.001) univar predictors of progr with log rank test. Detailed discussion of survival analysis .

Lerner SE et al. Combined laproscopic pelvic lymph node dissection + modified belt radical perineal prostatectomy for localized prostate adenocarcinoma. Urology, 1994

Treatment modality	RP + laporoscopic pelvic lymphadenectomy (LPLND)
Site	Montefiore Medical Center; Albert Einstein Coll of Medicine; Bronx, NY
Study design	series/ observational "report on the practical advantage of combining LPLND with RRP. "Evaluated based on total oper time, transfusion requirements, LOS, continence, + potency.
Sample Size	49 total. 4 LPLND only; 31 LPLND + RP; 14 RP alone.
Accrual dates	1990 - 1993
Patient stage	T1abc -T3. Comparisons of clinical + pathological findings
Patient age	mean= 63 years Range= 42-74
Duration of follow-up	6 to 36 months
Univar/Multiv Analyses (Covariates)	Calculated stat analysis of blood loss, total OR time, total transfusion req, LOS, + complications. Acct'd for learning curve by dividing into early (1st 15) + late (last 16) patients. Used 2 tail student t-test to eval diffs between means.
Outcome Definitions	Continence divided into 4 categories - complete = no urinary loss/no pads; minimal stress= total night cont + occ urin loss <2pads/day; stress incont= must wear pad when performing strenous activities; total incont= no urinary control. Erectile function divided into 3 categories - potent= sex active with suff for vaginal penetration; partial potency= req drugs for sex relations; complete impotence.
Incontinence	No patient was totally incontinent. 84% completely cont. 9%min stress incont. 7% stress incontinence.
Impotence	36 patients potent preop. Of those, 27 had ns surgery. Of the 27 prev potent ns patients, 22% are potent. An additional 30% are sexually active with pharmacotherapy + 48% are not sexually active.
Other outcomes/Results	Major complications include 1 MI + 1 partial small bowel obstruction. Mean OR time for LPLND with RP=4.5 hrs. Mean LOS=6 days. 26% combination pts required transfusion

Licht MR et al. Impact of bladder neck preservation during radical prostatectomy on continence and cancer control. Urology, 1994

Treatment modality	ns RP
Site	Cleveland Clinic Foundation. Cleveland, OH
Study design	Prospective anal of clin + path findings in 206 consec patients undergoing RP with surg tech emph bladder neck + to assess the effect of bladder neck preserv + other factors on rate of post-op urinary cont + CA control post RP.
Sample Size	206
Accrual dates	1989 - 1993
Patient stage	clinical T1- T2
Patient age	mean= 63. Range= 42-77
Duration of follow-up	6 months (for continence)
Univar/Multiv Analyses (Covariates)	Fisher's exact test + Wilcoxon rank sum test. Uni + multivar logistic regr used to id factors predicting continence
Outcome Definitions	Local recurrence positive vesicourethral anastomotic biopsy finding. PSA only failure= serum PSA >0.6 ng/mL with normal findings on a vesicourethral anastomotic biopsy specimen. Also provide basic defs of cont on pg.884
Method of Survival Analysis	Kaplan-Meier method used to estimate tumor recurrence rate as a function of preserv or resection of vesicle neck. Mantel-Haenszel log rank test used
Survival Curves	Survival estimates of time to local and/or PSA only failure as function of vesicle neck reconstruction.
Statistical Estimates Related to Survival Analyses	Pathologic anal based on all 206 patients. Found pos bladder neck margin in 6-8% of surg specimens + assoc with higher grade, advanced local stage, and other pos margins in all cases. Local recurrence + PSA only failure independent of vesical neck action. Preservation of bladder neck does not compromise CA control as assessed by local or PSA-only failure rates.
Incontinence	Continence data based on 1st 171 patients. Pts kept continence diary. Complete continence in 88% (150) patients, while 11% (20) had stress incontinence, & 6% (1) were totally incontinent. Continence achieved between 1-4 wks with 36%dry at 4 wks, 54% at 6 wks, + 77% at 3 months. Median time to continence = 6 wks. Bladder neck preservation has no impact on urinary control, but may be associated with lower risk of vesical neck contracture.

Light et al. The striated urethral sphincter: muscle fibre types and distribution in the prostatic capsule. Br J Urol, 1997

Treatment modality	nsRP
Site	Baylor College of Medicine; Houston, TX
Study design	N/A. Pathologic study of 23 prostates to clarify the muscle fibre types in the striated urethral sphincter and the pattern of distribution of this muscle in the prostatic capsule.
Sample Size	23 prostates
Other outcomes/Results	Various muscle types found - ideal for functioning as a sphincter muscle.

Maggio MI et al. Endoscopically controlled placement of urethrovesicle anastomotic sutures after radical retropubic prostatectomy. J Urol, 1992

Treatment modality	RP
Site	Walter Reed Army Medical Center - Washington, DC; Uniformed Services Univ of Health Sciences, Bethesda, MD
Study design	N/A. Technical paper describing how to put sutures into urethra using illuminators from cystoscope. Study assessing the use of 21 french cystoscope in selected patients to enhance quality of urethrally placed anastomotic sutures.

Appendix A. Outcomes Literature Table: Radical Prostatectomy

Menon M + Vaidyanathan S. The University of Massachusetts technique of radical retropubic prostatectomy. Eur J of Surg Oncol, 1995

Treatment modality	nsRP
Site	University of Massachusetts Medical Centre; Worcester, MA
Study design	Article describes a "modified RRP technique" that integrates Skinner's antegrade dissection + Walsh's early control of prostatic vasculature.
Sample Size	12
Duration of follow-up	3 months follow-up
Incontinence	At 3 months follow-up, all patients are continent with 3 patients (of 12) using protective pad for minimal stress incontinence.
Impotence	2 of 12 patients have partial potency - not suff for sexual activity. No formal eval of potency done. However, most patients in this series had marginal sexual function preop.
Other outcomes/Results	Integration of technique resulted in improved exposure + minimal blood loss. New technique average blood loss= 500ml vs. standard technique average blood loss= 1100ml. Average OR time = 150 mins. Technique is easy to teach. No intraop complications.

Mettlin et al. Results of hospital cancer registry surveys by the American College of Surgeons (ACS). Outcomes of Prostate Cancer treatment by radical prostatectomy. Cancer, 1997

Study design	Due to varying data + information on tx outcomes + need for additional tx, ACS conducted surveys of CA registries + reviewed the related data to gauge outcomes of RP tx. Phase 1: in 1993, hosp CA registries + progs sent survey forms req data on up to 5 patients tx by RP at the institution in 1990. Phase 2: in 1996, add data requested on tx administered to 1990 patients up to 5 years post surg + new data requested on patients dx post-1993.
Sample Size	482 hosps sub'd data for 2122 patients in 1990 + 265 hosps data for patients in1993. Follow-up data on 1076 of the 1990 patients provided by 258 hospitals.
Accrual dates	1990 to 1996
Patient stage	Range = <50 -75+
Duration of follow-up	3 + 5 years
Other Patient characteristics	1990: 92.8% white; 5.4% African-American; 1.8% unknown 1993: 89% White; 9% African-American; 2% unknown.
Method of Survival Analysis	Kaplan-Meier method + log rank test used to determine probability of additional therapy after RP.
Survival Curves	Cumulative 5 year prob of additional tx after RP in 1990 + 1993 - overall; by age; + by patholog reports of SV involvement.
Statistical Estimates Related to Survival Analyses	5 year cumulative probability of additional tx post-RP was 10.5%. Surg mortality rates <1% for 1990+93. Surg pathology reported for 1990+93 SVI, pos surg margins, LNI, capsular pen, high GI score, + high PSA all assoc with greater prob for additional tx. See pg. 1879. Table shows tumor features+ pathological results
Incontinence	81.3% (1990) + 79.8% (1993) of patients had complete control or occasional incontinence requiring no pads. Table reports incontinence post RP.
Impotence	Post-surg 27.5%(1990) + 29.7% (1993) patients maintained sufficient erectile function for intercourse. Table 2 reported potency post RP for 1990 and 1993.
Other outcomes/Results	Surgical mortality rates: 15 patients (0.7% died within 30 days of surg in 1990 vs 5 patients (0.4%) in 1993.

Miller JI and Larson TR. Simplified Technique for Improving Exposure of the Apical Prostate During Radical Retropubic Prostatectomy. Urology, 1993

Treatment modality	nsRP
Site	Mayo Clinic Scottsdale, Scottsdale, AZ; Univ of AZ Health Sciences Center, Tucson, AZ
Study design	N/A. Article describes a technique that assists in exposure of apical prostate during RRP - a modified " bunching" maneuver.
Other outcomes/Results	With increased exposure at apex, get decrease positive margins + decrease bleeding

Nadler RB + Andriole GL. Who is best benefited by radical prostatectomy? Hematol/Oncol Clin N Amer, 1996	
Treatment modality	RP and WW with delayed endocrine management
Site	Reiew article discussing which prostate cancer patients benefit from RP. Discussion of several studies within text.

Narayan et al. The role of TRUS - guided biopsy - based staging, preoperative serum PSA, and biopsy gleason score in prediction of final pathologic diagnosis of prostate cancer. Urology, 1995	
Treatment modality	RP (+ pelvic lymphadectomy pre-RP)
Site	6 sites
Study design	retrospective study of case records for 813 patients undergoing RP for clinically localized P CA intended to evaluate the role of u/s- guided systematic + lesion directed biopsies, biopsy preop id of risk and extraprostatic extension.
Sample Size	813
Patient stage	clinical T-t3 (localized + locally advanced
Other Patient characteristics	all patients had multiple systematic biopsies
Other Eligibility Criteria	Patients receiving preop hormonal therapy were excluded
Univar/Multiv Analyses (Covariates)	Logistic regression analysis with log likelihood chi sq test to define correlation between individual, as well as combo of preop variables + path stage. Regression showed combination of biopsy-based stage, preop serum PSA, + biopsy GI provided best production of final path stage. 58% of pts had organ-confined disease. 23% had ECE with or without pos surg margins. 9% had SVI. Probability plots prov significant information on risk of extraprostatic extension of individual patients. Tables show correlation of clin stage, biopsy based stages, preop PSA, and biopsy GI (all) with final pathologic stage.
Survival Curves	Figures depict plots representing probability of pathologic stages at various combinations of preop parameters

Ness PM et al. Prostate cancer recurrence in radical surgery patients receiving autologous or homologous blood. Transfusion, 1992

Treatment modality	nsRP
Site	Johns Hopkins University; Baltimore, MD
Study design	Study evaluates the effects of blood transfusion on recurrence + survival after RP for Pr CA. At time of surgery, no differences between the groups existed.
Sample Size	309 (Group 1= 94 homo Group 2= 215 autologous or none)
Accrual dates	1982 - 1986
Patient stage	A, B, + D (mostly A+B)
Patient age	mean= 59 years
Duration of follow-up	Most between 4 to 8 years. Followed annually by phys exam and PSA. Table 1
Other Patient characteristics	baseline clinical chars
Other Eligibility Criteria	no postop transfusion if hematocrit>32%
Univar/Multiv Analyses (Covariates)	Endpoints were time to recurrence, as defined by tumor recurrence or detection of elevated PSA and survival limit, defined by death. Tested association between homologous tranfusion with categorical outcome using chi sq + compared factors on continuous scale in blood comp groups using t-test. Also used Cox prop hazards model. Table shows chi sq analysis of associations between groups. Shows no sig association between homologous transfusion + any recurrence or PSA elevation.
Outcome Definitions	Perioperative transfusion= administration of any blood component within 1 month of surgery.
Method of Survival Analysis	Kaplan Meier method. Log rank statistic
Survival Curves	Figures show estimated survival time + recurrence free interval to tumor recurrence or any recurrence. Time to recurrence curves overlapped.
Statistical Estimates Related to Survival Analyses	No significant difference between patients receiving homol + autolog blood. Cancer recurr detected in 24.5% of Group 1 patients + 22.7% of Group 2 patients. Table shows groups post surg. Patients with SVI or LN involvement are at greater risk for recurrence endpoints. Table shows hazard ratio=0.925 for survival. In univar models, hazard est=0.874 for tumor recurrence + 0.76 for overall recurr. Preop GI sig prog factor for both recurr endpts - estimates shown for clinical and biochemical recurrence.
Impotence	Preop potency marginally associated with prolonged survival; hazard ratio 0.361, p=0.091

Norberg et al. 5 year followup after radical prostatectomy for localized prostate cancer - A study of the impact of different tumor variables on progression. Scand J Urol Nephrol, 1994

Treatment modality	RP
Site	Baylor College of Med; The Methodist Hospital; Houston, TX; Univ Hospital. Uppsala, SWEDEN
Study design	Retrospective study evaluating impact of age, caps pen, total tumor volume, GI score, SVI and LN metas on disease progression. Focus on tumor parameters possible to evaluate by TRUS-guided biopsies.
Sample Size	51
Accrual dates	1983 - 1986
Patient stage	Clinically localized stage A + B. Figures show clinical staging + classification
Patient age	mean= 62 Range= 50-74
Duration of follow-up	5 years (min). Mean observation time= 73 mo.
Other Patient characteristics	Clinical characteristics shown
Univar/Multiv Analyses (Covariates)	Cox proportional hazards model used for univar + multivar. Cox model findings similar to actuarial survical analysis findings, but tumor volume was only variable with independent stat sig influence on progression. Proportional hazard anal quantitative estimate on associations. Hazard rate for recurr was >100x higher for tumors with 2-4cc vol + approximately 90x higher for tumors with >4cc compared to tumors < 2cc.
Method of Survival Analysis	Kaplan Meier method used for progression free survival calculation + log rank test tested equality of surv curves for diff prog parameters.
Survival Curves	Figures show progression free survival by tumor volume, GI, and SV.
Statistical Estimates Related to Survival Analyses	During observation period 16 patients (31%) experienced progr. Tumor volume, GI grade, + SV were stat sig predictors of tumor progression. Age, preop stage, level of capsular penetration were not stat sig. 6 patients (12%) died; PC was cause of death in 2 (4%). Average progression occurred at 38 months

O'Dowd GJ et al. Update on the appropriate staging evaluation for newly diagnosed prostate cancer. J Urol, 1997

Treatment modality	RP
Site	UroCor, Inc. UroDiagnostics Path Dept. + UroSciences; Oklahoma City, OK; Michigan Prostate Institute; Ann Arbor, MI
Study design	N/A. Meta-analysis with update on "appropriate" staging for newly diagnosed PC pts, based on review of clin staging meths + decision support tools to assess accuracy of predicting path staging results + to determine appropriate clinical staging evaluation
Sample Size	Reviewed 142 articles
Other outcomes/Results	Decision support tools based on log regression had greater accuracy than any single staging method discussed. Most accurate decision support tools for clinical staging combined DRE (stage), systematic biopsy parameters (including GI scoring) + PSA.

Oesterling JE et al. Correlation of clinical stage, serum prostatic acid phosphatase and pre-operative gleason grade with final pathological stage in 275 patients with clinically localized adenocarcinoma of the prostate. J Urol, 1987.

Treatment modality	nsRP
Site	Johns Hopkins University; Baltimore, MD
Study design	Observational study to determine predictive value of 3 preop variables - clinical stage, serum prostatic acid phosphatase (PAP), and preop GI grade.
Sample Size	275
Accrual dates	1982 - 1986
Patient stage	Correlation between clinical + final stage shown in Figure and Table
Univar/Multiv Analyses (Covariates)	Logistic regr anal with liklihood ratio chi sq test - clin stage + GI grade had direct correlation with cap pen (p<0.0001 for both) SV (p<0.0001 for both) + pos LN (p<0.0001 + p<0.0002 respectively). Also, using logistic regr, determined best predictors of final path stage to be models using combinations of preop variables, not individual variables themselves. Models = p<0.00001 for 1) cap/serum PAP/GI 2) SV/clin stage/GI and 3) LV/clin stag/GI. Probability plots based on models allow preop prediction of final path stage. Correlation between clin + final stage presented. Correlation between serum PAP + final stage presented. Correlation between preop GI and final stage presented.

Oefliein et al. Survival after radical retropubic prostatectomy of men with clinically localized high grade carcinoma of the prostate. Cancer, 1995

Treatment modality	nsRP + surg with XRT
Site	Northwestern Memorial Hospital; Northwestern Univ; Chicago, IL
Study design	Retrospective observational study to evaluate efficacy of RP for men with localized, poorly differentiated PC and to characterize prognostic sig of traditional pathologic variables. Also assess efficacy of adjuvant XRT in sub-population where pathology suggests high risk of persistent disease
Sample Size	238 (74 were clinically localized, poorly differentiated)
Accrual dates	1980 - 1990
Patient stage	Clinical T1 - t3 (Mostly T1 +T2)
Patient age	mean= 63 years. Range= 40-76
Duration of follow-up	median= 6,2 years. 136 patients for 5 yrs, 26 for 10 yrs. Patient followup every 3 months in 1st year; semi-annually or annually thereafter.
Univar/Multiv Analyses (Covariates)	Pairwise comparisons + Cox proportional regression to determine which variables were independently correlated with progression + survival. Cox model included age, path stage, GI, and adjuvant therapy as predictors. Wald chi sq test to rank sig variables.
Method of Survival Analysis	Kaplan Meier method used + log rank test to test diffs between groups
Survival Curves	PSA progression free survival estimate stratified by GI to 14 years. Clinical progression-free survical curve stratified by GI to 14 years. Disease-specific survival curves stratified by GI to 14 years.
Statistical Estimates Related to Survival Analyses	5 yr disease-specific survival for 52 men with GI 7=92%; for 22 men with GI>=8= 79%. 5 yr likelihood of undetectable PSA if GI 7=50%; if GI>=8=38%. GI score was most powerful path predictor of disease progession + survival. Path stage associated with progression only for GI >7. Adjuvant XRT sig reduced risk of PSA progression (rel risk= 0.56), but XRT had no sig impact on disease-specific survival . At least 25% (8/32) of patients receiving adjuvant XRT had local recurr after undergoing RP.

Olsson CA. Staging lymphadectomy should be an antecedent to treatment in localized prostatic carcinoma. Urology (Suppl), 1985

Treatment modality	RP
Site	College of Physicians + Surgeons of Columbia University;New York.
Study design	Observational study of their own experiences looking at appropriateness of depending on primary lesion scoring alone to predict the incidence of prostatic nodes in PC pts.
Sample Size	120
Patient stage	GI 2-10; Stage A-C
Other outcomes/Results	Found no accuracy of GI score alone in prediction of lymph node metastases. Over 20% of patients with GI 2-4 had pelvic node spread. And close to 40% high grade (GI 8-10) patients were found free of regional metastases or LN spread.

Olsson CA et al. The use of RT-PCR for PSA assay to predict potential surgical failures before radical prostatectomy: molecular staging of prostate cancer. J Urol, 1996

Treatment modality	RP
Site	Dept of Urology; Columbia University; Squier Urol Clinic; Columbia Presbyterian Hosp; New York, New York
Study design	Study evaluating RT-PCR as a tool for staging patients with PrCA undergoing RP. Also evaluated role of preop endocrine therapy.
Sample Size	138 (34 patients received preop flutamide) Results based on 94 patients.
Accrual dates	1993 - 1995
Patient stage	Clinical T1-T2; Pathological T2 – T3.
Patient age	mean= 62.5 years Range= 49-7
Univar/Multiv Analyses (Covariates)	Compared sensitivity, specificity, positive predictive value, and negative predictive value of RT-PCR with surgical path results (ECE, pos margins, SVI) as gold standard. Odds ratios (associations between test result + pathol result) calculated. Final path analysis - correlation between RT-PCR + PSA and true path stage of dis. Influence of preop endocrine tx on final path stage evaluated. RT-PCR ability to predict potential surg failures compared to imaging, DRE, preop PSA, + GI score.
Outcome Definitions	Surgical failure = patients with pos surg margin and/or disease beyond SV
Other outcomes/Results	RT-PCR for PSA was best predictor of potential surgical failures. 70% patients with pos margins or SVI were identified preop by pos RT-PCR assay. RT-PCR able to identify patients preop with adverse pathol, despite low serum PSA values (<4.0 ng/ml). For patients with high PSA (>10ng/ml). RT-PCR discriminated between potentially curable patients + patients with extraprostatic disease. Conclusion: RT-PCR adds prognostic information for patients considering RP.

Partin et al. Evaluation of serum PSA velocity after radical prostatectomy to distinguish local recurrence from distant metastases. Urology, 1994	
Treatment modality	RP
Site	Johns Hopkins University; Baltimore, MD
Study design	Series/ observational study of preop data on rate of change of serum PSA levels as predictor of local vs distant disease recurrence following RP. Follow up consisted of PSA level and DRE.
Sample Size	1058
Accrual dates	1982 - 1991
Patient stage	T1-T3
Duration of follow-up	3,6,12 month 1st year; annually thereafter 542 patients for > 4 years 78 patients for >8 years.
Other Patient characteristics	Demographics, clin + path information shown. 51 patients with isolated PSA elevations followed expectantly until diagnosis of distant or local metastases.
Other Eligibility Criteria	Patients with stage 4 excluded
Univar/Multiv Analyses (Covariates)	Linear mixed effects regr anal used to model this data. Time to serum PSA of 0.5ng/mL, PSA level 1 year postsurg, path stage, Gl sum, + rate of change/PSAV tested as predictors of local vs distant metastases. Combo PSAV, path stage, + Gl best distinguished local from distant metas. Residual chi sq compared stat sig of uni + multi var combos of predictive factors. Also, chi sq goodness of fit stats show how well model fits the data. Figure 4 shows mixed effects regr estimate. Figures show likelihood of isolated postop elevated PSA rep local recurrence by logistic regression of serum PSA level and PSA velocity.
Outcome Definitions	Local recurr = either palpable induration at site of surg associated with elevated PSA + biopsy, chest xray, pelvic CT + bone scan or, >2 year follow-up with undetectable PSA post-RT to prostatic bed. Distant recurrence = evidence of metastases by bone scan with or without concurrent local recurrence
Method of Survival Analysis	Kaplan Meier method
Survival Curves	Progression free likelihood for overall prog, PSA delectability, + local and distant progression estimates for 10 yrs. 10 yr actuarial rates.
Statistical Estimates Related to Survival Analyses	10 yr actuarial recurr rate of 4% for loc recurr, 8% for distant metas; + 23% for isolated elev of serum PSA level only. Overall, 19% men have recurr post-surg. Overall actuarial 5+10 year progr free likelihood for any progr of 83% + 80%; PSA elevation 13% +23%; local recurr 3%+4%; and distant metas with or without local recurr 5%+ 8%. PSA recurrence. Longitudinal PSA data. Probability of local recurrence.

Paulson et al. Is grade or stage of primary importance in determining the outcome after radical prostatectomy for disease clinically confined to the prostate? Br J Urol, 1989.

Treatment modality	RP
Study design	Study assessing importance of grade or stage in determining post-surg outcome
Sample Size	145
Accrual dates	1973 - 1982
Patient stage	T1-T2, NOMO
Duration of follow-up	3 month intervals 1st year; 6 months intervals thereafter. Median follow-up= 4.98 years. Follow-up included: physical exam, acid phosph, occasional chest + full pelvic xrays.
Univar/Multiv Analyses (Covariates)	Univar anal of GI sum + distribution of disease. Multivar anal of GI sum after controlling for anatomical distribution of disease. Univar anal of failure as funct of GI sum p = 0.002 while univar anal of failure as function of disease not confined to prostate p = 0.014 Multivar anal p val= 0.0038 when GI adjusted for anatomical distribution but p = 0.033 when anatomical distrib of dis adj for GI sum. Shows GI sum better indicator of failure or recurr than anatomical distribution of disease
Outcome Definitions	Failure of tx indicated by elev acid phosphatase, biopsy with proven local disease or distant nodal disease, or by parenchymal or nodal disease by imaging modality.
Method of Survival Analysis	Kaplan Meier method to compare NED survival rates using time to first evidence of failure.
Survival Curves	Figures show survical + disease-free survical of pts at risk to 10 yrs. Figures show survival + disease-free survival stratified by organ confinement. Figure + Table show probability of relapse as function of SVI. Figure shows little difference between specimen confined and positive margin groups in pts with non organ-confined tumors.
Statistical Estimates Related to Survival Analyses	Overall survival for all pts was 95%, 93%, + 92% at 5,7,+10 yrs. Disease-free survival for all pts was 85%,72%,+62% at 5,7,+10years. Comparison of organ confined or not: confined showed little diff in survival (95,93,+92% at 5,7,+10years), but sig diff in disease-free survival - 92%,80%,+62% at 5,7,+10 yrs. Table and Figure show frequency of GI sum distribution, pt failures, time to failure in yrs. Non-confined tumors showed higher GI segregated according to local tumor extens (p<0.001) + higher the GI sum, the greater probability of failure.
Other outcomes/Results	Outcomes of surgical intervention related to anatomical extent of disease + predictied probability of disease outside the organ of origin.

Polasik TJ and Walsh PC. Radical retropubic prostatectomy: the influence of accessory pudendal arteries on the recovery of sexual function. J Urol, 1995

Treatment modality	nsRP
Site	Johns Hopkins University; Baltimore, MD
Study design	Study evaluates technique and its outcome, specifically looking at influence of accessory pudental arteries and influence of new surgical technique designed to preserve them on recovery of sexual function post RP.
Sample Size	835 potent men had RP. Identified accessory pudendal arteries in 33.
Accrual dates	1987 - 1994
Patient age	Range= 53-65
Duration of follow-up	>= 1 year (for 22 men)
Impotence	Of 835 potent men with RP, accessory pudendal arteries identified in 33 (4%). After developing new surg technique, were able to preserve arteries in 19/24 patients (79%). Potency sufficient for sexual activity occurred in 67% (8/12) for patients with preserved arteries and in 50% (5/10) in patients with "sacrificed" arteries.
Other outcomes/Results	Presence of accessory pudendal arteries rare (4%); Their existence can be associated with excessive bleeding. Potency rates similar in both groups, so procedure may not be worthwhile.

Pontes JE et al. Prognostic factors in localized prostatic carcinoma. J Urol, 1985

Treatment modality	Non nsRP
Study design	Prospective study to assess pathological factors influencing dissemination of PC.
Sample Size	54
Patient stage	clinical A1(5); B1(9); B2(40); GI 3-10
Incontinence	Only 5% of patients had severe stress incontinence
Other outcomes/Results	Path findings in accordance in 78% of pts with clin A2+B1. However, only 3 of 40 pts with clin B2 had path stage B2 disease. Comparison of surg path staging of primary tumor is shown. Comparison of surg/path staging of primary with the final path, including pelvic LN data also shown

Pound CR et al.. PSA after anatomic radical retropubic prostatectomy. Patterns of recurrence and cancer control. Urol Clin N Amer, 1997

Treatment modality	nsRP
Site	Johns Hopkins University; Baltimore, MD
Study design	Builds on 1993 series anal to include 1623 more men. Article "describes actuarial likelihood of undetectable PSA for men with surg @ JHU. Study also examines influence of clin + path parameters on actual rate of PSA recurr post-surg."
Sample Size	1699 (95% - 1623 are incl in this anal)
Accrual dates	1982 - 1995
Patient stage	T1, T2, T3a.
Patient age	mean= 59 years range= 34-76
Duration of follow-up	PSA + DRE every 3 months for 1st year; biannually for 2nd year; annually thereafter Average follow-up 5 yrs (1-13 yr range); 12% (193 patients) followed 10 yrs post-op.
Other Eligibility Criteria	Patients with inadequate postop PSA data, pre or immed post op adjuv XRT; pre or immed post op adjuv hormonal ther; or clin stage D0/D2 were excluded from analysis.
Univar/Multiv Analyses (Covariates)	Best path predictor of dis progression obtained using multivar model combining postop GI score, surg margin status, and presence or absence of and extent of capsular penetration.
Method of Survival Analysis	Kaplan-Meier method
Survival Curves	Provided
Statistical Estimates Related to Survival Analyses	Anatomic RP with preservation of neurovascular bundles had no effect on CA control. GI score of at least 8 or SVI is indicative of eventual failure from distant mets. In addition, timing of development of detectable serum PSA also is important in predicting local vs distant failure. 17% show recurrence after RP. Overall actuarial progression-free rate at 10 yrs was 68%. Actuarial rates at 10 yrs were 18% for development of isolated PSA recurrence; 8% for local recurrence; 9% for dist recurrence. No patient with T1a disease had detectectable post op PSA. Patients with T1c had 86% progession-free disease at 5 ys. Table shows comparison of GI, path stage, + timing of PSA recurrence by site. Overall actuarial cause-specific survival rates at 5 & 10 yrs were 99% & 93%, respectively. Table shows 5 & +10 year actuarial metastasis-free rates based on GI score + path stage.
Impotence	Preservation of potency did not influence CA control. Compared actuarial recurrence-free probabilities according to path stage + margin status between post-op potent + impotent patients. Found no diff in actuarial PSA recurrence rates after RP. Also found no diff in same rates for potent + impotent patients grouped by low or high grade (GI) disease.

Quinlan DM et al. Sexual function following radical prostatectomy: Influence of preservation of neurovascular bundles. J Urol, 1991

Treatment modality	nsRP
Site	Johns Hopkins University; Baltimore, MD
Study design	Series/ observational study analyzing the influence of preservation or excision of the neurovascular bundles on return of sexual function.
Sample Size	503 potent preop
Accrual dates	1982 - 1988
Patient stage	Table shows clin stage + operative technique. Majority were stage A1-2, B1-2, B1N
Patient age	mean= 59 years. Range= 34-72
Duration of follow-up	mean= 46 month follow-up range= 18 months to 8 years.
Statistical Estimates Related to Survival Analyses	Disease free survival - correlate potency sparing to risk of positive margin
Impotence	3 factors correlated with return of potency: patient age, surgical technique - ability to save nerves, and tumor stage. Of 503 preop potent patients, 68% (342) were potent postop. Preservation of 1 or both neurovasc bundles: preservation of both fared better. When adjusted for age, risk of postop impotence increased alot, if had capsular penetration ot SVI, or if 1 neurovasc bundle was removed.

Sall et al. Pelvic pain following radical retropubic prostatectomy: A prospective study. Urology, 1997.

Treatment modality	nsRP
Study design	Consec RP patients completed preop + postop (at 1,3,+ 6 mos) questionnaires on pain,QOL,+ incont. Prospective study to evaluate subacute +chronic pelvic pain by determining frequency, duration,+ severity of pain after RP for localized PC. Patients also wore pads for 24 hrs to measure urine loss before and after surgery. Also did retrospective chart review for other clin + path measures.
Patient age	mean= 61years. range= 51-73
Duration of follow-up	1,3, 6 month follow-up
Univar/Multiv Analyses (Covariates)	Fisher's exact test between ordered categories. Stnd ANOVA with student t test of continuos variables. Mann-Whitney rank sum test.
Outcome Definitions	Pain measurement using Wisconsin Brief Pain Inventory.
Incontinence	Strong relation between CA pain + incontinence at 1 month followup. Level of 496 ml/24hr in postop pain group compared with 90ml/24 hr in no pain group. Difference became insignificant at 3 months and 6 months.
Other outcomes/Results	3 patients had preop pain. 13(57%), 7(33%)+5(21%) had postop pelvic at 1,3, 6 months, respectively. Strong relation between pain + CA worry. Subacute postop pain that dissipates over time is common. Severe chronic pain is not. Effects of pain on QOL and physical functioning over time are shown. Greatest and fastest improvement seen in normal work + general activity. Emotional factors slower to improve.

Sanders H and Graham SD, Jr. Comparison of four automated prostate-specific antigen assays for detection of recurrence after radical prostatectomy. Urology, 1997

Treatment modality	RP
Study design	Observational study comparing 4 PSA assays - Abbott Imx, Tosoh, Chiron ACS PSA, + Chiron ACS PSA2 - on ability to detect PSA after RP. Collect serum samples from all postop RP patients attending urol clinic in March 1995.
Sample Size	22
Univar/Multiv Analyses (Covariates)	Linear regression to compare results of each assay. Table shows each assay's characteristics.
Other outcomes/Results	22 patients with undetectable PSA by Imx. PSA over RCDL of Tosoh in 5; over the ACS PSA in 15; + over the ACS PSA2 in 2 patients. Clearly diff in PSA assays + ability to detect low level PSA post RP. ACS PSA most sensitive; Imx least sensitive.

Appendix A. Outcomes Literature Table: Radical Prostatectomy

Schellhammer PF. Radical prostatectomy. Patterns of local failure and survival in 67 patients. Urology, 1998	
Treatment modality	Non nsRP; adjuvant hormone therapy
Site	Eastern Virginia Medical School; Norfolk, VA
Study design	Observational study assesses the results (local failure + survival) of RP without adjuvant hormone therapy for 67 patients. (22% of total patients at this institution presenting with localized PC between 1960 and 1974)
Sample Size	67 tx between 1960 - 1974 (7 lost to follow-up + 13 died on non PrCA causes) + 6 patients tx between 1975 and 1980.
Accrual dates	1960 - 1974 (began using more XRT for a while in 1975)
Patient stage	Tables outline clin and path staging
Duration of follow-up	15 years for 67. At least 5 years for 6.
Outcome Definitions	Local failure= biopsy documented recurr at vesicourethral anastomosis or prostatic bed. Distant failure= pos bone films or bone scan.
Method of Survival Analysis	Description of disease-free survival + overall survival calculations presented
Survival Curves	Figures show clin + path disease-free survival (5,10+15 yrs); time after tx to failure for 14 years. 5,10,+15 yr disease-free survival of evaluable patients by clin+path stage shown. 15 yr disease-free survival by stage+grade. Crude 15 yr survival among traced patients post RP for B1disease + path B disease. Tables show local failure by stage, local failure for stage B specifically, + failure related to pathologic extent.
Statistical Estimates Related to Survival Analyses	All statistics based on 15 yr follow-up: Crude or direct disease-free survival for patients with clin B1 nodules + B2 lesions followed for at least 15 yrs is 36% & 25%. Crude disease-free survival for path B & C is 31% & 8%. Local failure at 15 yrs for path stage B & C tumors is 17% & 31%, respectively. SVI associated with 44% local failure & 66% distant failure. Interval between RP + 1st failure averaged 69 months. And with hormone tx, interval between 1st failure + death averaged 70 months.

Schmidt JD et al. Trends in patterns of care for prostatic cancer, 1974-1983. Results of surveys by the American College of Surgeons. J Urol, 1986	
Treatment modality	RP; XRT; brachytherapy; hormone therapy
Site	Multi-institution survey of hospitals + tumor registries. Sponsored by American College of Surgeons.
Study design	Goal to compare patterns of diagnosis and tx of pts with PC in 1983 with patterns of care observed in a 1974 study. Article presents comparison andtrends in tx during this 10 year span.
Accrual dates	1983 - 1984
Other Patient characteristics	Study includes African-American + White patients.
Survival Curves	Provided
Statistical Estimates Related to Survival Analyses	5 year overall survival appeared to be improving for all stages for both racial groups. Survival of A-A patients, however, continues to lag, presumably due to later diagnosis and more advanced stage of disease at diagnosis.

175

Shir et al. Intraoperative blood loss during radical prostatectomy: epidural versus general anesthesia. Urology, 1995

Treatment modality	ns RP
Site	Johns Hopkins University, Baltimore, MD
Study design	randomized study to show effects of anesthetic technique on intraoperative blood loss in patients undergoing RP. 100 RP pts randomly assigned to Epidural Anesthesia (EA), Combination Epidural + General Anesthesia (EG), or General Anesthesia (GA) only.
Sample Size	100
Patient age	Mean = 63
Other Patient characteristics	demographic and anesthesia data shown
Univar/Multiv Analyses (Covariates)	3 groups compared with 1-factor ANOVA for continuous variables. Used ANOVA for repeated measures for variabless compared over time. Student-Newman-Keuls post hoc test used for analysis. Simple linear regression + 1 way ANOVA to identify univariate predictors of intraop blood loss. Multivariate regression with backward eliminationto identify important predictors of bleeding. Found correlation between intraop blood loss+ prostate weight for EA group on subanalysis. ($p=0.01$).
Other outcomes/Results	Calculated intraop blood loss by formal accounting for volume + HCT of fluid suctioned from surgical field, blood on pads + pt HCT (r=995) Mean blood loss in EA (1490 mL) sig < than mean blood loss in EG and GA groups. No difference in intraop blood loss between EG and GA. Found that GA increases bl loss.

Shrader-Bogen et al. Quality of life and treatment outcomes: Prostate carcinoma patients' perspectives after prostatectomy or radiation therapy. Cancer, 1997

Treatment modality	RP or XRT
Site	Healthsystem Minnesota, Minneapolis, MN. This institute includes a 425-bed community hospital with assoc. multispecialty clinics. It's an Amer College of Surgeons-approv Teaching Hosp CA Program that diagnosed &/or tx 1865 CA cases in 1995.
Study design	Patients from institutions' oncology registry. Data collected for this cross-sectional study by mailing patients self-administered survey with demographic items, FACT-G and PCTO-Q (Prostate Cancer Treatment Outcome Questionnaire).
Sample Size	354 sent survey > 306 returned > 274 eligible > 132 RP and 142 XRT
Accrual dates	1989-1994
Patient age	RP: mean= 66.2; SD=6.528 and XRT mean= 75.3; SD= 5.680
Duration of follow-up	Survey sent 1-5 years after diagnosis
Other Patient characteristics	Sociodemographics presented
Other Eligibility Criteria	Other eligibility: AJCC stage I or II dx, excluding capsular invasion (A or B); no tx other than RP or XRT; no other primary CA; alive; read & write in English; nurse access to charts.
Incontinence	Comparison of 7-day urinary symptoms (PCTO-Q) by tx (p values).
Impotence	Comparison of 7-day sexual function (PCTO-Q) by tx (p value).
Other outcomes/Results	Comparison of 7-d bowel symptoms (PCTO-Q) by tx (p value).

Soh et al. Has there been a recent shift in the pathological features + prognosis of patients treated with radical prostatectomy? J Urol, 1997	
Treatment modality	RP
Site	Matsunaga-Conte PC Research Cntr, Baylor College of Med, The Methodist Hospital, Houston, TX
Study design	observational study assessing changes in path stage or prognosis of patients with clinically localized PC undergoing RP between 1983-95. Analyzed diagnostic, path features and progression in PSA for 754 patients by 1 surgeon for clin stages t1 to 3NXMO by year of diagnosis.
Sample Size	3080 (2326 pts undergoing staging pelvic lymphadenectomy; 754 pts undergoing RP)
Patient stage	ct1 to t3. Path t2 to t4 + NO-N1. Tables show clinical features of patients and path features of specimens
Duration of follow-up	every 6 months for 5 years; annually thereafter
Other Patient characteristics	Table shows clinical features of patients tx with RP between 1983-95
Univar/Multiv Analyses (Covariates)	Grouped patients into 3 time periods (1983-87; 1988-91; 1992-95) to compare progression-free probabilities over time. Chi square test used to determine sig changes in proportion of patients detected with each technique, in path stage, or in prognostic category with time. Speaman's rank correlation coefficient to determine sig of trends in pt age, preop PSA, or tumor volume. Fisher's exact test to assess whether frequency of path features was sig different among the 3 periods. Non-parametric ANOVA to compare median values of tumor volume among the 3 periods.
Method of Survival Analysis	Kaplan Meier life table analysis used to calc actuarial non-progr rates for all patients + those treated in each of the 3 time periods
Statistical Estimates Related to Survival Analyses	Actuarial proability of progr after surgery was similar for pts teated from 1983-87, 1988-91, and 1992-95. In most recent group, proportion of pts with curable CA increased from 57% pre1992 to 64% since. For all ptswith mean probability of nonprogression was 85% at 2 years and 74% at 5 years. Compared actuarial probability of non-progression in pts treated in all 3 periods - no sig difference.
Other outcomes/Results	Fewer patients in recent years had advanced CA. Marked increase in number of RPs performed over time. Starting in 1990 nonpalpable CA detected by PSA increased substantially to 52% by 1995. However, no sig change in preop serum PSA, tumor volume, or path stage during study.

Stein et al. Predicting and monitoring results of therapy. Prostate specific antigen levels after RP in patients with organ confined and locally extensive prostate cancer. J Urol, 1992	
Treatment modality	RP
Site	UCLA School of Medicine, Los Angeles, CA
Sample Size	230:115 with organ confined; 82 with invasion into or through capsule; and 33 with SVI.
Accrual dates	1972 - 1989
Patient stage	t1-3 NO, MO. Preop clinical staging shown.
Patient age	mean= 64 Range= 44-80
Duration of follow-up	median= 48mo.
Other Patient characteristics	Summary based on degree of tumor shown
Other Eligibility Criteria	No pt in organ-confined group 1 received adjuvant XRT
Method of Survival Analysis	Time to clinical progression determined by cause specific Kaplan Meier analysis. Cox proportional hazard model used for group comparisons & covariate adjustment. Sig of comparison groups measd with log rank test or Cox model.
Survival Curves	Probability of dying with recurrent PC after RP to 12 years. Time to recurrence detected by clinical progression with & without consideration of PSA to 12 years. Time to clinical progression related to local tumor extension to 12 years.
Statistical Estimates Related to Survival Analyses	5 & 10 yr overall survivals for entire population were 95% & 77% respectively. Cause specific survivals were 99 & 91% respectively. For the 3 groups listed above, 10 yr cause specific survivals were 96%,90%, & 63% and 5 yr clinical disease-free survivals were 91%,79%, & 58%. When isolated detectable PSA also considered an indicator of progression, the 5 yr & 10yr disease-free survival rates were 61% & 41% respectively. RP was preferredd in pts with even minimal invasion into capsule, SVI is associated with greater clinical progression rate than in organ confined tumors. Table shows progression rate according to degree of tumor.
Incontinence	5 patients (2.2%) were severely incontinent postop, and 24 (10.5%) have stress incontinence.
Other outcomes/Results	Surgical complications shown

Tomic et al. Prognostic significance of transrectal fine-needle aspiration biopsy findings after orcheictomy for carcinoma of the prostate. Eur Urol, 1985	
Treatment modality	Medical hormone therapy and orchiectomy only
Site	Univ of Umea, SWEDEN
Study design	Series/observational study of PC cell changes after orchiectomy.
Sample Size	48
Patient stage	t1-t4 +M1. Table shows grade + stage pre- orchiec-tomy.
Patient age	mean= 74.2 range= 62-87
Duration of follow-up	6 and 12 mo.
Statistical Estimates Related to Survival Analyses	10% pts with regressively transformed CA cells and 41% pts with unmodified CA cells died of PC
Other outcomes/Results	Clinical regression at 36 mo sig more frequent in pts with regressively transformed CA cells at 6 and/or 12 months than in pts with unmodified CA cells: 73 & 32% respectively.

Vander Kooy et al. Irradiation for locally recurrent carcinoma of the prostate following radical prostatectomy. Urology, 1997.	
Treatment modality	XRT as salvage therapy for locally recurrent PC after RP
Site	Mayo Clinic, Rochester, MN
Study design	Reporting on a group of pts primarily treated with RP and pelvic LND for clinically localized PC who were subsequently managed by XRT with curative intent for an isolated prostatic fossa recurrence that was apparent by DRE, cytoscopy, or radiologic imaging.
Sample Size	35
Accrual dates	1979 - 1992
Patient stage	T1,T2,T3
Patient age	Median=64; range=47-74
Duration of follow-up	Median= 5.2 years; range=1.7-12.1
Other Patient characteristics	Preop clinical stage, path stage, Mayo tumor grade, pre-XRT PSA
Other Eligibility Criteria	Pts previously treated with hormones or with XRT in a primary or adjuvant setting or with a combined XRT-hormone tx program were excluded
Univar/Multiv Analyses (Covariates)	The association of pre-XRT PC-related characteristics with disease outcome were studied. The observed rate of relapse was obtained for each factor of interest, and univariate comparison of factors made by log-rank test.
Outcome Definitions	Outcomes include clinical relapse-free, any (clin or biochem) relapse-free, and overall survival. Tabulation of complications.
Method of Survival Analysis	Kaplan-Meier analysis. Time measured from initiation of XRT to date of event.
Survival Curves	Clin relapse-free, any relapse-free, and overall survival out 9 years. Number at risk provided for each year.
Statistical Estimates Related to Survival Analyses	8-yrr rates discussed. Disease outcome (8-yr clin relapse-free, any relapse-free, overall survival) according to pre-XRT disease-related characteristics (path stage, disease-free interval, pre-XRT PSA, tumor grade; p-value provided).
Other outcomes/Results	Briefly discusses chronic complications scored using RTOG and EORTC (e.g., bleeding of intestine/rectum (grades 1-2) that did not require intervention)

Velagapudi et al. Homologous blood transfusion in patients with prostate cancer: no effect on tumor progression or survival. Urology, 1994

Treatment modality	RP – surgery
Site	Mayo Clinic, Rochester, MN
Study design	Retrospective study to determine effect of perioperative transfusion in patients with RP recurrence. Comparing overall survival,cause-specific survival, and progression-free survival for pts with and without perioperative blood transfusion. Pts divided into 3 groups based on number of units transfused: Group 1=0 units(25%/440patients); Group2=1-2 units(42%/746patients); Group3=3+units (34%/599patients)
Sample Size	1785
Accrual dates	1966-1987
Patient stage	t1a-t13, NX; pt2c-pt3 N+; GI 2-10
Patient age	mean=63.8 range= 36-79
Duration of follow-up	mean= 7years range= 0-24.2years. 3 mo intervals for 1st 2years. Semi-annually for next 2-3 years. Annual thereafter. Pt characteristics and blood use shown in Table
Univar/Multiv Analyses (Covariates)	Chi square test used to compare the 3 blood use groups by stage + grade. ANOVA used to compare 3 groups by age.
Outcome Definitions	Periop transfusion= any blood transfused during hospitalization for the operation
Method of Survival Analysis	Kaplan Meier analysis. Survival from time of operation to endptoins of death, local, or systemic progression, & PC-specific death. Univariate comparison to determine sig of overall survival rates using log rank test. Adjusted for grade, stage, and use of hormone therapy; then used multivariate survival analysis. Cox model used to determine associations between blood use group + overall survival rate, cause-specific rate, or progression-free survival rate.
Survival Curves	Kaplan Meier survival curves from date of RP to date of death, cause-specific death, & progression-free death shown in Figures at 5, 10, and 15 yrs.
Statistical Estimates Related to Survival Analyses	Looked at correl between transfusion+ decr surv - none found. No statistically sig differences between groups for overall surv rate - 71, 75, 71% at 10 yrs (p=0.48) OR cause-specific survival rate - 89, 88, 86% at 10 yrs (p=0.36) OR progression-free survival rate - 61, 68, 68% at 10 yrs (p=0.83). Cox model found no sig association between blood use group to overall survival (p=0.45), cause-spec survival (p=0.17), or progression-free survival (p=0.34).
Other outcomes/Results	Estimated relative risk associated with blood transfusion (3+ units vs 0 units) was 1.03+0.76 to 1.38 for total mortality. 1.56+0.95 to 2.56 for cause-spec death. 1.20+0.91 to 1.57 for disease specific progression.

Wahle et al. Incidence of surgical margin involvement in various forms of radical prostatectomy. Urology, 1990.

Treatment modality	nsRP (20patients); standard RP (30patients); and Radical transperineal (14 patients)
Site	Univ of Iowa Hospitals and Clinics, Iowa City, Iowa
Study design	Retrospective review of pathol specimens of patients with RP + clinical stage A or B cancer for surgical margin involvement with CA
Sample Size	64
Accrual dates	1979 - 1992
Patient stage	clinically localized A, B1, B2. Path B, C, D1. Tables show distribution of clinical stage and path stage by surgical method.
Patient age	mean= 63 years. range= 48-73
Other outcomes/Results	78% of transperineal patients had resection margin involved vs 30% of standard RP cases and 45% of nsRP cases. Average tumor burden for transperineal group, larger than for other 2 groups. No sig difference in other characteristics for ns or standard RP. Margin rate same (p=0.28 using student t test). nsRP does not compromise surgical outcome compared to standard RRP. Tables showing tumor burden, positive resection margins, and mean Gleason in pts with positive and negative margins, compared by surg method.

Wasson et al. A structured literature review of treatment for localized prostate cancer. Arch Fam Med, 1993	
Treatment modality	RP; WW/EM; XRT; bracyther
Site	Dartmouth Medical School, Hanover, NH and several other research centers
Study design	Meta-analysis - structured literature review to define clinical course of localized PC, effectiveness of RP and XRT, + teratment complications. Primary goal to estimate mortality, occurence of distant metastases, and short term risks of surgery and XRT.
Sample Size	144 English Medline articles
Accrual dates	1966 - 1991
Patient age	mean range= 64-67
Other Patient characteristics	Patient characteristics and treatment outcomes shown.
Univar/Multiv Analyses (Covariates)	Snedecor + Cochran's method for range + Confidence Intervals for median correlations examined using Spearman's rank correlation coefficient. Statistical comparisons using Wilcoxon's rank sum test.
Statistical Estimates Related to Survival Analyses	Median annual risk for development of distant metastases = 2.6% and CA-related death = 1.0%. Controlling for grade, compared effectiveness of treatment tx. For overall survival, age was most sig (p=0.003). For annual metastatic rates and CA-related mortality, proportion of poorly differentiated CA was most sig in 27 (p=0.005) and 38 pts (p=0.004), respectively.
Incontinence	Table reports incidence and adverse outcomes of XRT + RP for articles between 1982 and 1991. RP had higher rates of urinary complications
Impotence	Brachytherapy may cause fewer cases of impotence, but is worse than XRT in all other ways. Very high rate of impotence after standard surgery. As few as 1/3 with nsRP suffered impotence. Sexual functioning effected by extent and grade of tumor.
Other outcomes/Results	Type of treatment correlated to disease control/ complication

Winter et al. Preoperative PSA in predicting pathologic stage and grade after radical prostatectomy. Urology, 1991	
Treatment modality	RP
Site	Memorial Sloan Kettering CA Center, New York
Study design	Retrospective chart review study of preoperative PSA and serum prostatic acid phosphatase (PAP) and their predictive value in patients undergoing RP.
Sample Size	63
Accrual dates	1987 – 1989
Patient stage	Clinically localized and advanced. pT1-T3. Figures summarize PSA values for each patient distributed according to path stage and grade.
Patient age	mean= 63 years. Range= 52-75
Other Eligibility Criteria	Pts receiving preop XRT or hormonal therapy were excluded. Also, pts with elevated preop PAP designated as stage D0 were excluded.
Other outcomes/Results	Path stage and grade were correlated to PSA values. Pts with organ-confined (p1+p2) and extracapsular (p3,p3N+) PC had elevated preoperative PSA levels (>4ng/mL) in 61+ 90% of cases, respectively. Pts with low grade high grade histology had elevated preop PSA levels in 62 and 80% of cases, respectively. No sig differences in preoperative PSA values with path stage and/or grade considered as a group or in determining stage and/or grade preoperatively on an individual basis. Median values and ranges of PSA by path stage shown in Table. No sig differences between PSA values between stage p2+p3 and no sig diffreences in PSA values between low and high grade tumor. Table shows preoperative PSA values in organ-confined CA. Table shows PSA preoperative staging differences between organ-confined and extracapsular CA.

Appendix A. Outcomes Literature Table: Radical Prostatectomy

Witherspoon LR. Early detection of cancer relapse after prostatectomy using very sensitive prostate-specific antigen measurements. Br J Urol, 1997	
Treatment modality	RP
Site	Ochsner Clinic, New Orleans, LA
Study design	Half review article. Half retrospective study of PSA levels in pts after RP (using frozen stored sera) comparing new ultrasensitive test (ImmuLITE 3rd Generation PSA Assay) with standard PSA tests. Study population divided into 3 Groups – outlined in article
Sample Size	127
Duration of follow-up	mean= 45 mo.
Other Patient characteristics	Group1= post surgical baseline PSA <0.01 ng/mL that did not change. Group2=PSA levels that clearly increased with time and were >0.01 by 30 mo. Group3= slowly increasing PSA levels - longer than Group 2.
Other outcomes/Results	All early (within 4 yrs of RP) clinical recurrences were in Group2. 1/3 of these were treated with XRT or hormonal therapy. Improved clinical detection provided clinically useful information not previously available. Correctly identified postoperatively 2/3 of pts not cured and destined for rising PSA by 2 years post surgery. Also, correctly identified pts at minimal or no risk for early recurrence. New test provides way to accurately assess risk of recurrence earlier than ever before.

Zagars et al. The source of pretreatment serum PSA in clinically localized prostate cancer - T,N, or M? Int J Rad Oncol Biol Phys, 1995.	
Treatment modality	Definitive XRT or RP (only XRT pts are summarized in table)
Site	University of Texas, MD Anderson Cancer Center, Houston, TX
Study design	Reporting on a group of PCpts who received definitive XRT as sole initial treatment
Sample Size	427
Accrual dates	1987-1991
Patient stage	T1 to T4
Patient age	mean= median= 68 years; range=47-84 years
Duration of follow-up	mean=33 mos; median=30; range=9-73
Other Patient characteristics	Stage distribution, MD Anderson grades, Gleason grades, and nodal status provided.
Other Eligibility Criteria	Patients selected beginning in 1987. PSA recorded.
Outcome Definitions	All outcomes limited to analyses of PSA levels, pre- and post-treatment. Most results combined for RP and XRT. Best-fit regression curves & back-extrapolated PSA values in patients who developed rising PSA profile after XRT.

182

Zeitman et al. Radical Prostatectomy for adenocarcinoma of the prostate: the influence of preoperative + pathologic findings on biochemical disease-free outcome. Urology, 1994	
Treatment modality	RP (with pelvic LN dissection)
Site	Boston University Medical Center + Massachusetts General Hospital, Boston, MA
Study design	Retrospective study evaluating outcomes for a cohort of men undergoing RP alone as primary tx for clinical t1-2 (localized) PC.
Sample Size	62
Accrual dates	1987 to 1992
Patient stage	Clin: t1-t2 clin localized. Table shows pt clinical + path characteristics.
Duration of follow-up	4-6 week follow-up, then 3-6 month phys exams
Other Eligibility Criteria	Pts with adjuvant or neoadjuvant endocrine therapy were excluded from study. Also, pts pre or post treatment PSA determine by the Hybritech assay were excluded. And, patients with clin t3 disease, nodal disease, immediate adjuvant therapy (within 3 months of surgery), or with no follow-up info also were excluded.
Univar/Multiv Analyses (Covariates)	Actuarial + multivariate analysis done of disease-free outcomes according to preoperative T stage, PSA, biopsy grade, + path findings at surgery. 52% pts had path t3 tumors. Of these, 81% had poitive surgical margins. Strongest predictors of pt3 disease were biopsy grade + initial serum PSA.
Outcome Definitions	Recurrence= persistence or recurrence of detectable serum PSA >= 4 wks post surgery Disease free= no detectable PSA
Method of Survival Analysis	Kaplan-Meier product method analysis. Determine likelihood of freedom from biochem failure (disease-free status) for univariate factors at 3 yrs. Cox proportional hazard regression analysis used to analyze impact of simultaneous variables.
Survival Curves	Influence of path findings on biochem failure to 5 yrs. Influence of preoperative PSA on likelihood of biochem failure to 5 yrs. Influence preoperative biopsy grade on biochem failure to 5 yrs. Influence of path evidence of SVI on biochem failure to 5 yrs.
Statistical Estimates Related to Survival Analyses	Actuarial analysis showed overall likelihood of remaining disease free at 4 yrs was 42% (75%for organ-confined + 27% for pT3) Poorest prognosis for patients with SVI - 0% vs 62% for patients without . Biopsy grade (Gleason grade >3 vs <=3) + initial PSA were independent preoperative predictors of biochem failure (+ dis free outcome) in Cox regression analysis. Likelihood of being biochem disease free at 4years >74% for pts with initial PSA <7.5ng/mL, but only 25% for pts with valPSA >15. Good prognosis for organ-confined. Likelihood of relapse for PSM + SVI.
Other outcomes/Results	Briefly discusses chronic complications scored using RTOG and EORTC systems

Zincke et al. Radical prostatectomy for clinically localized prostate cancer: long-term results of 1,143 patients from a single institution. J of Clinical Oncology, 1994	
Treatment modality	RP
Site	Mayo Clinic, Rochester, MN
Study design	Retrospective analysis of 1143 patients undergoing RP at Mayo. Complications for the population were compared with complications of a contemporary group of 1000 consecutive patients. Study intended to examine efficacy andcomplication rate of RP for localized PC.
Sample Size	Group1= 1143. Group2= 1000
Accrual dates	Group1= 1966 - June 1987. Group2 = 1989 - 1992
Patient stage	Clin t1-t2. Path 12% t3, N+. Clinically localized. Gleason 2-10. Clinical + path staging shown for patients in Tables.
Patient age	Mean= 64 years. range= 38-79
Duration of follow-up	Mean= 9.7 yrs; Group 1 minimum of 5 yrs; Group 2 minimum of 1 year.
Other Patient characteristics	17% received adjuvant XRT or androgen -deprivation therapy with in 3 mo of surgery.
Other Eligibility Criteria	Patients receiving prior androgen deprivation therapy or XRT were excluded.
Univar/Multiv Analyses (Covariates)	Charlson index used to determine comorbidity of population. Hazard rate calculation
Outcome Definitions	Crude survival = overall survival and includes death from any cause. Cause-specific survival = survival free of death rfom PC. Metastasis-free survival = survival free of clinically diagnosed systemic metastasis.
Method of Survival Analysis	Kaplan-Meier analysis. To determ crude, cause specific, and metastasis-free survival. Groups compared with log rank test. Multivariate survival analysis performed using Cox proportional hazard model with age, clinical stage (t2a vs t1 vs t2bc vs t1), biopsy grade, + adjuvant treatment as predictors.
Survival Curves	Survival estimates for RP plus adjuvant therapy. Survival estimates for RP only. Survival estimates for RP plus adjuvant therapy for clinical stage and Gleason score. Survival estimates for RP only for clinical stage and Gleason score.
Statistical Estimates Related to Survival Analyses	Survival at 15 yrs similar to expected survival rate. Low (median 7.5 yrs) mobidity and mortality associated with RP. 10% died of PC and 15% developed metastases. 10 and 15 yr crude survival rates were 75 and 60%, respectively. Cause-specific survival rates were 90 and 83%, respectively. Metastasis-free survival rates were 83 and 77%, respectively. 10 year survival rate for pts with Gleason >=7 were 74%. Tumor grade was only sig predictor for disease outcome.
Incontinence	Incontinence declined 1.4% for more recent 1000 patients. Rate of severe urinary incontinence at 1 year decreased to 1.4%.
Other outcomes/Results	Blood transfusion rate decreased from 77% in Group1 to 22% in Group2. Incidence of pulmonary embolism decreased 5-fold to 0.6%. Hospital mortality (death with in 30 days of RP) = 0.7% in Group 1and 0% in Group 2. Rectal injury rates decreased by half to 0.6%. Length of stay decreased from median of 12 to 6 days.

Abbreviations used in Appendices

adjuv, adjuvant
ADT, androgen deprivation therapy
anal, analysis
biochem, biochemical
bx, biopsy or biopsies
CA, cancer
Calc, calculated
cap, capsular
chemo, chemotherapy
CI, confidence interval
clin, clinical
Complix, complications
CRT, conformat radiation therapy
CT, computerized tomography
Cum, cumulative
DFS, disease-free survival
diff, difference
DRE, digital rectal examination
EM, endocrine management
ECE, extra-capsular extension
elev, elevated
er, endorectal
est, estimate or estimated
evid, evidence
Gl, Gleason
HRQOL, health-related quality of life
id, identify
incl, including
incont, incontinence
KPS, Karnofsky Performance Status
loc, location
LN, lymph node
LND, lymphadenectomy
mets, metastasis or metastases
MRI, magnetic resonance imaging
multivar, multivariate
NED, no evidence of disease
neg, negative
ns, nerve-sparing
PAP, prostatic acid phosphatase
path, pathological
PC, prostate cancer
pen, penetration
PFS, progression-free survival

PNBx, prostate needle biopsy
pos, positive
PSA, prostate specific antigen
PSM, positive surgical margins
pts, patients
QOL, quality of life
rad onc, radiation oncology
regr, regression
RP, radical prostatectomy
RTOG, Radiation Therapy Oncology Group
RT-PCR, reverse transcriptase polymerase chain reaction
SD, standard deviation
sig, significant or significance or significantly
sq, square
stat, statistical or statistically
surv, survival
SV, seminal vesical
SVI, seminal vesical invasion
TRUS, transrectal ultrasound
tx, treatment or treatments
undet, undetactable
unk, unknown
urin, urinary
univar, univariate
urol, urology or urological
var, variation
wk, week
wks, weeks
WW, watchful waiting
XRT, external beam radiation therapy

Appendix B. Outcomes Literature Table: Radiation Therapy

Amdur et al., The effect of overall treatment time on local control in pts w/adenocarcinoma of the prostate treated w/XRT.Int J Rad Oncol Biol Phys, 1990	
Treatment modality	XRT
Site	University of Florida
Study design	Retrospective analysis.
Sample Size	167
Accrual dates	1964-1982
Patient stage	A2-C2. A1 excluded
Patient age	mean at diagnosis 64, range 45-81
Duration of follow-up	All pts treated at least 5 yrs prior to analysis, 19% eligible for 10-yr follow-up
Other Patient characteristics	149 (89%) white, 17 (10%) black, 1 asian
Other Eligibility Criteria	Histologic proof of invasive adenocarcinoma, no evidence of regional or distant spread, initial tx only XRT using megavoltage teletherapy.
Univar/Multiv Analyses (Covariates)	Total tx time (wks), stage. Survival curves by stage, comparison between 2 tx time groups (>8 wks, <=8 wks). Tables give 5-yr local control by stage and grade in pts who received >=6500 cGy.
Outcome Definitions	2 methods of calculating local control were used - direct and life-table. Direct: local control only if prostate gland free of recurrent tumor >=5 yrs after XRT.
Method of Survival Analysis	Direct and life-table. For life-table the Cutler-Ederer method used with comparison using the Gehan test.
Survival Curves	5-yr local control rate for 5 stages and 2 XRT time treatment groups (>8 wks, <=8 wks) (% and p value given). Curves out as far as 8 yrs.
Statistical Estimates Related to Survival Analyses	Local control rate was 88% (<=8 wks) vs 55% (>8 wks) (p=0.002) for stage B2 who rec'd >=6500 cGy.

Anscher and Prosnitz, , Transurethral resection of prostate prior to definitive irradiation for prostate cancer: Lack of correlation with treatment outcome, Urology, 1991.	
Treatment modality	XRT with curative intent. Pts stratified into TURP and needle biopsy (PNBX) groups.
Site	Duke University Medical Center, Durham, NC
Study design	Records of all pts with newly diagnosed adenocarcinoma of the prostate treated with radiotherapy with curative intent were reviewed. All pts initially seen by a urologist.
Sample Size	107
Accrual dates	1970 - 1983
Patient stage	Staged retrospectively using the Whitmore system (A2,B,C, D1).
Patient age	mean= 65.8, range 52-81 for TURP; mean= 63.2, range 48-77 for PNBX
Duration of follow-up	64.6 months, range 16-152 for TURP; 63.9 months, range 6-164 for PNBX
Other Patient characteristics	Gleason groups: Well (2-4), Moderate (5-7), Poor (8-10). Clinical Characteristics
Univar/Multiv Analyses (Covariates)	Results all stratified by TURP and PNBX. Other covariates include age, TURP vs. needle biopsy, Stage (A2 and B vs C and D1), grade (well and mod vs poor), androgen ablation (yes/no), acid phosphatase (elevated vs normal).
Outcome Definitions	None given. Pts analyzed with regard to local control, survival, disease-free survival, and freedom from distant metastatses.
Method of Survival Analysis	Actuarial method. Pts lost to follow-up were censored at the date of last follow-up. Difference between curves assessed using log-rank test.
Survival Curves	4 figures compare survival, local control, disease-free survival, and probability of distant disease control for TURP and PNBX. Figures out to 10 yrs or more.
Statistical Estimates Related to Survival Analyses	Table of p values for each outcome and covariate (<=65 vs >65; TURP vs PNBX; A2&B vs C&D1; well & mod vs poor; hormone use; acid phos elevation also given

187

Appendix B. Outcomes Literature Table: Radiation Therapy

Arcangeli et al., Prognostic impact of transurethral resection on pts irradiated for localized prostate cancer, Radiotherapy & Oncol, 1995	
Treatment modality	Radical XRT. Pts stratified into TURP and needle biopsy (PNBX) groups.
Site	ITALY
Study design	Retrospective analysis of records of pts with carcinoma of the prostate localized to the pelvis treated with definitive irradiation.
Sample Size	264
Accrual dates	1974-1991
Patient stage	TNM classification for TURP and PNBX
Outcome Definitions	Survival curves and Cox proportional hazard analysis.

Asbell et al., Elective pelvic irradiation in Stage A2, B carcinoma of the prostate: Analysis of RTOG 77-06, Int J Rad Oncol Biol Phys, 1988	
Treatment modality	Randomized to receive only prostate bed irradiation or pelvic irradiation and a boost to the prostatic bed
Site	Case accrual from 34 sites (some outside US), randomized to 1 of 2 treatments
Study design	484 pts were entered into RTOG 77-06
Sample Size	445 analyzable, although only 413 pts treated per protocol.
Accrual dates	1978-1983
Patient stage	A2 or B according to Jewitt's modification or Whitmore staging (i.e., no clinical (lymphangiogram) or biopsy evidence of lymph node involvement).
Patient age	mean= 67.7 for prostate only; mean= 67.6 for prostate and pelvis
Duration of follow-up	min. follow-up=4.5 yrs, median=7 yrs
Other Patient characteristics	RTOG 7706 protocol: Analysis of tx arms for balance of pre-tx factors
Other Eligibility Criteria	Pts with prior XRT or potentially curative surgery and those with prior or concurrent CA other than skin CA were ineligible.
Univar/Multiv Analyses (Covariates)	Grade (1,2,3-4); Gleason score group (2-5, 6-7, 8-10), Stage (A2, B), no prior hormones, white race, normal/low acid phosphatase, No TURP/TURP, tumor size, laparotomy, lymphangiogram only.
Outcome Definitions	Local or regional failure defined as either progression of measurable dx at anytime or hist verification of tumor 2 y after completing XRT
Method of Survival Analysis	Kaplan-Meier method with comparison of tx arms by Mantel-Haenszel.
Survival Curves	Crude survival by tx arm (prostate vs prostate + pelvic);. Local or regional control; Distant metastases by tx arm; survival with no evidence of disease by tx arm. 5-yr % and p values given, curves out to 10 yrs.
Statistical Estimates Related to Survival Analyses	Tx arms compared at 5-y for all pts and for each covariate, p values provided (At 5-yrs, 88% prostate only vs 90% prostate + pelvic, p=0.15).

Asbell et al.,Impact of surgical staging in evaluating the radiotherapeutic outcome in RTOG phase III study for A2 and B prostate cancer, Int J Rad Oncol Biol Phys, 1989	
Treatment modality	Randomized to receive only prostate bed irradiation or pelvic irradiation and a boost to the prostatic bed
Site	Same study as above and reports same type of results but groups under study are those receiving lymphangiography (LAG) vs staging lymphadenectomy (SL)
Study design	Same as above
Sample Size	117 (26%) assessed by staging lymphadenectomy (SL); 328 (74%) lymphangiography (LAG)
Accrual dates	Same as above
Patient stage	Same as above
Patient age	mean= 67.9 (SL); mean= 67.0 (LAG)

Austin and Convery, Age-race interaction in prostatic adenocarcinoma treated w/external beam irradiation, Am J Clin Oncol, 1993	
Treatment modality	XRT
Site	CT SEER data
Study design	Analysis of SEER data.
Sample Size	1,435 cases selected, 521 excluded unk stage or grade, 914 cases for analysis
Accrual dates	1973-1987
Patient stage	Used AUA (A-D) staging system. Stages A1, A2, and D2 EXCLUDED b/c in a different study (see ref. 25 of paper), leaving B, C, and D1
Patient age	mean=69
Duration of follow-up	Survival curves out to 10 yrs
Other Patient characteristics	Grade I (well diff), II (mod well or mod diff), III (poorly diff), IV (undiff or anaplastic)
Other Eligibility Criteria	All black and white pts with primary adenocarcinoma of the prostate
Univar/Multiv Analyses (Covariates)	Stage, grade (I-IV), race, age, age and race. Cox proportional hazards model including Stage (B vs L/C, L/C vs D1), Grade (I vs II, II vs III&IV), Race, Age (decade)
Method of Survival Analysis	Used Kaplan-Meier method, censoring those living at last follow-up. Survival time calculated from diagnosis to date of last follow-up or death.
Survival Curves	10-yr overall survival (By stage, grade, race, and age (<=60, >60)

Austin et al., Effects of pretreatment transurethral resection on survival in prostatic carcinoma, J Natl Med Assoc, 1994	
Treatment modality	Definitive XRT. Stratified into TURP vs. PNBX groups
Site	SUNY-Health Science Center at Brooklyn and Kings County Hospital Center
Study design	Retrospective analysis of charts and slides
Sample Size	117; 64 TURP and 53 needle biopsy (PNBX)
Accrual dates	1970-1983
Patient stage	Staged using Jewett and Marshall system. Stages B, C, and D1.
Patient age	Not given
Duration of follow-up	Retrospective review of charts from 1970-83.
Other Eligibility Criteria	Local-regional adenocarcinoma of the prostate tx with definitive irradiation
Univar/Multiv Analyses (Covariates)	Method of diagnosis -- TURP vs. PNBX groups; Gleason group -- low (2 to 6) vs. high (7 to 10); race – black vs white
Outcome Definitions	Cancer-specific survival is the only outcome, adjusted for death due to other causes.
Method of Survival Analysis	Actuarial life table method used.
Survival Curves	Survival (Needle and TURP, out to 7 yrs). 5-yr survival rate by stage and PNBX & TURP. Survival high grade (7-10), PNBX & TURP. Survival low grade (2-6), PNBX & TURP.
Statistical Estimates Related to Survival Analyses	The 5-yr survival rate was 38% vs 46% (p=.29) TURP vs PNBX.
Other outcomes/Results	Table summarizes past studies comparing survival of TURP and PNBX groups.

Aygun et al., Long-term clinical and PSA f/u in 500 pts treated w/XRT for localized prostate cancer, MD Med J, 1995

Treatment modality	XRT with curative intent
Site	Radiation Oncology Affiliates of Maryland
Study design	Followed pts treated at one oncology facility.
Sample Size	500
Accrual dates	1975 - 1989
Patient stage	Whitmore-Jewett (A1, A2, B1, B2, C) and TNM (T1a-T4a)
Patient age	median= 69
Duration of follow-up	median=69 months
Other Patient characteristics	Histology, method of dx, race (white vs black), PSA (median pre-tx=16)
Other Eligibility Criteria	Excluded regional or distant metastases, prior tx with surgery, prior or concomitant hormonal tx, initial expectant management lasting months to yrs, locally advanced tumors trated with palliativel XRT
Outcome Definitions	Overall survival (death from any cause). Cancer-specific. Local failure: enlarging mass on rectal exam, + post-tx biopsy,or for 67 pts increasing PSA after tx.
Method of Survival Analysis	5-yr and 10-yr overall and cancer-specific survival Table. 5-yr and 10-yr local control rates by stage (T1a, T1b, T2a, T2b-T4, overall).
Survival Curves	89% (T1a) 5-yr overall survival. 100% (T1a) 5-yr cancer-specific survival. 82% (T1b) 5-yr local control (local failure based on abn rectal exam, +biopsy, or elev PSA) or 94% (local failure base on abnormal DRE or positive biopsy). Number at risk given.
Other outcomes/Results	% of pts with long-term XRT effects:self-limiting diarrhea, rectal bleeding, or hematuria or the same side effects requiring minor or major surg. 10-yr survival summary & 10-yr local control summary.

Beard CJ et al., Complications after treatment w/external-beam irradiation in early-stage prostate CA pts: A prospective multiinstitutional outcomes study, JCO, 1997

Treatment modality	XRT to whole pelvis (WP), small field (SF), conformal (C)
Site	Consult at either Dana-Farber, Brigham and Women's, or New England Deaconess
Study design	117-item self-administered questionnaire including POMS and SF-36
Sample Size	337 in original cohort study, 121 received XRT alone as primary tx and were eligible
Accrual dates	1991 - 1994
Patient stage	T1a-c, T2a-c, T3a-c
Patient age	mean= 70.1 (WP), 67.9 (SF), 67.3 (C)
Duration of follow-up	113 returned 3-month survey, 103 returned 12-month survey
Other Patient characteristics	Eduation level, income, employment status, marital status, median Gleason score, ICED score, treatment at academic center (44-100%)
Other Eligibility Criteria	All pts had clinically localized, biopsy-proven adenocar-cinoma of the prostate and hadn't received prior tx
Univar/Multiv Analyses (Covariates)	3 treatment groups (WP, SF, C)
Outcome Definitions	All HRQOL measures.
Incontinence	GI (e.g., diarrhea) and genitourinary (e.g., urine flow) symptoms over time (% with symptom pre-XRT, 3 months, 12 months with p-value at 12 months).
Impotence	Sexual symptoms (e.g., complete impotence, no sexual satisfaction) over time (% with symptom pre-xrt, 3 months, 12 months), p-value at 12 months.
Other outcomes/Results	HRQOL indicators (Profile of Mood States [POMS] and SF-36) by treatment group and time (mean baseline score, change at 12 months).

Appendix B. Outcomes Literature Table: Radiation Therapy

Beyer and Priestley, Biochemical disease-free survival following I125 prostate implantation, In J Rad Onc, 1997	
Treatment modality	Ultrasound-guided permanent I-125 brachytherapy
Site	One Arizona radiation oncology group in cooperation with several urologists
Study design	Followed pts who planned on receiving brachytherapy as sole tx
Sample Size	499 initially, 10 lost to follow-up within 1st year and excluded
Accrual dates	1988 - 1993
Patient stage	T1 and T2N0M0 only
Patient age	median=74 (range 51 to 95)
Duration of follow-up	34 months (range 3-70)
Other Patient characteristics	Gland size, Gleason (2-4, 5-6, 7-10, no grade), pre-tx PSA (median=7.3) at time of diagnosis 20% (95) of pts had a normal PSA (<=4)
Univar/Multiv Analyses (Covariates)	Cox multivariate analysis of biochem disease-free survival, local control, and disease-free survival using stage (T2C), grade (Cleason >=7), baseline PSA (>10), age (<65), or prior TURP
Outcome Definitions	Local failure = progressive, palpable disease or positive biopsy. Distant failure = clinical or radiographic progression outside prostate. Biochemical failure = PSA >4 ng/ml at most recent follow-up or at institution of any hormonal therapy.
Method of Survival Analysis	Kaplen-Meier method.
Survival Curves	5-yr local control survival by Gleason group or stage. 5-yr biochem disease-free survival by Gleason group or stage and by baseline PSA group
Other outcomes/Results	Comparisons among selected series for disease-free and biochem disease-free survival. Series limited to T1 or T2 using surgery, XRT, or Iodine seed implants.

Bolla et al., Improved survival in pts w/locally advanced prostate CA treated w/radiotherapy and goserelin, NEJM, 1997)	
Treatment modality	External irradiation alone vs external irradiation plus goserelin (hormone theray)
Site	Several EORTC Radiotherapy Cooperative Group institutions
Study design	Randomized, prospective trial
Sample Size	415 initially, data of 401 analyzed
Accrual dates	1987 - 1995

Borghede and Sullivan, Measurement of QOL in localized prostatic CA pts treated w/radiotherapy. Development of a prostate cancer-specific module supplementing the EORTC QLQ-C30, QOLR, 1996	
Treatment modality	Definitive XRT
Site	Sahlgrenska University Hospital, SWEDEN
Sample Size	214
Accrual dates	1987- 1992

Borghede et al., Analysis of the local control in lymph-node staged localized prostate CA treated by XRT assessed by digital rectal exam, serum PSA and biopsy, Br J Urol, 1997	
Treatment modality	External beam XRT
Site	Sahlgrenska University Hospital, Gothenburg, SWEDEN
Sample Size	175
Accrual dates	1987 - 1993

Appendix B. Outcomes Literature Table: Radiation Therapy

Centeno et al., Flow cytometric analysis of DNA ploidy,% S phase fraction, and total proliferative fraction as prognostic indicators of local control and survival following XRT for prostate carcinoma, Int J Rad Onc Biol Phys, 1994	
Treatment modality	Primary treatment of radical XRT
Site	Pts whose initial diagnostic procedure was at Mass General Hospital, Boston, MA
Study design	Retrospective analysis
Sample Size	77 identified, 7 excluded b/c of endocrine therapy leaving 70
Accrual dates	1976-1985
Patient stage	T1-4N0-XM0 (regionally confined prostate carcinoma)
Patient age	median=69 (range 52-82)
Duration of follow-up	median=5.8 yrs (0.3-13.4)
Other Patient characteristics	DNA ploidy, Grade (Gleason and categories of well, moderate, poor), and tumor size
Other Eligibility Criteria	No prior or concurrent endocrine therapy. Sufficient prostatic tissue available for flow cytometric analysis.
Univar/Multiv Analyses (Covariates)	DNA ploidy, grade, % S-phase, total proliferative fraction
Outcome Definitions	None.
Method of Survival Analysis	Kaplan-Meier method and log-rank tests.
Survival Curves	15-yr disease-free survival, local control, overall survival by DNA ploidy or grade. 15-yr local control by total proliferative fraction or % S phase.

Chodak et al., Results of conservative management of clinically localized prostate cancer, NEJM, 1994	
Treatment modality	Observation and delayed hormone therapy
Site	6: 1 Israel, 1 Scotland, 2 in US, 2 in Sweden. After adjustment for stage, pts with grade 1 tumors from each cohort had ns differences in disease-specific survival. The same was found for grade 2, but not 3. All cohorts analyzed together.
Study design	Pooled analysis of case records from 6 nonrandomized studies
Sample Size	828
Accrual dates	Medline articles published from January 1985 through July 1992
Patient stage	T0a, T01, A1 or focal; T0b, T0d, A2, or diffuse; T1 or B1; T2, B2, or B3
Patient age	mean= 69.6 +/- 7.8, median=69, range 37-93
Duration of follow-up	mean= 79.5 months +/- 49.9, median=78 months
Univar/Multiv Analyses (Covariates)	Grades 1-3, 4 staging systems were used TNM (1974 and 1978), Jewett-Whitmore, and Chisholm (comparable stages were identified except stages A1, focal, T01, and T0a).
Outcome Definitions	Disease-specific survival is survival among only those pts who did not die of causes other than prostate CA.
Method of Survival Analysis	Kaplan-Meier with log-rank or Mantel-Haenszel test.
Survival Curves	5-yr and 10-yr disease-specific and metastasis-free survival by grade (all stages), by grade 1 or 2 and age <61 or >=61, by grade 1 or 2 and stage. ~820 (gives number censored by grade and year). Figures out to 15 yrs.
Statistical Estimates Related to Survival Analyses	98% (95% CI 96-99) for 5-yr disease-specific, grade 1, all stages. 87% (95% CI 81-91) for 10-yr, grade 1, all stages. 93% (95% CI 90-95) for 5-y metastasis-free, grade 1, all stages. 81% (95% CI 75-86) for 10-yr, grade 1, all stages.

Appendix B. Outcomes Literature Table: Radiation Therapy

Coetzee et al., Postoperative PSA as a prognostic indicator in pts w/margin-positive prostate CA, undergoing adjuvant radiotherapy after radical prostatectomy, Urology, 1996

Treatment modality	Adjuvant radio-therapy within 6 months of radical prostatectomy
Site	Duke University Medical Center, Durham, NC
Study design	Evaluated 45 pts with MP (margin positive) disease who were pN0 after radical prostatectomy. Divided into 2 groups, initially undetectable PSA but later elevated, and persistently elevated.
Sample Size	45; Undet. PSA=30; Elev. PSA=15
Accrual dates	Unknown
Patient stage	T1-2 M0 and pN0
Patient age	Undetectable PSA mean=68.4, range=57.8-78.9; Elev. PSA mean=67.4, range=51-82
Duration of follow-up	mean since XRT=33 months
Outcome Definitions	Using post-op PSA levels, pts divided into 2 groups: those who initially attained undect. PSA levels but later had progressive PSA elev, and those in who the PSA level never reached undetectable levels.
Method of Survival Analysis	Kaplan-Meier method.
Survival Curves	Time to PSA failure by post-op PSA level out to 13 yrs (p. 233).
Statistical Estimates Related to Survival Analyses	Undet. PSA: Mean time to failure (elev. PSA) = 2.1 y; Median=3.31 year; range=4 mo-4.8 y. Elev. PSA: Mean time to failure (progressive increase in PSA) = 0.95 y; Median=0.92 y; range=4 mo-2.02 y

Critz et al., PSA nadir: The optimum level after irradiation for prostate CA, J CLin Oncol, 1996

Treatment modality	I-125 prostate implants followed by XRT
Site	Dekalb Medical Center, Atlanta, GA
Study design	Retrospective analysis of 538 consecutive pts irradiated for cure were identified. PSA measured every 6 months after tx.
Sample Size	536; 2 recurred before PSA levels were determined and were excluded
Accrual dates	1984 - 1994
Patient stage	T1T2N0 (11 T1a, 46 T1b, 119 T1c, 150 T2a, 156 T2b, 54 T2c)
Patient age	
Duration of follow-up	40 months; range=12-138 months
Other Patient characteristics	Mean pre-tx PSA=12.4; Median pre-tx PSA=8.4; range=0.3-188 (from 474 pts)
Univar/Multiv Analyses (Covariates)	Several figures of disease-free survival stratified by PSA nadir, "late" vs "early" nadir, pre-tx PSA< stage. Multivariate analysis including stage, grade, pre-tx PSA, prostate volume
Outcome Definitions	PSA nadir is the lowest PSA level at any time after tx. Recurrence is 2 consecutive increasing PSA values, but if incr less than 2 than 3rd reading required.
Method of Survival Analysis	Used life-table estimates method determined from date of implant.
Survival Curves	5-y Disease-free survival by PSA nadir level
Statistical Estimates Related to Survival Analyses	95% at 5-y for PSA nadir level of 0.2 ng/ml
Other outcomes/Results	Recurrences by PSA nadir level group. Fraction of pts, according to pre-tx PSA who achieved nadir<=0.5 using life-table method.

193

Critz et al., The PSA nadir that indicates potential cure after radiotherapy for prostate CA, Urology, 1997

Treatment modality	I-125 prostate implants followed by XRT
Site	Radiotherapy Clinic of Georgia, Atlanta, GA
Study design	Retrospective analysis of 660 consecutive men irradiated for cure. PSA measured every 6 months after tx.
Sample Size	598 (62 treated before use of PSA)
Accrual dates	1984 - 1995
Patient stage	T1T2N0
Patient age	
Duration of follow-up	median= 42 months; range=12-150; mean=48
Other Patient characteristics	Pre-tx PSA
Univar/Multiv Analyses (Covariates)	Pre-tx PSA
Outcome Definitions	Recurrence defined as PSA level, on 2 consecutive measurements, rising above lowest PSA level achieved by close of study. PSA measured every 6 months.
Method of Survival Analysis	Life-table estimates method determined from date of implant.
Survival Curves	Disease-free survival correlated with PSA nadir achieved after XRT (out to 10 y). % of men, according to pre-tx PSA and as a group, calculated to reach PSA nadir of 0.5
Statistical Estimates Related to Survival Analyses	Correlation of PSA nadir and disease-free survival in all men (min 60-monthfollow-up) 89% disease-free who have PSA nadir <=0.5. 96% disease-free at 7-y who had pre-tx PSA=0-4.

D'Amico and Propert, Prostate CA volume adds significantly to prostate-specific antigen in the prediction of early biochemical failure after XRT, Int J Rad Oncol Biol Phys, 1996

Treatment modality	XRT
Site	Joint Center for XRT, Boston, MA
Study design	Study of 227 consecutive pts, seen for follow-up at 1 month after XRT, and then at 3 month intervals up to a max of 5 yrs
Sample Size	227
Accrual dates	1990-1993
Patient stage	T1a,b,c (18%); T2a,b,c (71%); T3a,b,c (11%). This study did not limit its pts to localized prostate Ca (i.e., includes stage T3)
Duration of follow-up	Up to 5 yrs max, Kaplan-Meier curves go out to 2 yrs
Other Patient characteristics	PSA (10 & 20 ng/ml cutoffs); Gleason Sum (2-4, 5-6, 7-10); PSA density, Ca-specific PSA; Volume of Ca; Volume fraction Ca.
Other Eligibility Criteria	No patient received androgen ablative therapy or other systemic therapy prior to, during, or after XRT up to the time of their follow-up in this study
Univar/Multiv Analyses (Covariates)	Cox regression analysis of postradiation PSA failure with vars TRUS volume, stage, biopsy Gleason, PSA density, PSA, Ca-specific PSA, Ca vol, vol fraction of Ca. Univariate & multivariate p-values, and LL coeff.
Survival Curves	Time to PSA failure by volume of Ca; by % volume; by Gleason score. Two serial rising PSAs obtained 3 months apart after a nadir level were considered evidence of biochemical failure.
Statistical Estimates Related to Survival Analyses	See Figure (<=5, 5-4, >4; p=0.000042), Figure (>5% and <=5%; p=0.00086) and Figure 3 (2-4, 5-6, 7-10; p=0.037). Patient clinical characteristics and corresponding 20-month actuarial freedom from postradiation PSA failure.

Davies et al., Effect of blood transfusion on survival after radiotherapy as treatment for carcinoma of the prostate, 1991

Treatment modality	TURP and high dose radiotherapy
Site	Churchill Hospital, Oxford, UK
Sample Size	71
Accrual dates	1973-1986
Patient age	median=66; range=47-76
Survival Curves	5-yr survival
Other outcomes/Results	Recurrence

Diamond et al., The relationship between facility structure and outcome in CA of the prostate and uterine cervix, Int J Rad Oncol Biol Phys, 1991

Treatment modality	XRT
Site	Patterns of Care Study. Gives 2 references for description of methodology of PCS.
Study design	Used outcome data (recurrence, cx, overall survival) for pts treated in 1978 for cervical or prostate CA and data from a survey sent to all facilities in the US which provided structure info regarding equipment, personnel, & new patient load.
Sample Size	770
Accrual dates	1978
Duration of follow-up	Treated 1978, survey 1983
Other Eligibility Criteria	Pts were part of the Patterns of Care Study (PCS)
Univar/Multiv Analyses (Covariates)	Table 4. p-values from logistic regression, adenocarcinoma of the prostate. Covariates technologists per machine, new pts per technologist, new pts per MD, new pts per physicist, stage.
Survival Curves	Crude outcome by stage-adenocarcinoma of the prostate. Gives the % alive, in-field failure, any failure, and major complications by stage.

Duncan et al., Carcinoma of the prostate: Results of radical radiotherapy (1970-1985), Int J Rad Oncol Biol Phys, 1993

Treatment modality	XRT
Site	Princess Margaret Hospital, Toronto, Ontario, CANADA
Study design	Retrospective review of 999 pts with histologically confirmed prostate adenocarcinoma
Sample Size	999
Accrual dates	1970-1985
Survival Curves	5 and 10 year overall survival reported by stage
Other outcomes/Results	5 and 10 year relapse rates and complication rates

Duncan et al., The influence of transurethral resection of prostate on prognosis of pts w/adenocarcinoma of the prostate treated by radical radiotherapy, Radiotherapy & Oncol, 1994

Treatment modality	Radical radiotherapy with pretreatment TURP or needle biopsy
Site	Princess Margaret Hospital, Toronto, Ontario, CANADA
Study design	999 consecutive pts
Sample Size	999; 427 PNBX, 541 TURP
Accrual dates	1970-1985
Patient stage	T1, T2, T3, T4

Egawa et al., Detection of residual prostate cancer after radiotherapy by sonographically guided needle biopsy, Urology, 1992

Treatment modality	Definitive XRT
Site	Scott Department of Urology, Baylor College of Medicine, Houston, TX
Study design	Between 1987 and 1989, 73 pts with prostate cancer treated with radiotherapy had transrectal ultrasonagraphy (TRUS) at least once after treatment.
Sample Size	56
Accrual dates	1987-1989
Patient stage	Of the 27 pts who had an US-guided biopsy: A2 (7), B1(9), B2(5), C1(6)
Duration of follow-up	US performed 9-154 months (mean=39) after XRT; Biopsies performed 11-131 months (mean=27) after XRT
Other Eligibility Criteria	Of the 73 eligible pts, 12 sought a 2nd opinion for a biopsy-proven recurrent prostate CA, and 5 others got add'tl therapy, these 17 were excluded.
Outcome Definitions	Outcomes limited to the effectiveness of TRUS and US-guided biopsy with PSA measurement and DRE in aiding detection of residual cancer after definitive XRT

Fowler et al., Outcomes of external-beam XRT for prostate cancer: A study of Medicare beneficiaries in 3 surveillance, epidemiology, and end results areas, JCO, 1996	
Treatment modality	High-energy XRT compared to radical prostatec-tomy sample
Site	3 SEER sites (XRT); 5% sample of Medicare (radical prostatectomy)
Study design	Sample of 799 eligible XRT pts. drawn from 3 SEER regions (GA, CT, MI). 5% sample of all Medicare beneficiaries used to ID men who had undergone radical prostatectomy during a 3-y period plus MA sample. Survey in Appendix A.
Sample Size	621 XRT, 373 surgery
Accrual dates	Diagnosis 1989-1991 (XRT), Claim 1988-1990 (surgery)
Patient stage	Not reported: "local or regional prostate CA"
Patient age	At TX: 37% 70-74 y XRT; 41% 70-74 surgery
Duration of follow-up	N/A; survey of pts
Other Eligibility Criteria	All pts with XRT eligible except those with confirmed distant metastases
Incontinence	Self-report of dripping, leaking urine in past month by Tx group
Impotence	Self-report of sexual functioning in past month by Tx group
Other outcomes/Results	Self-report of BM problems, follow-up Tx, perceived Ca status, worry, and more

Forman et al. Frequency of residual neoplasm in the prostate following 3-D conformal radiotherapy, The Prostate, 1993	
Treatment modality	Definitive XRT. All tx fields were designed with a CT-based 3-D tx planning system, resulting in a static conformal radiotherapy plan (3D-CRT)
Site	Department of Radiation Oncology, Providence Cancer Center, Southfield, MI
Study design	Sample of 30 consecutive pts with localized adenocarcinoma of the prostate
Sample Size	30
Accrual dates	1988-1989
Patient stage	26 stage T1, T2NxMo, and 4 T3NxMo
Patient age	ave=70; range= 54-82
Duration of follow-up	median= 36 months; max=48 months; eval 1-month posttx, quarterly for 1st year, semiannually thereafter
Other Patient characteristics	16 needle bx, 14 TURP. Ave pre-tx PSA=26.7; range=1.9-128
Outcome Definitions	2 yrs following completion of tx, all pts had digital rectal exam (DRE), transrectal ultrasound with multiple biopsies, bone scan, and serum PSA
Method of Survival Analysis	None
Other outcomes/Results	Residual CA by bx in 6/30 (20%) pts 2 yrs after completion 3D-CRT. 4 pts abn DRE 2 yrs following CRT, but only 1 had pos bx. Transrectal us abn in 9 pts, bx confirmed in 1. PSA correlated with post-tx bx results.

Appendix B. Outcomes Literature Table: Radiation Therapy

Forman et al., Neoadjuvant hormonal downsizing of localized carcinoma of the prostate: Effects on the volume of normal tissue irradiation, Cancer Investigation, 1995

Treatment modality	3 months of leuprolide prior to definitive XRT. Purpose to reduce morbidity by downsizing prostate and reducing vol bladder and retum receiving hi dose XRT.
Site	Harper Hospital, Wayne State University, Detroit, MI
Study design	Sample of 20 pts with localized adenocarcinoma of the prostate entered on prospective phase II study evaluating effects Lupron (3 monthly injections) prior to XRT.
Sample Size	20
Accrual dates	1992-1993
Patient stage	T1 or T2 (A, B)
Other Patient characteristics	Pre- and posthormone (PSA, testosterone, prostate vol., prostate shrinkage)
Other Eligibility Criteria	No evidence of extracapsular extension
Univar/Multiv Analyses (Covariates)	Varying XRT doses
Outcome Definitions	The vols of the prostate, seminal vesicle, bladder, and rectum from both pre- and posthormone tx planning CT were entered onto a 3-D tx-planning system. Ave vol of the prostate and rectum the outcomes of interest.
Method of Survival Analysis	None
Other outcomes/Results	Cumulative dose-vol histograms (CDVH) of the rectum in 1 pt before and after 3 months of leuprolide. CDVH of bladder in 1 pt before and after 3 months of leuprolide

Forman et al. Definitive Radiotherapy following prostatectomy: Results and complications, Int J Rad Oncol Biol Phys, 1986

Treatment modality	XRT after prostatectomy
Site	Division of Radiation Oncology, Johns Hopkins Oncology Center, Baltimore, MD
Study design	Retrospective analysis of 34 pts with localized carcinoma of the prostate who had been treated with prostatectomy (radical or simple) and postop XRT
Sample Size	34
Accrual dates	1975-1984
Patient age	age at tx=67.3; range=55-78
Duration of follow-up	median=4 yrs; range=1-4; 1 months post-tx, quarterly for 3 yrs, twice yearly for 2 yrs, and yearly thereafter
Other Patient characteristics	Grade I-III, lymph node pos/neg/unk, 3 groups: 1 (rad prost with extracap ext, 2 (simple prost with extracap ext), 3 (palpable local recur after rad prost)
Outcome Definitions	Survival calculated from the date of first radiation tx. Pts scored as relapsed if palpable local recurrence detected on rectal exam or metastatic dx found on physical exam or radiographic studies. Comparisons using Gehan's gen. Wilcoxan 2-sided test.
Method of Survival Analysis	Kaplan - Meier actuarial method.
Survival Curves	Actuarial survival for 3 groups out 8 yrs with table of pts at risk. Disease-free survival for 3 groups out 8 yrs with table of pts at risk.
Statistical Estimates Related to Survival Analyses	5-year actuarial survival and disease-free survival for all pts were 82 and 72%, respectively. Survival sig worse for pts irradiated for recurrence (group 3) compared with groups 1&2 (p=0.002).
Incontinence	% affected overall and by group. 5 pts (15%) had urinary stress incontinence (3 of 5 incontinent prior to XRT). 2 pts (6%) had urinary outlet obstruction.
Impotence	17 ot 19 pts (89%) who had radical prostatectomy were impotent before and after XRT. 2 of 6 pts who were potent following simple prostatectomy were impotent after XRT.
Other outcomes/Results	Tx-related complications. Number (%) of total and by group who had edema, urinary incontinence., urinary obstruction, proctitis. Complications by tx modality (Surg only vs XRT only).

197

Fukunaga-Johnson et al. Results of 3D conformal radiotherapy in the treatment of localized prostate cancer, Int J Rad Oncol Biol Phys, 1997	
Treatment modality	3D conformal radiotherpy (3D CRT)
Site	University of Michigan (Ann Arbor, MI) and Providence Hospital (Southfield, MI), Dept. of Radiation Oncology
Study design	Retrospective analysis of pts with localized prostate cancer treated with 3D CRT
Sample Size	707
Accrual dates	1987-1994
Patient stage	603 T1-T2; 98 T3-T4
Patient age	median=72; range=44-87
Duration of follow-up	median=36 months; up to 8 yrs ; 10% followed beyond 5.5 yrs; PSA and DRE every 3-6 months following tx
Other Patient characteristics	Patient characteristics (bNED at 5-yrs, stage, preXRT PSA, Gleason, age group, white/black, total dose, boost tech, pelvic field, favorable, surg status
Other Eligibility Criteria	Pts with pathologically-confirmed pelvic lymph node metastasis, treated with preXRT androgen ablation, or treated postprostatectomy were excluded
Univar/Multiv Analyses (Covariates)	bNED survival curves according to preXRT PSA, Gleason, preXRT PSA and T-stage, favorable (PSA<=10, Gleason<7, T1-T2)/unfavorable status
Outcome Definitions	Biochemical failure defined as (1) 2 consecutive PSA rises >2.0 if nadir PSA <=2.0, (2) 2 consecutive rises in PSA over nadir if nadir PSA >2.0, (3) start of hormonal tx after XRT. Time of PSA failure the date of confirmatory PSA rise. Biochemical surv date of end of XRT to date of PSA failure or last PSA for censored pts
Method of Survival Analysis	Distribution of bNED (biochem control) surv est non-parametrically by Kaplan-Meier method. Length of bNED surv comopared between pts groups with log rank test. Multivar analyses using Cox regression.
Survival Curves	bNED at 5 yrs, 95% CI, p value. Best predictive Cox model of bNED, risk ratio, 95% CI, p value. bNED curves out to about 100 months according to preXRT PSA, Gleason, pre-XRT PSA and T-stage, favorable/unfavorable status. Short discussion of 5-year overall survival
Statistical Estimates Related to Survival Analyses	88% pts biochem NED at 5-yrs with a pre-XRT PSA <=4
Other outcomes/Results	Complix graded using RTOG scale. Complix with tech: 3% actuarial risk at 7 yrs of grade 3-4 rectal complix and 1% actuarial risk at 7 yrs of grade 3 bladder complix.

Fuks et al. The effect of loca l control on metastatic dissermination in carcinoma of the prostate: Long-term results in pts treated w/125I implantation, Int J Rad Oncol Biol Phys, 1991	
Treatment modality	Brachytherapy: Retropubic 125I implantation. During procedures had radical or modified lymph node dissection.
Site	Memorial Sloan-Kettering Cancer Center (MSKCC), New York
Study design	Probability of distant metastatses studied in 679 pts with stage B-C/N0 carcinoma of prostate treated at MSKCC. Total of 1013 pts with biopsy-proven adenocarcinoma of prostate treated from 1970-1985.
Sample Size	679/1013
Accrual dates	1970-1985
Patient stage	MSKCC staging system: 191 B1, 328 B2, 71 B3, 87 C.
Patient age	mean=61.5 +/- 6.5; range=36-79. No sig diffs in age among stage or grade subgroups.
Duration of follow-up	median=97+ months among survivors; 2-6 month intervals until death
Other Patient characteristics	249 grade I, 362 grade II, 41 grade III, 27 unknown.
Other Eligibility Criteria	Of the 1013 pts treated, only the 679 whose lymph node dissection showed node neg were included, other 334 with pos lymph nodes excluded
Univar/Multiv Analyses (Covariates)	Cox proportional hazard analysis of covars (local failure, grade, stage, implant vol, implant dose, age) affecting DMFS.
Outcome Definitions	Local failure: bladder outlet obstruction req. TURP, evid of tumor progress on successive DRE, pos biopsy at >=1 year after implant. Distant failures usually involved bone.
Method of Survival Analysis	Survival curves calculated as time-adjusted rates from date of 125I implant by the Kaplan-Meier product-limit method adj denominator at every time pt for pts at risk.
Survival Curves	Overall surv, distant metastases free surv (DMFS), & local relapse free surv (LRFS). Figures of K-M survival curves out to 20-yrs with stratification by stage, grade, implant dose. Also looked at pts with local failure and distant metastatses.
Statistical Estimates Related to Survival Analyses	The time adj DMFS for locally controlled pts at risk at 15 yrs was 77%, corresponding rate for pts who developed local recurrence was 24% (p<0.00001). % reported in text generally 10 or 15 yrs.

Geara et al. Influence of initital presentation on treatment outcome of clinically localized prostate cancer treated by definitive XRT. Int J Rad Oncol Biol Phys, 1994.	
Treatment modality	Definitive XRT.
Site	University of Texas MD Anderson Cancer Center, Houston, TX
Study design	Retrospective analysis of 427 men with clin localized prostate CA and known pre-tx PSA levels who recv'd XRT as sole initial tx at MD Anderson. Initial presentations: abn "routine" PSA, abn "routine" DRE, Symptoms (largely urinary obstructive).
Sample Size	427
Accrual dates	1987-1991
Patient stage	122 T1, 147 T2, 152 T3, 6 T4
Patient age	mean=median=68; range=47-84
Duration of follow-up	mean=33 months; median=30 months; range=9-73 months; only 8 pts followed < 1 yr.
Other Patient characteristics	7 Grade2, 46 G3, 97 G4, 91 G5, 77 G6, 70 G7, 24 G8, 6 G9, 9 unassigned. Stage, grade, pre-tx PSA by initial pres. Initial presentation: 54 PSA, 173 DRE, 200 Symptoms.
Other Eligibility Criteria	No clinical radiographic evididence of nodal or hematogenous metastases. No pt received adjuvant androgen ablation.
Univar/Multiv Analyses (Covariates)	Pts stratified by initial presentation (PSA, DRE, symptoms) for all analyses since purpose to address whether init pres should influence choice of WW vs TX. Multivar propotional hazards regression: initial presentation, pre-tx PSA, grade, TURP in T3&T4.
Outcome Definitions	PSA values rising if 2 or more consec values rising, or if most recent value appeared to have risen, PSA scored as rising if this value was higher than prior by 1 ng/ml or factor of 1.5. Timing and intensity of follow-up of pts with rising PSA up to MD. Pts clin free of dx if no clin-rad evid of metastases & no evid of local recurrence. Local recurrence confirmed by biopsy.
Method of Survival Analysis	Actuarial incidence curves calc using Berkson-Gage and Kaplan-Meier methods. Test of sig diffs between curves using log rank.
Survival Curves	Relapse or rising PSA. Incidence of relapse or rising PSA by initial presentation (trended p=0.71) out 60 months after XRT. Incidence of relapse or rising PSA by stage (T1b, T1c, T2a, T2b, T2c) out 60 months after XRT.
Statistical Estimates Related to Survival Analyses	Acturarial outcome at 5 yrs according to presentation (trended log rank p value for all endpts >0.5). E.g., 29% relapse, 36% rising PSA, 42% relapse or rising PSA for the DRE groups.

Gervasi et al. Prognostic significance of lymp nodal metastases in prostate cancer. J of Urology, 1989	
Treatment modality	Combination of gold seed implants and XRT (started 2-3 wks after seeds).
Site	Department of Radiotherapy, Baylor College of Medicine and Methodist Hospital, Houston, TX
Study design	Retrospective analysis of records. 511 pts identified with biopsy-proven adenocarcinoma of prostate, stages A2-C1, who underwent pelvic lymph node dissection and radioactive gold seed implantation, and who completed XRT.
Sample Size	511
Accrual dates	1966-1979
Patient stage	130 A2, 25 B1N, 140 B1, 100 B2, 116 C1
Patient age	mean=64; range=43-82
Duration of follow-up	mean=8.6 yrs; range=2.5-17.5; 500 followed at least 5 yrs; 282 at least 10; 225 at least 15 or until death
Other Patient characteristics	grade I, II, or III; frequency and extent of nodal metastases; acid phosphatase elevated in 9% before tx.
Other Eligibility Criteria	No evid of distant metastases at tx and no hormones or chemo prior to recurrence.
Univar/Multiv Analyses (Covariates)	Results analyzed by stage, grade, and presence and extent of lymph node metastases (neg/pos and 1,2, or 3 pos nodes). Significance of cross-tabs tested with chi-square.
Outcome Definitions	Local recurrence: clin phenonmenon with discrete signs or symptoms (e.g., palpable regrowth causing pain confirmed by tissue diagnosis. Pos post-irradiation biopsy or palpable abn on rectal exm along did not count. Distant recurrence: persistantly elev acid phos, pos bone scan, blastic lesion seen on skeletal radiographs or biopsy proved soft tissue metastasis.
Method of Survival Analysis	Life-table analysis with sig diffs tested using Lee-Desu statistic.
Survival Curves	Actuarial rate of recurrence, distant metastases, and all cause & cancer-specific survival rates by presence and extent of nodal metastases out to 15 yrs. P-values and 95% CI error bars.
Statistical Estimates Related to Survival Analyses	Actuarial rate of recurrence, all cause & CA-specific survival at 5, 10, 15 yrs by extent of nodal metastases (% +/- 2 std errors). E.g., 86% recurrence +/- 10 at 10 yrs for the 1 node positive group.
Other outcomes/Results	Comparison to 2 other studies (Zincke & Utz,1984 -- prostatectomy with orchiectomy; and Smith & Middleton, 1985 -- XRT or hormones) which included pts with a single positive node.

Glick et al. Are three substages of clinical B prostate carcinoma useful in predicting disease-free survival. Urology, 1990.

Treatment modality	Definitive XRT using either I-125 interstitial radiotherapy or XRT. No sig diff in disease-free survival for the 2 tx and therey were combined for analysis.
Site	Eastern Virginia Graduate School of Medicine, Norfolk, VA
Study design	Retrospective analysis of records between 1974 and 1985. Identified 249 pts who recv'd XRT (84 125I and 165 external beam) with stage B.
Sample Size	176
Accrual dates	1974-1985
Patient stage	46 B1N, 78 B1, 52 B2
Patient age	mean=65.7
Duration of follow-up	mean=55 months; range=3-135
Other Eligibility Criteria	Needed detailed pre-tx DRE, CA proved by biopsy, neg metastatic workup, no therapy prior to XRT.
Univar/Multiv Analyses (Covariates)	Survival curves stratified by stage, grade (well, mod, poor), acid phosphatase (abn/norm).
Outcome Definitions	No definition, only looked at disease-free survival (DFS).
Method of Survival Analysis	"Using survival analysis in SPSS, disease-free survival curves were ocmputer-calculated for each tumor stage, grade, pre-tx acid phosphatase, adn stage under anesthesia."
Survival Curves	Probability of DFS by 2 substages (B1N, B2), 3 substages (B1N, B1, B2), tumor grade, acid phosphatase, acid phosphatase for B1N, acid phosphatase for B1. All curves out to 8 yrs, p value given.
Statistical Estimates Related to Survival Analyses	Tend to discuss p values and not report %. E.g., B1N vs B1, p=0.28; B1 vs. B2, p=0.13
Other outcomes/Results	Pts treated with 125I implants were staged by rectal exam and again under anesthesia at time of implant. Stage change (none, upstaged, downstaged) under anesthesia (chi-square analysis).

Hanks et al. Outcome for lymph node dissection negative T-1b, T-2 (A-2, B) prostate cancer treated with external beam XRT in RTOG 77-06, Int J Rad Oncol Biol Phys, 1991.

Treatment modality	XRT and elective nodal irradiation
Site	It appears several US centers/hospitals were involved
Study design	RTOG #77-06 was a prospective randomized trial to evelute ELECTIVE NODAL IRRADIATION in pts with T1b & T2 prostate CA whose nodal status was deter. by lymphangiogram (LAG), CT scan, or dissection (LND). NO OUTCOME differences in arms, so combined.
Sample Size	104 pts; 51 of 104 pts also had nodal irradiation
Accrual dates	Not reported in this article
Patient stage	16 T1b (A2), 88 T2 (B)
Patient age	mean=67; range=50-81; 325 >70 yrs
Duration of follow-up	median=7.6 yrs; range=0.1-11.1; continous follow-up
Other Patient characteristics	grade (well, intermediate, poor, unk)
Outcome Definitions	Local failure (prostate only): incomplete regression following tx or incr in size of prostate after init complete response (rarely confirmed by biopsy). Isolated local failure (LF) is LF in absence of concurrent metastasis. Distant or metastatic failure determined by clin eval (e.g., imaging, incr in acid phophatase to abnormal levels). Cause specific surivival (pts dying of cancer).
Method of Survival Analysis	Kaplan-Meier actuarial analysis. Pts censored at the time of 1st failure and no. pts available for follow-up indicated on figure. 1st tx day was starting patient for all analyses. No statistical analyses, descriptive.
Survival Curves	Survival, local control, metastasis, any failure, and cause specific survival after XRT out to 10 yrs from onstudy.
Statistical Estimates Related to Survival Analyses	Usually 5 and 10 year % reported. E.g., 96% free of isolated local recurrence, 93% free of local recurrence with or without metastasis. 87% free of isolated local recurrence at 10 yrs, 84% free of local recurrence with or without metastasis at 10 yrs

Hanks et al. A ten year follow-up of 682 pts treated for prostate cancer w/radition therapy in the United States. Int J Rad Oncol Biol Phys, 1987.

Treatment modality	XRT using a variety of techniques and doses.
Site	106 US facilities randomly sampled
Study design	Patterns of Care Study. The initial review took place in 1978 in 106 facilities. 682 records reviewed. Treated between 1973-75. In 1983 contacted the same facilities for update.
Sample Size	Initially 682; follow-up on 78% pts (532)
Accrual dates	1973-5; followup study in 1983
Patient stage	A, B, C
Duration of follow-up	3-5 yrs for study, this study is a 10 year follow-up
Other Patient characteristics	Table 3. Distribution of grade by stage (p. 502). The authors state, "As grade was an independent var, this distribution must be compored when comparing the outcomes obs in this series to any other."
Other Eligibility Criteria	
Univar/Multiv Analyses (Covariates)	Cox regression of factors (time, age, stage, grade) influencing survival after 1st recurrence (stratified infield and metstatic). P values reported
Outcome Definitions	
Method of Survival Analysis	Actuarial analysis according to Kaplan and Meier out to 10 yrs. Both observed and expected survival estimated.
Survival Curves	Survival. Stages A, B, C. Actuarial analysis of infield recurrence-free rate for stages A-C. Actuarial analysis of free from any recurrence for stages A-C. Actuarial analysis of free of major cx for 682 pts. Actuarial analysis of survival for stage B&C following 1st recurrence at metastatic site. Actuarial analysis of surival for stage B&C following first recurrence in treatment field.
Statistical Estimates Related to Survival Analyses	Report 5 and 10 year rates. E.g., Local recurrence-free rates by stage at 5 yrs are 97% A, 85% B, 72% C.
Incontinence	Table 1. Complication severity in 682 pts. Gives the No. pts who had a bowel, bladder, or soft tissue complication that resulted in (1) hospital admission, no surgery; (2) hospital admission, surgery; (3) death.

Hanks et al. Patterns-of-failure analysis of patents w/high pre-tx PSA levels treated by XRT: The need for improved systemic and locoregional tx. J Clin Oncol, 1996

Treatment modality	Conformal or conventional external beam XRT
Site	Fox Chase Cancer Center, Philadelphia, PA
Study design	508 pts with prostate CA were tx with conformal or conventional XRT, 459 had pre-tx PSA. 129 pts were then identified for this analysis. Arbitrarily grouped by PSA: (1) 20-29.9; (2) 30-49.9; (3)>=50
Sample Size	129
Accrual dates	1988-1993
Patient stage	T1, T2C, T3
Patient age	median for group 1=69.5; 2=70; 3=68.
Duration of follow-up	median=34; range=4-77; median for group 1=34 months; 2=32 months; 3=40 months. Seen at 3 and then 6 months intervals
Other Patient characteristics	Gleason 2-6 and 7-10 by pre-tx PSA.
Other Eligibility Criteria	Pts who recv'd any irradiation as an adj to surgery or irradiation combined with hormonal mgmt, T4 pts, and histologically proven node pos were excluded.
Univar/Multiv Analyses (Covariates)	Cox proportional hazards model using palpation tumor stage (T1, T2, T3); Gleason score (2-6,7-10); pre-tx PSA group, central dose (continuos), age (continuous), tx technique (prostate only vs whole pelvis).
Outcome Definitions	Freedom from any failure (no evidence of biochemical disease (bNED). Freedom from distant metastases (fdm) as shown from imaging evidence.
Method of Survival Analysis	bNED and fdm were calc from start of XRT to the occurrence of the event ot date of most recent follow-up. Estimates of cNED and fdm calc using Kapln-Meier method. Univariate comparisons made using log rank.
Survival Curves	bNED and fdm for pts with pre-tx PSA >=20 out to 80 months from onset of tx. Number at risk given at yearly time points.
Statistical Estimates Related to Survival Analyses	Table 2. Outcome by pre-tx PSA lvel. Provide the N, fdm at 36 months, bNED at 24 months for the 3 groups.
Other outcomes/Results	Univariate and multivariate analyses of bNED and fdm. p values for each covariate.

Appendix B. Outcomes Literature Table: Radiation Therapy

Hanks et al. Patterns of radiation treatment of elderly pts with prostate cancer. Cancer, 1994.	
Treatment modality	Conformal or conventional external beam XRT
Site	Many US facilities including Fox Chase Cancer Center, Philadelphia, PA.
Study design	Patterns of Care Study. 4 national surveys conducted in 1973, 1978, 1983, and 1989. Also used Dept. of Radiation Oncology prostate CA dbase of pts treated at Fox Chase.
Sample Size	2210
Accrual dates	1973, 1978, 1983, 1989
Patient stage	A(T1), B(T2), C(T3,4)
Patient age	stratifies by age <, >=70 and shows shift in age groups over time.
Method of Survival Analysis	Used "standard" survival analysis. All analyses are compared for pts younger than 70 and those 70 and older.
Survival Curves	5-year outcomes (local control, NED survival, free of CA death, free of intercurrent death, survival): All stages pooled by year of tx for 1973, 1978, 1983, all.
Statistical Estimates Related to Survival Analyses	For the pts <70 the local control rates were 78%, 78%, 91%, and 79% in 1973, 1978, 1983, and overall, respectively.
Incontinence	
Impotence	
Other outcomes/Results	Several tables of % over the yrs of the study (1973, 1978, 1983, 1989, all) for the 2 age groups to examine the age of the pts, late morbidity of tx, local control, clinical NED, cause-specific death, survival, dose, XRT tx vol.

Hanks et al. Patterns of care and RTOG studies in prostate CA: Long-term survival, hazard rate observations, and possibilities of cure. Int J Rad Oncol Biol Phys, 1993.	
Treatment modality	XRT
Site	Many US facilities. Survival and freedom from recurrence (sometimes disease free survival or NED surival) at 10 and 15 yrs by stage for pts at Stanford, MD Anderson, Wash U.
Study design	Patterns of Care Study and two groups of pts from RTOG studies (7706 and 7506)
Sample Size	1973 PCS N=668, 1978 PCS N=728, RTOG 7706 N=84, RTOG 7506 N=503
Accrual dates	PCS 1973, 1978; RTOG 7706 1978-1983; RTOG 7506 1976-1983.
Patient stage	T1 Nx M0 (A), T2 Nx M0 (B), T3/4 Nx M0 (C)
Duration of follow-up	Continuous follow-up at each institution
Outcome Definitions	Survival, NED survival, freedom from local recurrence
Method of Survival Analysis	Survival estimates from life tables. Hazard rate plots. All out 13-16 yrs.
Survival Curves	Survival and Hazard Rates for T1NxM0 pts in PCS and RTOG 7706 compared to expected. Survival and Hazard Rates for T1NxM0 in PCS. Survival and Hazard Rates for T3/4NxM0 in PCS and RTOG 7506.
Statistical Estimates Related to Survival Analyses	5, 10, 15 year survival, freedom from local recurrence, and NED survival for different stages and year of tx.

204

Hanks et al. The outcome of treatment of 313 pts w/T1 (UICC) prostate cancer treated w/external beam irradiation. Int J Rad Oncol Biol Phys, 1988.

Treatment modality	XRT
Site	Many US facilities
Study design	Patterns of Care Study. All XRT facilties in the US were identified and stratified (e.g., size, hospital affiliation). 2-stage random sampling so that representative of US. 1973/4 N=682; 1978=713
Sample Size	313 pts with T1N0M0 treated with XRT
Accrual dates	1973/4 and 1978
Patient stage	T1N0M0
Duration of follow-up	up to 10 yrs for 1973, 3.5-5.5 for the 1978 group
Other Patient characteristics	Table 1. Characterization of 1973/4 and 1978 PCS surveys; T1N0M0. Includes age group, Karnofsy, grade, central prostate dose.
Outcome Definitions	Survival, infield recurrence, distant metastases.
Method of Survival Analysis	Actuarial survival with expected survival for age matched controls from US life tables. Mantel-Haenszel test to test dose/complications sig. Chi-square test for linear trend.
Survival Curves	Observed vs expected survival for those treated in 1973, treated in 1978, combined. Freedom from recurrence. for 1973 and 1978 pts.
Statistical Estimates Related to Survival Analyses	Influence of grade on survival, infield recurrence, and distant metastases. Provide the % alive at 5 yrs for 1973 &1978 groups, and combined w/p value. E.g., 84% grade 1 alive at 5-yrs who were treated in 1973.
Other outcomes/Results	Radiation dose and major complications. Provides the 5-year rates and p values suing Mantel-Haenszel and Chi-square.

Hanks et al. Conformal technique dose escalation for prostate cancer: biochemical evidence of improved cancer control w/higher doses in pts w/pre-tx PSA >=10. In J Rad Oncol Biol Phys, 1996

Treatment modality	XRT of the whole pelvis with prostate or prostate + seminal vesicle boost using 4-field conformal tech
Site	Fox Chase Cancer Center, Phildelphia, PA
Study design	375 pts treated with conformal tech between 1989 and 1993. This includes 233 consecutive pts treated in a formal dose escalation study between 3/89-10/92 and 142 consecutive pts treated to dose >72 Gy between 10/92-12/93.
Sample Size	375
Accrual dates	1989-1993
Patient stage	T1, T2, T3
Duration of follow-up	median=21 months; range=3-67 months. All alive pts had >18 months follow-up
Other Patient characteristics	Gleason score group and stage N and % given for 3 PSA groups in Table 1.
Outcome Definitions	Biochemical freedom from disease (bNED). Failure defined as PSA >=1.5 and rising on 2 consecutive values. Time measured from onset of XRT to date of failure or last follow-up.
Method of Survival Analysis	Kaplan-Meier product-limit methods. All curves out to 36 months. Log rank test used to test diffs in bNED by dose groups.
Survival Curves	bNED for all pts by dose above or below 71 Gy and above or below 73 Gy. bNED for pts with pre-tx pSA 10-19.9, dose above/below 71 and above/below 73. bNED for pts with pre-tx PSA 20+, dose above/below 71 and above/below 73.
Statistical Estimates Related to Survival Analyses	P values provided and 24 and 36 months bNED survival rates presented when there are adequate nos. of pts at risk (see Table 3). E.g., 94% 24-month bNED for <71 Gy and pre-tx PSA <10 ng/ml.

Appendix B. Outcomes Literature Table: Radiation Therapy

Hanks et al. Patterns of Care Studies: Dose-reponse observations for local control of adenocarcinoma of the prostate. In J Rad Oncol Biol Phys, 1985	
Treatment modality	XRT
Site	163 randomly selected faciltities in the US
Study design	Patterns Care Study from 1973-5. 682 pts records reviewed at 163 facilities randomly selected from the 1000 present at the time. 108 excluded
Sample Size	574
Accrual dates	1973-5
Patient stage	55 T0, 147 T1, 133 T2, 163 T3, 76 T4
Other Eligibility Criteria	108 excluded: 37 with pos lymph nodes, 14 with missing dose, 57 with unknown stage
Univar/Multiv Analyses (Covariates)	All analyses stratified by radiaiton dose
Outcome Definitions	4-year In-field failure rate. In field failure is the clinical impression recorded in the record by the MD following the patient.
Method of Survival Analysis	Kaplan-Meier actuarial method. Sig calc for whole curve comparisons and linear trend.
Survival Curves	Several tables of the 4 year free recurrence rates for different primary doses and para-prostatic doses (number of pts at each dose provided). P values for whole curve and linear trend provided for each table/analysis.
Statistical Estimates Related to Survival Analyses	Table 3a gives the N & 4-year free recurrence rates for 6 primary dose groups (<5000, 5000-5499, 5500-5999, 6000-6499, 6500-6999, >=7000). E.g., 23 pts (55 total) rec'vd 6500-6999 rad with 100% 4-year free of recurrence. Whole curve/linear trend NS.

Hanks et al. The effect of dose on local control of prostate cancer. Int J Rad Oncol Biol Phys, 1988.	
Treatment modality	XRT
Site	Many US facilities
Study design	Patterns of Care Study. Three surveys analyzed in this paper: Nat'l (tx 1973, 74), 5 large facilities (tx 1973), Nat'l survey (tx 1978)
Sample Size	1516
Accrual dates	1973-4, 1978
Patient stage	168 A, 724 B, 624 C
Outcome Definitions	Infield recurrence determined by DRE and/or pelvic imaging tech
Method of Survival Analysis	Kaplan-Meier curves compared for several dose ranges by linear trend and Mantel-Haenszel tests.
Survival Curves	Dose-response for infield recurrence, stage B, p=0.004 M-H, p=0.004 linear trend, out 10 yrs from start of tx. Effect of grade (well, mod, poor) on infield recurrence for stage C, p=0.001.
Statistical Estimates Related to Survival Analyses	Relation of dose to infield recurrence for all pts, stage A, B, and C. Provides #failed/total, 3, 5, and 7 year actuarial rates, linear trend, and mantel p values. Relation of grade to infield recurrence.
Other outcomes/Results	Relation of hormones to infield recurrence. Effect of photon energy on infield recurrence. 3, 5, and 7 year actuarial free recurrence, M-H p provided.

Hanks et al. Analysis of independent vars affecting survival after recurrence of prostate cancer. Int J Rad Oncol Biol Phys, 1989.

Treatment modality	XRT
Site	Many US facilities
Study design	Patterns of Care Study. pts treated in 1973 and 1974 and analyzed in a national survey. Orig survey conducted on 608, 75% follow-up.
Sample Size	266 recurrences
Accrual dates	1973-4
Patient stage	stage B and C
Duration of follow-up	approximately 10 yrs
Univar/Multiv Analyses (Covariates)	Grade (well, mod, poor), site (local, distant), stage (B,C), year (1st, 2nd). Cox regression was tabulated on cases with complete date to ascertain which factors were stat sig independent predictors.
Outcome Definitions	Survival calculated from the point of recurrence following initial therapy.
Method of Survival Analysis	Kaplan-Meier curves out to 108 months
Survival Curves	Survival from time of recurrence (STR) for B&C combined, and by stage. STR for local recur. vs local metastases. STR for loca recur. by stage. STR for distant metastases by stage. STR for combined stages B&C by time of recurrence after tx. STR for stage B, stage C by time of recurrence after tx. STR combined B&C by grade. STR for combined B&C after distant metastases by grade.
Statistical Estimates Related to Survival Analyses	Of 608 pts, 266 recurred, they have median survival=30 months, 5-year actuarial survival=22%, 8-year actuarial survival =13%.
Other outcomes/Results	STR for calculated "best," "average" and "worst" combinations of independent var

Harlan et al. Geographic, age, and racial variation in the treatment of local/regional carcinoma of the prostate, J Clin Oncol, 1995.

Treatment modality	Radical prostatectomy, XRT, other treatment
Site	SEER Data (9 geographic areas)
Study design	Population-based cancer registry that began in 1973. It covers approx 10% of the US pop.
Accrual dates	1984-1991
Outcome Definitions	There are NO OUTCOMES. This is an analysis of variation in txby geography, age, and race. E.g., Age-adjusted proportion of men (age 50+) with local/regional prostate CA who rev'd radical prostatectomy or XRT by year of diag & registry (9 sites).

Appendix B. Outcomes Literature Table: Radiation Therapy

Jonler et al. Sequelae of definitive XRT for prostate cancer localized to the pelvis. Urology, 1994.

Treatment modality	Definitive XRT
Site	University of Wisconsin, Madison, WI
Study design	Retrospective; obtained the names and addressed of 133 consecutive pts who had XRT and mailed survivors (18 dead) and those not lost to follow-up (4) a questionnaire.
Sample Size	98 of 111 returned the questionnaire (88%)
Accrual dates	1989-1992
Patient stage	T1a-T4, 72% T2a-T2b
Patient age	57% were 70-79 at diagnosis; median at XRT=71; range=52-87; median at follow-up=74; range=55-89
Duration of follow-up	median time from XRT to follow-up=31 months; range=14-60 months
Other Patient characteristics	Data for 98 pts at time of XRT (age group, marital status, educ status, tumor grade, PSA group, TURP, clin stage, pelvic irradiation). 5% pts had surgery /dilation due to bladder neck contractures or urethral strictures.
Other Eligibility Criteria	Few eligibility criteria. 8 pts (8%) had adjuvant tx: 1 orchiectomy, 5 hormones, 2 had both.
Outcome Definitions	Used the questionnaire of Fowler et al. (1993) except sub. "XRT" for "prostate surgery" and added 3 questions.
Method of Survival Analysis	No survival analysis, but used Fisher's exact test (2 tail) and sig level of 5% to test differences between groups.
Incontinence	Survey (e.g., dripping at least some urine daily). Table III gives % from this study and a study of radical prostectomy pts answering same questions. Table reports questions stratified by pt characteristics.
Impotence	Survey contains questions on impotence (e.g., no erection in past month). Table III gives % from this study and a study of radical prostatectomy pts answering same questions. Table gives % to questions stratified by patient characteristics.
Other outcomes/Results	16 of 96 (17%) pts thought their CA had spread or recurred. Give % that have had bowel problems. Some general health questions (e.g., 25% rated their health as excellent or good).

Kabalin et al. Identification of residual cancer in the prostate following XRT: Role of transrectal ultrasound guided biopsy and prostate specific antigen. J of Urology, 1989.

Treatment modality	XRT
Site	Stanford University Medical Center, Stanford, CA
Study design	27 men who had undergone transrectal ultrasound exam of the prostate and biopsy during routine clinical follow-up after XRT were identified.
Sample Size	27
Accrual dates	1987-1988
Patient stage	A1-D1
Patient age	mean=70 at biopsy
Duration of follow-up	min 18 months since completion fo tx required
Outcome Definitions	Outcomes are limited to identifying which pts had residual cancer as identified thru techniques including by transrectal u/s biopsy and to try and relate this to PSA level.
Other outcomes/Results	Results are descriptive and largely patient by patient. Some cross-tabs.

Kaplan et al. The importance of local control in the treatment of prostate cancer. J of Urology, 1992.	
Treatment modality	XRT
Site	Stanford University Hospital, Stanford, CA
Study design	Retrospective analysis of the data base of the Division of XRT at Stanford
Sample Size	946
Accrual dates	1958-1989
Patient stage	319 Stanford stage T1, 227 T2, & 400 T3.
Duration of follow-up	mean=7.1 yrs; follow-up every 3-4 months for 2 yrs after XRT, then every 6 months
Other Eligibility Criteria	No patient rec'vd hormonal therapy or chemo before evid of progression.
Outcome Definitions	Clinical local control (CLC), disease-specific survival (DSS), & survival after XRT were the outcomes. Clinical local recurrence defined as enlarging nodule or area of induration det. by DRE. Initiation of XRT the start patient for survival curves.
Method of Survival Analysis	Actuarial method of Kaplan & Meier out 25 yrs. For DSS pts censored at last follow-up or time of intercurrent death. For CLC cases scored as events at time of relapse, or censored at death or last follow-up. Gehan stat to test sig diff between patient groups.
Survival Curves	CLC for T1avs T1b,T1c,&T1d and T1 vs T2 vs T3. DSS for T1,T2,T3 with or without clin local recurrence(CLR). Surv for T1,T2,T3 with or without CLR. DSS for T1,T2,T3 without CLR, with or without pos transrectal biopsy (PTRB).
Statistical Estimates Related to Survival Analyses	Survival for T1,T2,T3 without CLR with or without PTRB. Discuss 10 and 15 yr rates. E.g., DSS in t1 pts with clin local recurrence was 52.4% +/-7.7% at 10 yrs.
Other outcomes/Results	PSA and post-irradiation biopsy. Status (NED, local relapse, distant metasatsis) of biopsy pos cases. Trend of PSA level and biopsy results for selected pts for whom serial PSA values were available.

Kaplan and Bagshaw. Serum prostate-specific antigen after post-prostatectomy radiotherapy. Urology, 1992.	
Treatment modality	XRT after radical prostatectomy
Site	Stanford University Hospital, Stanford, CA and its satellite facility
Study design	Reporting on the 39 post-prostatectomy pts who were subsequently treated with XRT between 1985- 1991
Sample Size	39
Accrual dates	1985-1991
Patient age	Mean at time of XRT=65; range=46-78
Duration of follow-up	Time between surgery and XRT range=6 wks-7 yrs. In 20 pts XRT begun within 6 months, in 19 XRT after >6months. Exams every 3-4 months after XRT
Other Patient characteristics	Define 3 risk groups bases on PSA level and changes in PSA (see Table III)
Other Eligibility Criteria	Table I provides no. of pts who had det/undet PSA, neg DRE, local tumor recurrence, pos margins, pos seminal vesicles, pos node, Gleason category. Table II describes dose to pelvis and prostatic fossa.
Outcome Definitions	"Outcomes" ltd to changes in PSA level over time. Table IV reviews the incidence of surgical upstaging in the literature. Table V reviews the results of post-radical prostatectomy radiotherapy , including % local tumor control and DFS (year varies).
Other outcomes/Results	PSA trend (log PSA) after postrad prostatectomy irradiation for low risk, 3 indeterminate risk pts, 4 high-risk pts

Appendix B. Outcomes Literature Table: Radiation Therapy

Kaplan et al. Radiotherapy for prostatic cancer: Pt selection and the impact of local control. Urology, 1994.	
Treatment modality	XRT
Site	Dept. of XRT at Stanford University, Stanford, CA
Study design	They identified a group of 178 pts from 1,118 pts who rec'vd XRT between 1956-1990.
Sample Size	54 <60 yrs with Stanford stage T1a&b (B1) vs 75 60-70 yrs with similar stage; 17 lymph node dissection T1a&b N0M0 (B1) vs 30 T3N0M0 (C)
Accrual dates	1956-1990
Patient stage	Stanford T1a, T1b, T3. Table 1 provides urologic stage equivalents (A-C)
Patient age	Comparison among <60 and 60-70
Duration of follow-up	follow-up every 3-4 months after XRT for 2 yrs and then every 6 months for 5 yrs, then yearly. mean and median=10.2 & 9.8 yrs; range=0.25-18.6 for T3N0 pts.
Other Patient characteristics	Gleason score (3-5, 6-7, 8-10, unknown)
Outcome Definitions	Local control: absence of recurrence det. by DRE. Pts scored as events at time of local relapse, or censored at last follow-up or death. For metastatic control, pts scored as events at time of metastatic relapse or censored at time of last follow-up or death. For cause-specific survival, pts scored as events at time of death dur to prostate CA, or censored at time of last follow-up or intercurrent death. For survival, pts scored as events at time of death due to any cause or censored at time of last follow-up.
Method of Survival Analysis	Actuarial method of Kaplan and Meier. Sig diffs between groups analyzed using Wilcoxon method Gehan.
Survival Curves	(a) Metastatic control and (b) clinical local control for T1a&b, younger vs older. Cause-specific, expected, and overall survival for T1a&b, (a) young vs (b) older. Curves out 25 yrs. Figures also show (a) clin local control, (b) metastatic control, (c) cause-specific survival, and (d) survival for surgically staged node neg pts T1a+b N0 vs T3N0. Curves out 15 yrs.
Statistical Estimates Related to Survival Analyses	Figures report multiple rates. E.g., Rates of local control at 10, 15, and 20 yrs were 94.1+/-3.3%, 87.0+/-5.0%, and 87.0+/-5.0%, respectively, for pts <60 and 95.1+/-2.8%, 90.8+/-4.0%, and 83.2+/-5.6%, respectively for 60-70 (p=0.89).

Kavadi et al. Serum prostate-specific antigen after XRT for clinically localized prostate CA: Prognostic implications. Int J Rad Onocl Biol Phys, 1994.	
Treatment modality	Definitive XRT
Site	MD Anderson Cancer Center, Houston, TX
Study design	Reporting on group of pts who had XRT as sole initial treatment and had pre-tx and posttx PSA values.
Sample Size	427
Accrual dates	1987-1991
Patient stage	Clinical stages: 122 T1, 147 T2, 152 T3, 6 T4
Patient age	mean=median=68; range=47-84
Duration of follow-up	mean=33 months; median=30 months; range=9-73 months; 8 pts followed <1year; follow-up every 3 months
Other Patient characteristics	Distribution. of Gleason score
Univar/Multiv Analyses (Covariates)	Proportional hazards model with log-linear relative hazard function. Sequential PSA changes eval using paired t-test on log PSA values. Data not shown, but summarized
Outcome Definitions	Incidence of clinical relapse, which can be represented by rising PSA.
Method of Survival Analysis	Actuariral curves using the Berkson-Gage and Kaplan-Meier methods. Log rank to test sig Curves plotted only for time intervals where >8 pts at risk.
Survival Curves	Incidence of relapse or rising PSA according to nadir PSA (nPSA; 4 groups); p<0.00001 Incidence of relapse or rising PSA according to nPSA, all<1.0 (N=182 pts);trended p=0.308. Both out 60 months. after XRT.

210

Kearsley JH. High-dose radiotherapy for localized prostatic cancer: An analysis fo treatment results and early complications. Med J Australia, 1986.

Treatment modality	Definitive high-dose XRT within 6 months diagnosis
Site	Queensland Radium Institute, Brisbane, AUSTRALIA
Study design	Retrospective analysis of medical records
Sample Size	477 consecutive pts
Accrual dates	1970-1983 (inclusive)
Patient stage	T0-T4
Patient age	mean=64.4; range=45-88
Method of Survival Analysis	5 and 10 year actuarial survival rates.
Other outcomes/Results	Some local recurrence and failure rates; early complications.

Keisch et al. Preliminary report on 10 pts treated w/radiotherapy after radical prostectomy for isolated elevation of serum PSA levels. Int J Rad Oncol Biol Phys, 1990.

Treatment modality	XRT for persistently elev PSA after prostatectomy
Site	Radiation Oncology Center, Mallinckrodt Institute of Radiology, Washington University Medical Center, St. Louis, MO
Study design	Identified pts with persistently elev PSA 3-43 months post-prostatectomy who then received irradiation to limited pelvic volume
Sample Size	10
Accrual dates	1987 - 1990
Patient stage	preop A2-B2; postop A2-C2
Patient age	mean=63.4; range=45-72
Duration of follow-up	time since XRT ranges from 1-10 months
Other Patient characteristics	One patient rec'vd adj hormonal therapy (megesteral acetate) following comopletion of XRT for cont rising PSA levels. Provide grade, acid phosphatase, margin info.
Other Eligibility Criteria	All pts had radical prostatectomy with staging lymphadenectomy at initial tx. None had previous irradiation. None had any pos finding other than PSA elev.
Outcome Definitions	NO OUTCOMES. Report is descriptive, providing PSA levels over time.

Kuban et al. The effect of TURP on prognosis in prostatic carcinoma. Int J Rad Oncol Biol Phys. 1987

Treatment modality	Definitive XRT
Site	Department of Radiation Oncology and Biophysics, Eastern Virgina Medical School, Norfolk, VA
Study design	Identified those pts treated with definitive XRT and had min follow-up 4 yrs. 287 or 533 pts treated between 1976-1986.
Sample Size	287; 162 TURP 4-6 wks prior to XRT; 125 no TURP
Accrual dates	1976-1986
Patient stage	staged using Fowler-Whitmore (A-D) det by DRE
Patient age	mean=66; range=48-85
Duration of follow-up	median=59 months; min 4 yrs
Other Patient characteristics	Histologically graded by modified Gleason (well diff, mode-well diff, poorly diff)
Other Eligibility Criteria	Wanted to look at those with TURP (162) and those without (125).
Outcome Definitions	Local recurrence: progressive, prostatic enlargement, induration, or asymmetry on serial DRE with histologic confirmation by rebiopsy in all equivocal cases.
Method of Survival Analysis	Berkson-Gage method; curves out 5 yrs. Chi square and Fisher's exact tests.
Survival Curves	Actuarial survival by stage (B2,C) with and without TURP. Actuarial survival by tumor grade, with and without TURP. Actuarial survival with and without local recurrence and with and without TURP.
Statistical Estimates Related to Survival Analyses	5 year rates reported. E.g., 68% vs 38% 5-year survival for stage C pts, No TURP vs TURP (p=0.003).
Other outcomes/Results	Comparison of incidence of bony metastasis with or without TURP by stage (p value), Table 3. by grade. Similar tables for local recurrence and combination of 2

Kuban et al. The significance of post-irradiation prostate biopsy w/long-term follow-up. Int J Rad Oncol Biol Phys, 1992.

Treatment modality	Definitive XRT or 125I interstitial implantation
Site	Eastern VA Medical School, Norfolk, VA
Study design	Reviewing cases from 1975-1981
Sample Size	309; 200 XRT, 109 implants; 94 biopsy and studied here (55 implants, 39 XRT)
Accrual dates	1975-1981
Patient stage	A2-C
Duration of follow-up	range=26-14.5 yrs
Other Patient characteristics	Histologically graded according to modified Gleason (well diff, mode-well diff, poorly diff)
Outcome Definitions	Clin local failure: progr. prostatic induration, nodularity, incr size of asymmetry, or obstructive sx at ureterovesical junction or bladder outlet. Clin suspicion conf. by biopsy. Distant failure: bone scan or other diag. study. Hormonal tx only used only after documentation of tx failure.
Method of Survival Analysis	Kaplan-Meier use to calc. LF and DFS. Lee-Desu stat applied to assess diffs in outcomes. Sig diffs in proportions tested using Chi-square and Fisher's exact.
Survival Curves	Clin local failure , pos vs neg biopsy. DFS, pos vs neg biopsy. Out 12 yrs.
Statistical Estimates Related to Survival Analyses	Usually 5 and 10 year discussed. E.G., Actuarially, local failure at 5 & 10 yrs was 8% and 24%, resp., in the biopsy neg group with median survival=152 months and 44% and 75%, resp., with median survival=72 months for biopsy-pos group (p=0.0001).

Lai et al. Prognostic significance of pelvic recurrence and distant metastasis in prostate carcinoma following definitive radiotherapy. Int J Rad Oncol Biol Phys, 1992

Treatment modality	Definitive radiotherapy, but since looking at recurrent cases only, 2/3 pts rec'vd hormones, including bilateral orchiectomy.
Site	Radiation Oncology Center, Mallinkrodt Institute of Radiology, and affiliate hospitals,Washington University School of Medicine, St. Louis, MO
Study design	Retrospective analysis of 317 pts with recurrent prostate carcinoma, following definitive XRT to 738 pts with histologically confirmed, clin stage T1b-T4(A2-D1) adenocarcinoma of the prostate The study in this paper also required: (1) min dose at least 6500 cGy, (2) no endocrine tx
Sample Size	317
Accrual dates	1967-1988
Patient stage	T1b-T4 (A2-D1). Initially staged AUA, and gives corresponding ACJ-TNM. See p. 424 for specific note about D1(T4).
Patient age	median=67; range=42-82
Duration of follow-up	median=6 yrs
Univar/Multiv Analyses (Covariates)	Mantel-cox used to test for potentially sig factors for survival.
Outcome Definitions	Time of recurrence is the disease-free interval from initial tx.
Method of Survival Analysis	Actuarial life table as applied by Cutler and Ederer. curves out to 10 yrs. Variety of test stats and trend analysis.
Survival Curves	Prob pelvic recurrence by stage. Cumulative time course of recurrence by site. Overall survival with recurrent CA after XRT. Cause specific surv, stage T1b&T2, T3. Surv by site of recurrence, stage T1b&T2, T3.
Statistical Estimates Related to Survival Analyses	Table provides 5-year NED survival and pattern of failure (pelvic, pelvic & distant metastasis, distant metastasis). Report 5, 8, and 10-year rates in text.

Lai et al. The effect of overall tx time on the outcome of definitive radiotherapy for localized prostate CA: The XRT oncology group 75-06 and 77-06 experience. Int J Rad Oncol Biol Phys, 1991

Treatment modality	Pelvic and prophylactic periaortic irradiation Elective pelvic irradiation in pts without evid of spread beyond prostate
Site	2 prospective studies of the RTOG
Study design	RTOG 75-06. Aim to test the value of pelvic and prophylactic periaortic irradiation in pts in whom there was evid of tumor extension beyond the prostate, but ltd to pelvis RTOG 77-06. Aim to test the value of elective pelvic irradiation in pts without evid of spread beyond the prostate (T1b(A2) & T2(B)) and no evid of lymph node involvement (LAG or LAP) The study in this paper also required: (1) min dose at least 6500 cGy, (2) no endocrine tx
Sample Size	607; 484; 1091 from 2 studies; 780 eligible
Accrual dates	1976- 1983 & 1978-1983
Patient stage	T1b, T2, T3,4
Duration of follow-up	median=9 yrs; 6 yrs 5 months-13 yrs 3 months
Other Patient characteristics	Pts divided into 3 groups based on total # elapsed days while on tx: within 49 days; 50-63 days; >=64 days. Distribution of pts by stage, Gleason, and XRT duration
Other Eligibility Criteria	Stage T3,4(C) were eligible whether or not pelvic lymph nodes involved. Stage T1b(A2) and T2(B) were eligible only if there was pelvic lymph node involvement conf. by LAG or histologically. Evaluation of regional lymphatics was mandatory Pts divided into 3 groups based on total # elapsed days while on tx: within 49 days; 50-63 days; >=64 days. Distribution of pts by stage, Gleason score, and XRTduration
Survival Curves	Survival from time of recurrence by disease-free interval from initial tx: (a) pelvic recurrence only, (b) pelvic recurrence and distant metastasis, (c) distant metastasis only. Actuarial Kaplan-Meier analysis. Comparisons made using log-rank or Mantel-Haenszel. See p. 927, "Details of protocol design, work-up, patient char, stratification criteria, part. institutions, XRT tech, and endpts have been reported."
Statistical Estimates Related to Survival Analyses	Overall survival by stage. NED survival by stage. Local/regional control by stage. Local/regional control by Gleason score group (2-5,6-7,8-10). Curves out 10 yrs.
Other outcomes/Results	Incidence of tx-related GI or GU complications. Further analyzed local/regional failure by stage and Gleason score using scatterplots.

Movsas et al. Analyzing predictive models following definitive radiotherapy for prostate carcinoma. Cancer, 1997

Treatment modality	Definitive XRT
Site	Fox Chase Cancer Center, Phildelphia, PA
Study design	Retrospective analysis of 551 pts with clin localized prostate CA that rec'vd XRT. Id 421 that had sufficient info. to calc. several values that are part of their models. Purpose to predict outcome accurately following XRT.
Sample Size	421
Accrual dates	1988-1994
Patient stage	332 T1-T2ab, 89 T2c+
Duration of follow-up	median=34 months; range=2-87; all cont. monitored at 3 to 6 months intervals; no pts lost to follow-up
Univar/Multiv Analyses (Covariates)	Estimated 6 different models. The std model is a multivar Cox proportional hazard analysis using the forward stepwise log rank test of assoc of the covars: PSA density, pre-tx PSA, dose, Gleason, palpation stage, perineural invasion.
Outcome Definitions	Biochemical failure: PSA >=1.5 and rising in 2 consec values. Pts free of clin and PSA evid of dx were termed bNED. Follow-up calculated from 1st day of radiotherapy
Method of Survival Analysis	Kaplan-Meier product-limit method.
Survival Curves	bNED control rates according to the risk breakpts of Pisansky et al. Curve out to 60 months from onset of tx. No. at risk given for each year. P-value provided for 3 risk groups

O'Dowd et al. Update on the appropriate staging evaluation for newly diagnosed prostate CA. J Urology, 1997.

Study design	Searched MEDLINE. Refs. selected compared results of the clin staging method being eval to the path staging outcomes of RP or pelvic lymphadenectomy
Sample Size	140 articles
Accrual dates	1975-1997
Outcome Definitions	NO OUTCOMES. Purpose to predict path stage.

Perez et al. Factors influencing outcome of definitive radiotherapy for localized carcinoma of the prostate. Radio and Oncol, 1989

Treatment modality	Definitive XRT
Site	Mallinckrodt Institute of Radiology Radiation Oncology Center and affiliated hospitals, St. Louis, MO
Study design	577 pts with histologically proven adenocarcinoma of the prostate localized to the pelvis and treated with XRT
Sample Size	577
Accrual dates	1967-1983
Patient stage	A2,B,C, D1
Patient age	Number in each age category (<=60,>60) for each stage
Duration of follow-up	median=6.5 yrs; min=3
Other Patient characteristics	Degree of differentiation (4 categories). Some pts recv'd hormones
Univar/Multiv Analyses (Covariates)	Mantel-Cox use to test for potentially sig factors for survival
Outcome Definitions	Actuarial survival, disease-free survival (NED)
Method of Survival Analysis	Actuarial life table as applied by Cutler and Ederer
Survival Curves	Several figures out to 10 yrs of actuarial survival and NED survival by stage, histological grade, race. Also surv after failure/recurrence.
Statistical Estimates Related to Survival Analyses	Several tables report the 5-year actuarial and NED survival rate

Perez et al. Technical and tumor-related factors affecting outcome of definitive irradiation for localized carcinoma of the prostate. Int J Rad Oncol Biol Phys, 1993

Treatment modality	Definitive XRT
Site	Mallinckrodt Institute of Radiology Radiation Oncology Center and affiliated hospitals, St. Louis, MO
Study design	Retrospective analysis of records. Pts had histologically proven adenocarcinoma of the prostate localized to the pelvis and treated with XRT
Sample Size	738
Accrual dates	1967-1988
Patient stage	A2(T1b), B(T2), C(T3), D1(T4)
Patient age	
Duration of follow-up	median=6.5 yrs;range=3-22; follow-up obtained for 98%
Other Patient characteristics	Causes of death
Univar/Multiv Analyses (Covariates)	Mantel-Cox use to test for potentially sig factors for survival. Multivar analysis of clin stage, hist grade, TURP, diefld size, central axis tumor does, lymph nodes tx, CT scan tx, LND
Outcome Definitions	Disease-free survival (DFS), pelvic failure rate
Method of Survival Analysis	Actuarial life table as applied by Cutler and Ederer
Survival Curves	Several figures of actuarial pelvic failure rate out to 10 yrs.
Statistical Estimates Related to Survival Analyses	DFS at 5 yrs was 76% for A2 and B, 57% for C, and 20% for D1. Corresponding rates at 10 yrs were 62%, 38%, and 0%, respectively. Actuarial surv 5-10% higher b/c pts survived for several yrs after recur.
Other outcomes/Results	Annual incidence of distant metastases correlated with pelvic tumor control/failure for A2&B, and C

Perez et al. Definitive XRT in carcinoma of the prostate localized to the Pelvis: Experience at the mallinckrodt institute of radiology. NCI Monographs, 1988. SAME PTS AS PEREZ ET AL. 1989

Treatment modality	Definitive XRT
Site	Mallinckrodt Institute of Radiology Radiation Oncology Center and affiliated hospitals, St. Louis, MO
Study design	577 pts with histologically proven adenocarcinoma of the prostate localized to the pelvis and treated with XRT
Sample Size	577
Accrual dates	1967-1983
Patient stage	A2,B,C, D1
Duration of follow-up	median=6.5 yrs; min=3; follow-up obtained for 98%
Other Patient characteristics	Degree of differentiation (4 categories). Some pts recv'd hormones
Method of Survival Analysis	Actuarial life table as applied by Cutler and Ederer. Curves out 10 yrs.
Survival Curves	Tumor-free actuarial (NED) surv by stage for 577 pts. Actuarial and NED surv for 185 stage B pts (a) & 328 stage C(b) & comparison with normal life expectancy. Tumor-free actuarial surv by hist grade for B & C dx. Relapse free actuarial surv by lymph node status (-/+) in 37 B and 38 C pts. Actuarial surv after failure for pts with B and C cancer. Tumor-free surv for B and C pts correlated with concomitant hormonal tx.
Statistical Estimates Related to Survival Analyses	5-year direct surv and % adj surv. 10 y direct surv and % adj survr.
Incontinence	Major definitive complications from XRT in 577 pts. Minor definitive complix from XRT in 577 pts

Peschel et al. The effects of advanced age on the efficacy of XRT for early breast cancer, local prostate cancer and grade III-IV gliomas. Int J Rad Oncol Biol Phys, s1993

Treatment modality	XRT
Site	Yale University School of Medicine Therapeutic Radiology Program, New Haven, CT
Study design	Retrospective analysis of XRT charts
Sample Size	294
Accrual dates	1975-1990
Patient stage	A2,B,C
Other Patient characteristics	Divide into <70 (NGCP) and >=70 (GCP) groups for analysis
Method of Survival Analysis	Life table method used to calc actuarial overall survival rates, cause specific disease-free (NED) survival rates, and local control rates with assoc std errors.
Survival Curves	None
Statistical Estimates Related to Survival Analyses	Table provides the 5 and 10 year NED and overall survival rates for the NGCP and GCP groups. Table provides the 5 and 10 year NED surv rates for the NGCP and GCP groups by stage.

Pilepich MV. XRT oncology group studies in carcinoma of the prostate. NCI monographs, 1988. SEE LAI ET AL.

Treatment modality	XRT
Site	XRT Oncology Group (RTOG)
Study design	RTOG 75-06; RTOG 77-06
Sample Size	607 accrued; 566 analyzable; 484 accrued; 444 analyzable
Accrual dates	1976-1983 & 1978-1983
Patient stage	3 A2, 63 B, 500 C; 84 A2, 360 B
Outcome Definitions	Largely a report on tx-related morbidity using a grading system from 1 (minor sx requiring no tx) to 5 (fatal).
Method of Survival Analysis	
Survival Curves	Incidence of local-regional recur as a fn of tumor size expressed as product of tumor dimensions.
Incontinence	Table 2. Summary of tx-related morbidity. Graphs of the pattern of resolution of proctitis, diarrhea, and cystitis.
Other outcomes/Results	Correlation of prostate boost dose and incidence of diarrhea and incidence of rectal bleeding.

Pilepich et al. Phase III trail of androgen suppression using goserelin in unfavorable-prognosis carcinoma of the prostate tx w/definitive XRT: Report of RTOG 85-31. J Clin Oncol, 1997

Treatment modality	Adjuvant goserelin in definitively irradiated pts. About 15% of each arm had RP as well.
Site	RTOG
Study design	RTOG 85-31 was designed to eval the relative effectiveness of elective (adjuvant) vs therapeutic androgen suppression with goserelin on dx progression and survival in a hi risk pop.
Sample Size	977 accrued; 488 adj G; 489 observation
Accrual dates	1987-1992
Patient stage	T3 or T1&2 if radiographic or histologic evid of spread to reional lymph nodes
Other Patient characteristics	Gleason, nodal status, acid phosphatase, prostatectomy
Univar/Multiv Analyses (Covariates)	Interaction between Gleason sum & tx for local failure, time to distant metastases, NED surv, and absolute surv tested using Cox proportional hazards regression.
Outcome Definitions	Disease-free surv (NED) : absence of local or reg. failure or distant mestases, PSA failure. Local failure: persistance of palpable tumor >24 months after entry, reappearance of palpable tumor, or biopsy-proven CA >=2yrs after entry.
Method of Survival Analysis	NED and absolute survival estimated according to Kaplan-Meier method. Log -rank test.
Survival Curves	15 figures with curves out 7 yrs from date of randomization.
Statistical Estimates Related to Survival Analyses	Summary of efficacy end points (provides the estimated 5-year rate for local failure, distant metastatses, NED surv, NED surv with PSA<4, NED surv with PSA<1.5, and absolute surv) as well as p values for the 2 tx arms.

Pilepich and Hederman. Prognostic significance of the pattern of tumor regression following definitive radiotherapy for carcinoma of the prostate. Am J Clin Oncol, 1986.

Site	Div of Radiation Oncology, Washington University School of Medicine in St. Louis, MO
Study design	Retrospective analysis of pts meeting the following criteria: definitive tx given (min 6,000 rad), palpable tumor present at initial visit, 3 yrs min follow-up
Sample Size	262
Accrual dates	1967-1981
Patient stage	B1, B2, C1, C2
Duration of follow-up	median=51.6 months; min=36 months; seen every 3 months 1st year; every 3-4 months 2nd year; 2x 3rd, 4th, 5th year; once a year thereafter
Other Eligibility Criteria	Excluded postprostatectomy pts and stage A
Outcome Definitions	Pattern of tumonthr response: (1) degree of tumor regression at 90 d after end of tx, expressed as %tumor size, (2) time to complete regression. Endpts: tumor control, patterns of relapse, disease-free (NED) survival. Local failure: progression of clin detect. dx or biopsy-proven tumor beyond 2nd year. Pts who developed distant metastases as the 1st site of failure were censored from locoregional control analyses.
Survival Curves	Several figures of the time to complete resolution of the palpable tumor and the incidence of locoregional failure
Statistical Estimates Related to Survival Analyses	Tumor regression at 90 days by stage and histological grade. Tables 3&4. Sites of failiure by regression at 90 days

Pilepich et al. Phase II RTOG study of hormonal cytoreduction w/flutamide and zoladex in locally advanced carcinoma of the prostate treated w/definitive radiotherapy. Am J Clin Oncol, 1990

Treatment modality	Hormonal cytoreduction (induction regimen) using goseralin (LH-RH agonist) and flutamide (anitandrogen) and XRT initiated 2 months after drug administration
Site	RTOG
Study design	The primary aim of RTOG 85-19 was to evalute the effectiveness and toxicity of the combined (hormonal cytoreduction+definitive radiotherapy) regimen.
Sample Size	31 accessioned; 30 analyzable
Accrual dates	1986-1986
Patient stage	8 T2(B), 22 T3(C)
Other Patient characteristics	Table 1. Histological grade (well, mod, poor). Nodal Status (4 pos, 26 neg). Method of Nodal evaluation (laparotomy, lyphagiogram, CT scan)
Other Eligibility Criteria	KPS >=60; pts with evid of distant metastasis, hx of previous or concurrent CA other than basal ceel carcinoma were not eligible. Pts w.involved para-aortic lymph nodes were not eligible.
Outcome Definitions	Not really a study of XRT and no XRT related outcomes.
Other outcomes/Results	Table 4. DRUG-related morbidity. Diarrhea a side effect of XRT. 2 pts died the 1st year & had palpable abn at last follow-up. Tumor clearance (according DRE) was observed in all other pts. No local failures. 2 pts had DM. 3 died of non-CA-related causes.

Pilepich et al. Extended field (periaortic) irradiation in carcinoma of the prostate- analysis of RTOG 75-06. Int J Rad Oncol Biol Phys, 1986.

Treatment modality	Extended field XRT
Site	RTOG
Study design	The aim of RTOG 75-06 was to test the value of elective periaortic irradiation in pts with locally advanced disease, clinically confined to the pelvis.
Sample Size	607 entered; 523 analyzable; 448 known to have rec'vd tx per protocol
Accrual dates	1976-1983
Patient stage	A2, B, C
Duration of follow-up	median=4 yrs and 3 mos
Other Eligibility Criteria	Stage C pts without lymph node involvement & those with A2 or B with evid of lymph node involvement were eliglble. Pts with lymph node involvement beyond pelvis, previous XRT or curative prostatic surgery, previous or concurrent CA other than skin were not eligible.
Outcome Definitions	Incidence of distant metastases, NED survival, and survival for pelvic tx vs extended field tx. Fail=death or relapse.
Method of Survival Analysis	Kaplan-Meier with comparison of tx arms (pelvic field vs extended field) by Mantel-Haenszel. All curves out 96 months from onset of tx
Survival Curves	Incidence of distant metastases (p=ns). Survival (p=ns). Disease-free survival (p=ns)
Statistical Estimates Related to Survival Analyses	Tx comparisons (N=523). Tx comparisons (N=448). Tx comparisons by grade, hormonal tx, Gleason, stage, age, TURP, and nodal status (C only). Each table gives the 3 & 5 year rate, Failures/total for each group (with p-values).

217

Appendix B. Outcomes Literature Table: Radiation Therapy

Pilepich et al. Androgen deprivation w/XRT compared w/XRT alone for locally advanced prostatic carcinoma: A randomized comparative trial of the XRT oncology group. Urology, 1995.	
Treatment modality	Goserelin and flutamide 2 months before and during XRT vs XRT alone
Site	RTOG
Study design	The study was designed to test the potential value of a combination of goserelin acetate (LHRH analogue), and flutamide (antiandrogen), used as cytoreductive agents prior to and during XRT in locally adv (bulky) carcinoma of the prostate
Sample Size	471 enrolled; 456 analyzable; 226 on tx and 230 controls
Accrual dates	1987-1991
Patient stage	T2b, T2c (B2) and T3, T4 (C)
Patient age	median=70 , range=50-88 (hormone+XRT); median=71, range=49-84 (XRT alone)
Duration of follow-up	median potential follow-up=4.5 yrs
Other Patient characteristics	Pre-tx char (age, KPS, differentiation, Gleason, nodal status, acid phosphatase, stage)
Other Eligibility Criteria	No evid of osseous metastasis
Outcome Definitions	Local control rates, progression-free survival, and survival. Local progression (LP): PSA>4 at 1 year or more from rand. or addt'l hormone tx in absence of metastasis., incr o f>50% in tumor size, recurrence of palpable tumor, pos biopsy >=2 yrs after entry. Regional metastasis (RM): clin or rad evid of tumor in pelvis with or without palpable tumor (DRE). Distant metastasis (DM): clin or rad evid of dx beyond pelvis. Failure in progress-free surv: failure in surv, local progress, or RM or DM.
Method of Survival Analysis	Kaplan-Meier method with comparisons using the log-rank stat in the case of censored data or by the proportional hazards model. Stat comparisons for cum incid of local progression or DM made using Gray's test. Curves out 5 yrs.
Survival Curves	Cumulative incidence of LP by Tx group; Cumulative incidence of DM by Tx group; Progress-free surv by Tx group; Surv by Tx group (p value provided for all figures and no. at risk at each year)
Statistical Estimates Related to Survival Analyses	5-year rates and p values of differences between tx arms discussed. E.g., the cum inc of local progression at 5 yrs was 46% for the hormone+XRT group and 71% for the XRT alone group (p<0.001).
Impotence	There was no diff in freq or time of return to sexual potency in the tx groups
Other outcomes/Results	Summary of toxicities presented

Pisansky et al. An enhanced prognostic system for clinically localized carcinoma of the prostate. Cancer, 1997.	
Treatment modality	XRT alone
Site	Mayo Clinic, Rochester, MN
Study design	Reporting on pts treated exclusively with external beam XRT. Purpose to develop criteria to be used to id prognostic groupings based on independent covars predictive of clin relapse or any relapse
Sample Size	500
Accrual dates	1987-1993
Patient stage	T1-4, N0 or NX, M0 CaP
Duration of follow-up	median=43 mos; mean=46; range=4-103; every 3-4 months for 2 yrs; 6-12 months thereafter
Other Patient characteristics	Had pretherapy PSA determinations and Gleason grading applied to biopsy
Other Eligibility Criteria	Pts treated with androgen deprivation before or during XRT and postprostatectomy were excluded.
Univar/Multiv Analyses (Covariates)	Logistic regression for estimation of risk score. The prob of any relapse within 5 yrs was estimated as a function of pretherapy factors using logistic reg. Both jackknife and split-sample cross-validation were used to develop and validate the models.
Outcome Definitions	Sites of initial tumor relapse were classified as local (prostate or contig tissues), regional nodal, or distant). Local tumor recurrence: primary tumor regrowth (serial DRE). Simultaneous locoreg & distant relapse was classified distant. Biochem relapse: 2 or more consec PSA that rose >=1 from posttx nadir PSA without subsequent spontaneous decline)
Method of Survival Analysis	Kaplan-Meier. Time intervals were measured from XRT initiation date to the date of event under consideration.
Survival Curves	Freedom from any relapse according to risk group (out 6 yrs)
Statistical Estimates Related to Survival Analyses	Multivar logistic reg of pre-tx factors assoc with disease relapse within 5 yrs (stage, Gleason, OSA). Risk of relapse within 5 yrs of RT for localized CaP according to prognostic group. (#,%,95%CI, p value)
Other outcomes/Results	Probability of any relapse within 5 yrs of XRT according to comb. of tumor stage & Gleason as fn of pre-tx PSA.

Pisansky et al. A multiple prognostic index predictive of disease outcome after irradiation for clinically localized prostate carcinoma. Cancer, 1997.

Treatment modality	XRT alone
Site	Mayo Clinic, Rochester, MN
Study design	Same group as above
Sample Size	500
Accrual dates	1987-1993
Patient stage	T1-4, N0 or NX, M0 CaP
Patient age	median=74; range=56-84
Duration of follow-up	median=43 mos; mean=46; range=4-103; every 3-4 months for 2 yrs; 6-12 months thereafter
Other Patient characteristics	Had pretherapy PSA determinations and Gleason grading applied to biopsy
Other Eligibility Criteria	Pts treated with androgen deprivation before or during XRT and postprostatectomy were excluded.
Univar/Multiv Analyses (Covariates)	Table 3. Multivar logistic regression of pretherapy factors assoc with any disease relapse within 5 yrs (RR, 95% CI, p value).
Outcome Definitions	Any relapse: clinical or biochemical.
Method of Survival Analysis	Kaplan-Meier analysis of outcomes for the entire study group. Time intervals were measured from XRT initiation date to the date of event under consideration.
Survival Curves	Overall survival and clin relapse-free and any relapse-free estimates. The figure provides the 3 curves (no numbers) out 6 yrs.
Statistical Estimates Related to Survival Analyses	Univar analysis of pretherapy factors assoc with disease relapse (clinical; any) within 5 yrs. Table gives the # pts, %, and p value for diffs between groups (stage, Gleason, PSA, elective nodal radiation)
Other outcomes/Results	Risk of any relapse within 5 yrs according to pre-tx PSA and Gleason for (2) T1a-2a pts, (3) T2b-c pts, (4) T3-4

Ploysongsang et al. Comparison of whole pelvis vs small-field XRT for carcinoma of prostate. Urology, 1986

Treatment modality	XRT to whole pelvis and boost to prostate
Site	Christ Hospital, Good Samaritan Hospital, and University Hospital in Cincinnati, OH
Study design	Reporting on pts evaluated and treated in the department of radiation oncology at 3 hospitals over an 8 year time period.
Sample Size	136
Accrual dates	1975-1983
Patient stage	A2-D2
Patient age	1 40-49; 20 50-59; 73 60-69; 38 70-79; 4 >80 at diagnosis
Duration of follow-up	median=32 mos; range=6 months to 8 yrs; 18 pts lost to follow-up
Other Patient characteristics	91 TURP; 41 Needle Biopsy; 1 patient suprapubic prostatectomy prior to XRT; 26 received DES
Outcome Definitions	Failure: local (progressive enlarge. of primary prostate CA with or without histologic confirm, lymph node enlarge. in pelvis) or systemic (bone, lung, or other soft tissue metastases). Routine biopsies not performed after tx.
Method of Survival Analysis	Overall and disease-free surv calc using actuarial or life table methods out 5 yrs.
Survival Curves	Survival by stage (A2,B1,B2; C; D). Disease-free surv by stage (A2; B1,B2; C, D). E.g., 5-year actuariral DFS for A2 100%; B1&B2 76%, C 42%, D1&D2 28%.
Statistical Estimates Related to Survival Analyses	Surv (5-year) and pattern of failure by mode of diagnosis(TUR vs PNBX) in Stage C. Compar. prostatic irrad vs whole pelvis & boost (% DFS at 3 yrs, overall surv at 5 yrs, local control)
Incontinence	Radiation reaction (e.g., % cystitis, incontinence, diarrhea) in relation to sequence of boost XRT

Pollack et al. Relationship of tumor DNA-ploidy to serum PSA doubling time after radiotherapy for prostate CA. Urology, 1994.	
Treatment modality	Definitive XRT
Site	MD Anderson Cancer Center, Houston, TX
Study design	Identified the pts treated with definitive XRT who had adequate formalin-fixed paraffin-embedded tissues for flow cytometry. Purpose to examine prognostic ability of DNA ploidy and the relationship to PSA-DT, another prognostic indicator.
Sample Size	76 out of a possible 314, but only 24 had sufficient info to calc PSA doubling times (PSA-DT)
Accrual dates	1987-1991
Patient stage	6 T1b, 2 T2a, 2 T2b, 1 T2c, 3 T3a, and 10 T3c; stages T1 and T2 pooled for analyses
Patient age	Whole group (n=76): mean=67.3, median=68; PSA-DT (n=24) median=66
Duration of follow-up	Whole group: median=37 mos, range=18-68 and PSA-DT: median=45; range=24-66; follow-up at 3 monthintervals
Other Eligibility Criteria	314 pts comprised this cohort, tissue blocks for flow cytometry obt from 50%, approx 25% had sufficient material. Of these 76, 27 had rising PSA, and sufficient info to calc OSA-DT in 24.
Univar/Multiv Analyses (Covariates)	Correlation of PSA-DT with different parameters (stage, grade, pre-tx PSA, ploidy, local relapse, metatstases, any relapse; p value provided). Actuarial analyses by 2 groups (PSA-DT <=10 mos; PSA-DT >10)
Outcome Definitions	Free of dx until clin or radiographic evid of local or metastatic failure. Local control: palapble normal prostate or biopsy prompted by rising PSA is neg. Biopsy conf of local recurrence obt in all pts scored as having failure locally. Post-tx rising PSA: 2 or more consec values that incr and with last value >1. Onset of PSA rise: ave time between nadir PSA and 1st elevated.
Method of Survival Analysis	Actuarial curves calc using the Berkson-Gage method. Actuarial calculations begun at completion of radiotherapy out 40 months.
Survival Curves	(A) Actuarial local control, (B) Freedom from metastases, and (C) Disease freedom. Actuarial disease freedom in pts having nondiplod tumors by PSA-DT (<=10 (n=11) vs >10 (n=3). (p<0.05 using log-rank).
Statistical Estimates Related to Survival Analyses	Minimal discussion of 3-year (36 mos) rates

Prestidge et al. The clinical significance of a positive post-irradiation postatic biopsy w/o metastases. Int J Rad Oncol Biol Phys, 1992.	
Treatment modality	Primary XRT
Site	Stanford University Medical Center, Stanford, CA
Study design	Reporting on a subset of pts (264) who rec'vd XRT and who underwent prostatic biopsy 12 months of greater post-tx.
Sample Size	139 pos biopsy and 64 neg out of orig cohort of 1,070
Accrual dates	1956-1989
Patient stage	T1(A); T2a (B1); T2b (B2); T3/4 (C)
Patient age	median= 64 for pos; median= 61 for neg
Duration of follow-up	Follow-up after XRT: median= 11.5 yrs; range=1.2-29.8 for pos; median= 9.6 yrs; range=1.2-22.9 for neg. Follow-up after Bx: med=4.9; range=0.3-19.2 for pos; med=6.3; range=0.4-21.5 for neg
Other Patient characteristics	Char of post-irradiation prostatic biopsy pts (stratified pos/neg). Secondary therapies used among 99 pts.
Other Eligibility Criteria	264 of 1,070 had biopsy >=12 months post-tx. Of 264, 188 had pos biopsy, 61 had distant metastases, resulting in 139 pos
Method of Survival Analysis	Cause-specific surv (CSS) and metastatic control calc. from initiation of XRT and time of biopsy using Kaplan-Meier actuarial method. For CSS, pts censored at last follow-up or at time of intecurrent death. Curves out to 20-30 yrs. Gehan p value provided.
Survival Curves	(a) Surv according to post-XRT biopsy status from init XRT compared to an age-matched control group. (b) CSS from init XRT. (a) Surv from time of biopsy compared to age-matched controls. (b) CSS, from time of post-irrad biopsy. Freedom from distant relapse from time of post-XRT biopsy. CSS from time of pos post-XRT biopsy according to tx-to-biopsy interval.
Statistical Estimates Related to Survival Analyses	Discussion in terms of 10- and 15-year survival. E.g., pts with pos biopsy had a 10- and 15-year surv of 61% and 41% (median follow-up=11.5 yrs).

Radge et al. Interstitial I125 radiation w/o adjuvant therapy in the treatment of clinically localized prostate CA. Cancer, 1997.	
Treatment modality	Iodine-125 interstitial radiation
Site	Northwest Hospital, Seattle, WA
Study design	126 consecutive pts treated with I125. 4 died of intercurrent illness within 1 year postimplant, leaving 122 for study.
Sample Size	122
Accrual dates	1988-1990
Patient stage	23% T1 and 77% T2. Clinical T classification at presentation (T1a-T2c)
Patient age	median= 70
Duration of follow-up	median= 69.3 mos
Other Patient characteristics	Gleason's score at diagnostic biopsy. PSA at presentation.
Outcome Definitions	PSA failure: PSA progression (i.e., 2 consec incr from nadir or failure to attain an arbitrary PSA of 1.0 or 0.5 at last follow-up.
Method of Survival Analysis	Kaplan-Meier with survival rates calc from date of implant. Time to PSA event measured from time of implant to 2nd PSA elev in case of PSA progress., and to last follow-up for pts whose PSA exceeded 1 or .5 cutoffs.
Survival Curves	PSA progr free surv. Freedom from PSA > 1 failure. Freedom from PSA >0.5 failure (out 7 yrs, # at risk provided)
Statistical Estimates Related to Survival Analyses	All K-M results discussed at 7 yrs. E.g., Actuarial freedom from PSa >0.5 rate of 79% at 7 yrs, with 23 pts at risk at that time.
Incontinence	Kaplan-Meier analysis of % continent between 48 TURP and 70 non-TURP pts (out 7 yrs). Late complications (n=118, % provided, all relating to incontinence).
Other outcomes/Results	RTOG morbidity grades 1-5.

Ritter et al. PSA as a predictor of radiotherapy response and patterns of failure in localized prostate CA. J Clin Oncol, 1992.	
Treatment modality	Definitive XRT
Site	University of Wisconsin, Madison, WI
Study design	Reporting on (prior to exclusions) 82 pts with stages A2-C (modification of AUA, p. 1209) who rec'vd curative XRT. Purpose to examine relationship between pre and posttx PSA & outcome. Bulk of analysis looks at baseline and half-life PSA values between failing and non-failing (NF) pts. Outcomes ltd.
Sample Size	63; 41 recurrence-free, 22 recurred clinically
Accrual dates	1987-1989
Patient stage	A-C. Clinical status by stage and grade in 63 pts
Duration of follow-up	median=25 months in disease-free; range=10-49. Follow-up time to failure ranged 4-43 mos; median=16 mos.
Other Patient characteristics	Distribution of pre-tx PSA. Pre-tx PSA by (A) stage and (B) grade. Clin status by stage and grade.
Other Eligibility Criteria	13 pts who had <3 serial PSA values, or, for nonfailing <10 months posttx follow-up and 4 pts who rec'vd hormonal tx before failure were excluded
Univar/Multiv Analyses (Covariates)	Prognostic factors for failure (Univar and Multivar results).
Outcome Definitions	Distant failure: bone or CT scan. Local: either new, palpable prostatic nodule or bipsy conf, or serial incr in PSA and neg metastatic workup that led to confirmed bipsy.
Method of Survival Analysis	None
Statistical Estimates Related to Survival Analyses	Table provides the median pre-tx PSA, pre-tx % elev alkaline phosphatase, median half-life follow-up PSA, median baseline or nadir follow-up PSA for 3 types of failure (disease-free, local, metastatic +/- local).
Other outcomes/Results	PSA trends in NF pts as fn of time after XRT. Distribution of (A) half-lives for PSA decr or (B) PSA baseline after XRT in 32 NF pts. Patterns of PSA incr in (A) 15 distant and (B) 7 local failures.

Roach et al. The prognostic significance of race and survival from prostate cancer based on pts irradiated on XRT oncology group protocols (1976-1985). Int J Rad Oncol Biol Phys, 1992.

Treatment modality	Radomization between pelvic & prostate or pelvic & prostate, plus para-aortic irradiation Randomized to receive prostate irradiation only or pelvic plus prostate irradiation. Radomized to receive neoadjuvant megesterol and DES 2 months prior to and during XRT.
Site	RTOG. This article reports on 3 RTOG studies, 2 of which have been reported on above. ALL results are stratified by race (Black/white).
Study design	RTOG 7506 (this study has been reported on above). RTOG 7706 (this study has been reported on above) RTOG 8307
Sample Size	571; 64 coded black; 487 coded white; 1294 among all 3 studies 484; 35 black; 419 white 203; 21 black; 173 white
Accrual dates	All 3 trials occurred from 1976-1985
Patient stage	T3-4 Nx M0 or T1b or T2N1-2 T1b or T2, Nx or N0 T2b-T4 Nx M0
Other Patient characteristics	Presented for each trial
Other Eligibility Criteria	
Univar/Multiv Analyses (Covariates)	Distr of nodal status by race RTOG 75-06 (p value). Distr of pre-tx SAP by race for each trial. (p value). Distr of pre-tx Gleason by race for each trial (p value).
Outcome Definitions	For this articles, survival was measured until death from any cause & disease-free (NED) surv was measured as time to 1st failure (local, regional, distant, death). Local or reg failure: progress. of measureable disease at any time or verif. Of tumor presence 2 yrs after completion of XRT.
Method of Survival Analysis	Methods not very detailed.
Survival Curves	Surv by race. NED surv by race. (curves out 15 yrs;# at risk provided every 3 yrs; p value). Surv by race. NED surv by race. (curves out 15 yrs;# at risk provided every 3 yrs; p value). Surv by race. NED surv by race. (curves out 15 yrs;# at risk provided every 3 yrs; p value).
Other outcomes/Results	Selected series suggesting a difference in surv by race. Selected series suggesting no diff in surv by race.

Roach et al. A pilot survey of sexual function and quality of life following 3D conformal radiotherapy for clin localized prostate CA. Int J Rad Oncol Biol Phys, 1996

Treatment modality	3-D conformal XRT
Site	University of California, San Francisco.
Study design	Reporting on consecutive pts with localized prostate CA who were treated with 3D CRT at UCSF. Each of these pts were mailed questionnaires, and were given the option of involving their partners.
Sample Size	124 pts treated; 60 potent or marginally potent prior to XRT
Accrual dates	1991-1993
Patient stage	T1,T2,T3
Patient age	median=72.3; range=48-87
Duration of follow-up	median=21 mos; range=7-40
Other Patient characteristics	Pts treated with radical prostatectomy were NOT excluded, but rec'vd lower doses.
Impotence	Patient responses to questions regarding sexual fn. Tx self-image and/or relationship with partner
Other outcomes/Results	Partner reponses to questions regarding sexual function

Rosen et al. Radiotherapy for prostate carcinoma: The JCRT experience (1968-1978). II. Factors related to tumor control and complications. Int J Rad Oncol Biol Phys, 1985

Treatment modality	XRT
Site	Joint Center for Radiation Therapy, Boston, MA
Study design	Reporting on pts who rec'vd definitive XRT for pathologically proven prostate CA
Sample Size	229
Accrual dates	1968-1978
Patient stage	modification of AUA. 25 A, 85 B, 88 C, 18 D1.
Patient age	median=66 at time of initiation of tx
Duration of follow-up	median=5 yrs
Other Patient characteristics	12 pts rec'vd XRT after radical prostectomy, and one preop XRT
Univar/Multiv Analyses (Covariates)	local-regional recurr as fn of conedown field size and stage. Table 2. local-reg recurr as fn of initial field size. local-regional recurr as fn of conedown field tech.
Outcome Definitions	Local Recurr.: Pts with progressive prostatic enlargement or nodularity on exam, pelvic mass, ureteral obstruction, or reappear. of obstr symptoms with pos biopsy.
Method of Survival Analysis	Actuarial surv according to Berkson and Gage.
Survival Curves	Relapse-free surv as fn of TURP performed prior to XRT. Relapse-free surv as function of size of initial field. Relapse-free surv as function of adjuvant hormonal tx. (out 8 yrs; # at risk every 2 yrs).
Other outcomes/Results	Complix of XRT (+surgery). Urinary or bowel complix as fn of size of initial field. Very brief results. Complix as fn of field size & tx tech. Complix as fn of surg procedures.

Russell et al. PSA in the management of pts w/localized adenocarcinoma of the prostate tx w/primary XRT. J of Urology, 1991.

Treatment modality	XRT
Site	5 institutions in the greater Seattle metro area (U of Washington Med Center, VA Mason Med Center, Overlake Hospital, Providence Hospital, and Evergreen Hospital).
Study design	Medical records of pts with localized prostate CA treated with primary XRT at 5 institutions in greater Seattle area were reviewed.
Sample Size	143
Accrual dates	1985-1987. Although pts from U of Wash Med Center treated <1985 in phase I and II dose-searching clin trials involving fast neutron XRT were reviewed.
Patient stage	A1,A2,B1,B2,C,D1
Patient age	median=70; range=52-85
Duration of follow-up	median=27 mos; range=18-91; follow-up 1 month after completion tx, every 3 months thereafter until 2 yrs after tx. Then every 4 to 6 mos.
Other Patient characteristics	Distribution of pre-tx PSA in 50 pts by stage and Gleason sum
Univar/Multiv Analyses (Covariates)	Logistic regression used to det effect os PSA on outcome while controlling for other factors.
Outcome Definitions	At last follow-up pts categorized as: (1) complete response, (2) clin failure, or (3) chem failure. Complete responders: no clin evid of recurrent prostate CA and normal PSA. Clin failiures had recurrent tumors. Chem failures were clin normal, but elev PSA.
Method of Survival Analysis	None. Largely Chi-square and t-tests. All end pts. timed from conclusion of therapy. End pts for clin failures included development of local tumor recurrence or distant metastases.
Statistical Estimates Related to Survival Analyses	Outcomes by stage and Gleason sum. Table 3. Outcomes as related to pre-tx PSA in 50 pts. Tx outcome correlated to normalization of PSA within 6 &12 months after tx. (Chi-square).
Other outcomes/Results	Post-radiation biopsies in 19 pts correlated with PSA.

Schellhammer et al. PSA levels after definitive irradiation for carcinoma of the prostate. J Urology, 1991	
Treatment modality	Definitive irradiation therpy either by I125 implantation or XRT
Site	Eastern Virginia Medical School, Norfolk, VA
Study design	PSA levels were determined in 78 pts judged clinically to be free of disease at intervals of 36 months or more after completion of irradiartion therapy.
Sample Size	34 XRT; 44 I125
Patient stage	A1-D2
Duration of follow-up	XRT follow-up range=38-127 mos; I125 follow-up range=40-186 mos
Outcome Definitions	Outcomes in this study are limited to tabulations of PSA levels for pts at least 3 yrs after tx. Not all info. is stratified by tx type
Other outcomes/Results	PSA levels in 78 pts clin free of dx more than 3 yrs after irradiation. Pts with undetectable PSA by pre-tx clin grade & stage. Table 3. Present PSA vs past biopsy results. Pre-tx PSA by clin stage

Schellhammer et al. PSA to determine progression-free surv after XRT for localize carcinoma of prostate. Urology, 1993.	
Treatment modality	XRT and interstitial brachytherapy
Site	Eastern Virginia Medical School, Norfolk, VA
Study design	918 with clin stage A-C treated . 792 with XRT and 126 with I125. 123 I125 pts treated and followed by an author. 317 of XRT pts treated and followed by an author
Sample Size	123 I-125; 311 XRT
Accrual dates	1975-1990
Patient age	I-125 mean=62.7; XRT mean=68.9.
Duration of follow-up	median follow-up of 317 XRT=51 mos; range=12-178
Other Eligibility Criteria	3 of I125 pts and 6 XRT pts rec'vd hormonal therapy prior to clin appearance of failure and were excluded.
Outcome Definitions	Local failure: (1) persistent induration during & after tx, (2) bleeding or obstructiv sx treated by TURP and yielding malignant tissue, or (3) evid of ureterovesical junction obstr. Distant failure: id by bone scan or rising PAP. Pts clin progress-free if DRE ok, bone scan neg, no sig clin complaints.
Method of Survival Analysis	Actuarial progression-free surv curves constructed using Kaplan-Meier. All curves out 10 yrs or more
Survival Curves	Prob of nonprogress. by stage based on clin status or PSA marker level among XRT pts. Prob of nonprogress. by grade based on criterion of clin status or PSA marker level among XRT pts. Prob of nonprogress. by clin stage based on clin status or PSA marker level among I-125 pts. Prov of nonprogress by grade based on clin status or PSA marker level among I-125 pts.
Statistical Estimates Related to Survival Analyses	E.g., using normal PSA marker criterion, the 10-year progress-free surv of XRT-treated pts fell from 65-35% for A2, 40-20% B1, 35-20% B2, 25-10% C. Regardless of stage,grade, tx modality, progress-free survival at 10-year <10% when undetectable PSA used.
Other outcomes/Results	Observed outcomes: Clin and PSA prgoress-free surv (10-year min follow-up). Provides the % by stage and grade.

Schmidt et al. Adjuvant therapy for clinical localized prostate cancer treated w/surgery or irradiation. European Urology, 1996.	
Treatment modality	Adjuvant therapy after surgery or irradiation
Site	National Prostate Cancer Project (NPCP) initiated 2 protocols. Authors from La Jolla, CA; Seattle, WA; Birmingham, Alabama
Study design	Protocol 900: Following radical surgery or cryosurgery, pts were randomized to receive either cyclophosphamide, estramustine, or observation. Protocol 1000: Following definitive XRT, pts were randomized to receive either cyclophosphamide, estramustine, or observation
Sample Size	184 (170 evaluable) 253 (233 evaluable); 403 pts total
Accrual dates	1978-1985
Patient stage	B2,C,D1
Duration of follow-up	mean=132 months or 11 yrs; range=92-172 mos; for BOTH protocols; info collected thru 1993
Other Eligibility Criteria	All pts underwent staging pelvic lymph node dissection
Univar/Multiv Analyses (Covariates)	Impact of prognostic factors (tx, age, stage, grade, % pos lymph nodes, cadiovascular and respiratory statue, alkaline & acid phosphatases) on PFS and survival were studied (chi-square given)
Outcome Definitions	Recurrence, median progression free survival (PFS) and overall (CA-specific) survival. Recurrence (dx progression) defined according to NPCP criteria. In most cases recurrence reflected appearance of distant metastatic dx by bone scan.
Method of Survival Analysis	Curves out 140-180 mos. None given.
Survival Curves	PFS by adjuvant tx. PFS for stage C pts. PFS for C pts in BOTH protocols. PFS for grade 3 pts in BOTH protocols. PFS for D1 N+ pts in BOTH protocols. PFS by adj tx. Fig 10. PFS for D1 N+ pts. PFS for D1 N+ pts with extensive nodal metastases. PFS for C pts 900 VS 1000. Survival for C pts 900 VS 1000.
Statistical Estimates Related to Survival Analyses	Recurrent dx according to initial stage & assigned adj (n & % pts). Table 2. Recurrent dx according to grade of tumor & assigned adj (n & % pts). Recurrent dx according to initial stage & assigned adj (n & % pts). Table 4. Recurrent dx according to grade of tumor & assigned adj (n & % pts).
Other outcomes/Results	BOTH protocols combined: Recurrent dx in D1, N1-3 pts by degress of metastases

Schneider et al. The prognostic value of PSA levles in XRT of pts w/carcinoma of the prostate: The UCLA experience 1988-1992. Am J Clin Oncol, 1996

Treatment modality	Definitive radiation including intersitital implant (7); photon (81); neutron (13)
Site	Department of Radiation Oncology and Jonsson Comprehensive Cancer Center Tumor Registry, University of California, Los Angeles, CA
Study design	Retrospective review of the records of all pts with histologically proven adenocarcinoma of the prostate, who rec'vd definitive XRT at UCLA.
Sample Size	116 charts reviewed; 101 evaluable
Accrual dates	1988-1992
Patient stage	4 A; 77 B; 16 C; 4 D
Patient age	mean=69.7; median=71; range=51-81
Duration of follow-up	mean=32.9 mos; median=28 mos; range=1.8-68.6 mos
Other Patient characteristics	86 white, 8 black, 6 hispanics, 1 asian. 18 Gleason2-4; 68 Gleason 5-7; 13 Gleason 8-10. Table 1. Patient char by tx modality. Table 3. Pre-tx PSA by stage and Gleason (Tukey's).
Other Eligibility Criteria	Eligibility: pre-tx PSA, rec'vd XRT at UCLA, no androgen ablation therapy prior to XRT
Univar/Multiv Analyses (Covariates)	Multivar used logistic regression. Multivar analysis of potential prognostic factors (age, clin stage, Gleason, PSA nadir, pre-tx PSA, PSA normalization by 6 mos, PSA normalization by 12 mos) for disease outcome. Provides coefficient., SD, p value.
Outcome Definitions	Disease-free (DF) and overall survival. Free of dx: no evid of clin or biochem failure. Clin failure: metastatic dx by bone scan, biopsy-proven local recurrence; change in rectal exam prompted intervention. Chem failure: 2 consec rising PSA, each at least 0.3 greater than previous, PSA nadir >4.
Method of Survival Analysis	Kaplan-Meier. In addtn, separate 1-way ANOVA used to compare mean pre-tx PSA levels stratified by AUA stage and Gleason score. Freq of norm & abn PSA at 6 & 12 months compred to stage and outcome by chi-square. Also used Tukey's and t tests.
Survival Curves	Actuarial overall surv (out 6 yrs). Actuarial survival free of clin or chem relapse (DF surv; out 5 yrs). Surv free of clin or chem relapse based on pre-tx PSA (out 3-5 yrs). 4-year act overall surv 85%; 4-year DF surv 32% (p 67).
Statistical Estimates Related to Survival Analyses	Pre-tx PSA by outcome (NED, chem failure, clin failure; ANOVA and chi-square. Outcome by stage and Gleason (chi-square). Postirradiation PSA norm and outcome (chi-square).
Other outcomes/Results	Postirradiation PSA noramlization and relationship to stage and Gleason (chi-square). Relationship between PSA nadir and outcome (2-sample t test)

Shaeffer et al. Nuclear roundness factor and local failure from definitive XRT for prostatic carcinoma. Int J Rad Oncol Biol Phys, 1992.

Treatment modality	Definitive XRT; I-125 and external beam
Site	Eastern Virginia Medical School, Norfolk, VA
Study design	Reporting on a series of 375 pts with prostatic CA treated definitively with xRT and having a min of 5-yrs' follow-up. Match pts into 2 groups (
Sample Size	375, but then match 23 local failure only (LF0) pts with 23 NED pts and report on these 2 groups (22 pts each b/c of slide availability).
Patient stage	A2 (but then they don't report of A2),B1,B2,C
Patient age	mean LF=66.2 and mean NED=68.4 at diagnosis
Other Patient characteristics	Table 2. Char of study pop (stratified by 22 LF and 22 NED). 18 of each group rec'vd XRT and 4 of each group rec'vd I125.
Outcome Definitions	None really, know that 220 had no evid of disease (NED), 72 had distant metastasis only, 60 had distant metastasis and local failure, and 23 had local failure only (LFO). Metastasis and local failure by grade and stage (provides the n & %).
Method of Survival Analysis	None. Data limited to t tests of differences in nuclear char of LFO and NED groups.
Other outcomes/Results	Summary of nuclear morphometric data for LFO and NED (p value). Tumor nuclear roundness factor for LFO and NED (p value). Nucleolus/normal cell nucleus for LFO and NED (p value).

Schrader-Bogen et al. Quality of life and treatment outcomes: Prostate carcinoma pts' perspectives after prostatectomy or XRT. Cancer, 1997	
Treatment modality	Prostatectomy or XRT
Site	Healthsystem Minnesota, Minneapolis, MN. This institute includes a 425-bed community hospital with assoc. multispecialty clinics. It's an Amer College of Surgeons-approv Teaching Hosp CA Program that diagnosed &/or tx 1865 CA cases in 1995.
Study design	Pts id in the institutions' oncology registry. Data collected for this cross-sectional study by mailing pts self-admin survey with demographic items, FACT-G and PCTO-Q (Newly developed Prostate Cancer Treatment Outcome Questionnaire).
Sample Size	354 sent survey; 306 returned; 274 eligible; 132 RP;142 XRT
Accrual dates	1989-1994
Patient age	RP: mean=66.2; SD=6.528 and XRT mean=75.3; SD=5.680
Duration of follow-up	Survey sent 1-5 yrs after diagnosis
Other Patient characteristics	Sociodemographics
Other Eligibility Criteria	Other eligibility: AJCC stage I or II dx, excluding capsular invasion (A or B); no tx outside RP or XRT; not other primary CA; alive; read & write in English; nurse access to charts.
Incontinence	Comparison of 7-day urinary symptoms (PCTO-Q) by tx (p values).
Impotence	Comparison of 7-day sexual function (PCTO-Q) by tx (p value).
Other outcomes/Results	Comparison of 7-d bowel symptoms (PCTO-Q) by tx (p value).

Soffen et al. Conformal static field XRT tx of early prostate CA vs non-conformal tech: A reduction in acute morbidity. Int J Rad Oncol Biol Phys, 1992	
Treatment modality	Definitive XRT using either four field box, bilateral arcs, or rotational field tech.
Site	Fox Chase Cancer Center, Philadelphia, PA
Study design	Reporting on morbidity of consecutive pts treated with XRT. Table 2 provides the tx parameters
Sample Size	20 noncoformal XRT (NCG), 26 conformal XRT (CG)
Accrual dates	1985-1989 & 1989-1991
Patient stage	T1b(A2), T2a (B1), T2b(B2)
Patient age	median= 71; range=56-84; median= 71; range=52-81
Duration of follow-up	wksly during tx; 1,3, and 6 months after.
Other Patient characteristics	Patient Char (age, KPS, stage, Gleason)
Outcome Definitions	Outcomes ltd to acute morbidity: urinary symptoms. rectal symptoms. urinary & rectal symptoms, urinary or rectal symptoms, symptoms persisting > 1month. Symtoms quantified in severity as to whether meds and/or tx interruption required.
Incontinence	Acute Morbidity; urinary and/or rectal symptoms (n and % provided)

Talcott et al. Patient-reported symptoms after primary therapy for early prostate CA: Results of a prospective cohort study. J Clin Oncol, 1998

Treatment modality	XRT; radical prostatectomy; other
Site	Dana-Farber Cancer Institute's Genitourinary Oncology Clinic, Divisions of Urology at Brigham & Women's and New England Deconess Hospital, & Joint Center for Radiation Oncology
Study design	Survey of pts going for consultation on primary therapy of early prostate CA. Patient-completed questionnaire about symptoms and quality of life.
Sample Size	428 asked to participate; 30 ineligible; 80 refused; 29 incomplete; 287 of 398 eligible (72%) ; 3-monthdata from 241; 12-monthfrom 223
Accrual dates	1990-1994
Patient stage	T1a-c, T2, T3 for RP and XRT group and all pts given in Table 3.
Patient age	RP: median=62; mean=60.9; range=41-72; XRT: median=68; mean=68.0; range=49-86
Duration of follow-up	3 month and 12 month questionnaires
Other Patient characteristics	Sociodemographic char of 260 pts choosing RP or XRT as initial tx. Table 3. Clin char of pts choosing RP or XRT as initial tx.
Other Eligibility Criteria	Pts who did not receive either XRT or RP were excluded.
Outcome Definitions	Outcomes are related to morbidity and QOL.
Incontinence	Symptoms of bowel & bladder irritation by tx. Symptoms of urinary incontinence (UI) by tx. Symptoms of UI, by age (<=64, >=65). (for each table: % men with complaint at baseline, 3-mo, 12-mos)
Impotence	Symptoms of sexual dysfunction (SEXD). Freq of patient-reported SEXD before RP or XRT at 3 and 12 months. Symptoms of SEXD among pts reporting erections before tx.
Other outcomes/Results	Symptoms of SEXD among pts who rec'vd RP or XRT as initial therapy for early prostate CA, stratified by age. (for each table: % men with complaint at baseline, 3-mo, 12-mos)

Teshima et al. Rectal bleeding after conformal 3D tx of prostate CA: Timr to occurrence, response to tx and duration of morbidity. Int J Rad Oncol Biol Phys, 1997.

Treatment modality	3-Dimensional conformal radiation therapy (3DCRT)
Site	Fox Chase Cancer Center, Philadelphia, PA
Study design	Reporting on a group of pts with prostate cancer treated with 3DCRT. In particular, examining rectal bleeding by grade (II-V)
Sample Size	670
Accrual dates	1989-1995
Patient stage	89 T1, 421 T2, 147 T3, 12 unknown
Patient age	median= 70; range=49-89
Univar/Multiv Analyses (Covariates)	A stepwise Cox regression model was calc to examine the effect of prognostic indicators upon complications. Covars: dose, hormones prior to XRT, age, TUPR, diabetes, hypertension, tx tech, obstruction symptoms at presentation.
Outcome Definitions	Late radiation GI morbidity scales. Outcome measured from date of completion of XRT to onset of Grade 2 or 3 bleeding or date of last follow-up. Diffs in latency and duration were eval using nonparametric Wilcoxon.
Method of Survival Analysis	Estimates of rates for Grade 2&3 bleeding were calc. using Kaplan-Meier product-limit method. Log rank used to test diffs.
Survival Curves	Cum occurrence % of late rectal bleeding by Grade (2 or 3) (p=0.09; out 50 mos). Cum occurrence curves of Grades 2&3 rectal bleeding by dose (p value; # at risk each year; out 6 yrs).
Statistical Estimates Related to Survival Analyses	Cum duration curves of late rectal bleeding >Grade 1 after tx by Grade (2 or 3) (p value; out 50 mos). E.g., The 3 year actuarial rate of Grade 2 rectal bleeding was 11% in pts who rec'vd <73 Gy and 22% in those >=73 Gy, respectively (p=0.005).
Other outcomes/Results	Cox analysis: Predictors of Grade 2&3 bleeding (p value). Tx method & improvement to <Grade 2 GI bleeding. Time to return of symptoms to <Grade 2 with tx.

Watkins-Bruner et al. RTOG's first quality of life study - RTOG 90-20: A phse II trial of XRT w/etanidazole for locally advanced prostate CA. Int J Rad Oncol Biol Phys, 1995

Treatment modality	Radiotherapy and etanidazole
Site	RTOG
Study design	RTOG 90-20 eligibility included men with Stage T2b or higher, previously untreated adenocarcinoma of the prostate, KPS >=70%. 3 QOL instruments used: FACT, SAQ, Changes in Urnary Function (CUF)
Sample Size	36 accrrued to RTOG 90-20, 26 filled out baseline FACT, 26 filled out baseline SAQ, 24 filled out both.
Patient stage	Stage T2b or higher
Patient age	57% > 70 yrs
Duration of follow-up	Compliance as % of all eligibles ranged from 22-72%, QL questionnaires administered pre-tx, end of tx, 3 months follow-up, 12 mos, then annually until death
Outcome Definitions	All outcomes are related to QOL.
Incontinence	Comparison of patient self-reports of dysuria and diarrhea to med professional rating
Impotence	Comparison of patient self-reports of erectile inability to med professional rating of NO erection. Comparison of patient self-reports of erectile ability to med professional rating of YES erection.
Other outcomes/Results	Table 5Institute of Canada)

Weyrich et al. I125 seed implants for prostatic carcinoma: 5 and 10 yr follow-up. Urology, 1993

Treatment modality	interstitial implantation of I125 and pelvic lymphadenectomy; includes pts on hormone therapy
Site	Depts of Urology and XRT, West Virginia University Med Center, Morgantown, W VA
Study design	Reporting on pts treated with I125 with clinical Stage A2,B, or C carcinoma of prostate
Sample Size	132
Accrual dates	1975-1985
Patient stage	11 A2, 32 B1, 54 B2, 12 C1, 23 D1
Patient age	mean=64; range=50-75
Duration of follow-up	mean=9.2 yrs; follow-up included 1 and 2 year postimplantation transrectal needle biopsies of the prostate
Other Patient characteristics	Number of pts per histologic grade at implantation (72 I, 42 II, 18 III)
Outcome Definitions	Disease-free: negative rectal exams, transrectal needle biopsies, and normal (<4.0) PSA.
Method of Survival Analysis	None, reporting No. of pts alive, disease-free, on hormone therapy at 5 and 10 yrs.
Statistical Estimates Related to Survival Analyses	Disease-free rates. Table VII. Survival rates (5 and 10 yrs; n and %).
Incontinence	Short-term complications (48 hrs - 3 months postop). Table III. Long-term complications (>3 mos). These tables include no. of pts with urinary problems
Other outcomes/Results	Operative complications (within 48 hours of surgery)

Vander Kooy et al. Irradiation for locally recurrent carcinoma of the prostate following radical prostatectomy. Urology, 1997.	
Treatment modality	XRT as salvage therapy for post-prostatectomy locally recurrent prostate CA
Site	Mayo Clinic, Rochester, MN
Study design	Reporting on a group of pts primarily treated with RP and pelvic LND for clinically localized CaP who were subsequently managed with curative-intent XRT for an isolated prostatic fossa tumor recurrence that was apparent by DRE, cytoscopy, or radiologic imaging.
Sample Size	35
Accrual dates	1979-1992
Patient stage	T1,T2,T3
Patient age	median=64; range=47-74
Duration of follow-up	median= 5.2 yrs; range=1.7-12.1
Other Patient characteristics	Patient characterisitcs (preop clin stage, path stage, Mayo tumor grade, preXRT PSA)
Other Eligibility Criteria	Pts previously treated with hormones or with RT in a primary or adjuvant setting or with a combined RT-hormone tx program were excluded
Univar/Multiv Analyses (Covariates)	The assoc of preXRT CaP-related characteristics with disease outcome were studied. The observed rate of lreapse was obt for each factor of interest, and univariate comparison of factors made by log-rank test.
Outcome Definitions	Outcomes incluide clinical relapse-free, any (clin or biochem) relapse-free, and overall survival. Tabulation of complications.
Method of Survival Analysis	Kaplan-Meier analysis. Time measured from initiation of XRT to date of event.
Survival Curves	Clin relapse-free, any relaspe-free, and overall survival out 9 yrs. Number at risk provided for each year.
Statistical Estimates Related to Survival Analyses	8 year rates discussed. Disease outcome (8-year clin relapse-free, any relapse-free, overall survival) according to preXRT disease-related char (path stage, dx-free interval, preXRT PSA, tumor grade; p value provided).
Other outcomes/Results	Briefly discusses chronic complications scored using RTOG and EORTC. E.g., bleeding of intestine/rectum (grades 1-2) that did not require intervention.

Zagars et al. The prognostic importance of Gleason grade in prostatic adenocarcinoma: A long-term follow-up study of 648 pts treated/XRT. Int J Rad Oncol Biol Phys, 1995

Treatment modality	Definitive external beam photon XRT
Site	University of Texas, MD Anderson Cancer Center, Houston, TX
Study design	Reporting on a group of pts who rec'vd definitive XRT. "This series is proper subset of that reported by us earlier." (p 238).
Sample Size	648
Accrual dates	1966-1988
Patient stage	Stages T1 to T4, NO or NX, MO
Patient age	mean=65; median=66; range=44-81
Duration of follow-up	for 402 pts alive at last contact; median=6.5 yrs; mean=7 yrs; range=20-239 mos. 70 pts were followed for less than 4 yrs.
Other Patient characteristics	Distribution of Gleason grades
Other Eligibility Criteria	Pts were eligible if they rec'vd NO androgen ablation therapy and all pathology slides were reviewed and assigned a Gleason grade.
Univar/Multiv Analyses (Covariates)	Multivar actuarial regression using Cox proportional hazards model with the log linear function. Sig of coeffs tested with likelihood ratio. Table 6. Stat sig of vars predicting metastases, any relapse and survival.
Outcome Definitions	Local control: prostate gland normal to palpation except when TURP prompted by obstr. sx, or PNBX prompted by rising PSA were pos. Disease free: clin-radiographic evid of metastases and no local recurrence.
Method of Survival Analysis	Life-table or product-liimit methods. Time from the end of radiation. All curves out 120 months (# and p values provided). Log-rank test used to test stat sig.
Survival Curves	Actuarial incid of local recurr according to 4-tier grade grouping. Actuarial incid of any dx relapse according to 4-tier grade grouping. Actuarial surv according to 4-tier grade grouping.
Statistical Estimates Related to Survival Analyses	Actuarial local recurr. Actuarial incid of DM . Actuarial incid of any dx relapse. Actuarial surv. All tables by grade,univar analyses (log rank p value), 5 & 10 year % and initial n provided.
Other outcomes/Results	Actuarial outcome (local recurrence, DM, any relapse, surv) by grade for grading base on PNBX only (5 & 10 yrs, p value by trended log rank).

Zagars et al. The source of pretreatment serum PSA in clinically localized prostate cancer - T,N, or M? Int J Rad Oncol Biol Phys, 1995.

Treatment modality	Definitive radiotherapy or radical prostatectomy (only the XRT pts are summarized here)
Site	University of Texas, MD Anderson Cancer Center, Houston, TX
Study design	Reporting on a group of CaP pts who rec'vd definitive XRT as their only initial tx.
Sample Size	427
Accrual dates	1987-1991
Patient stage	T1 to T4
Patient age	mean= median= 68 yrs; range=47-84 yrs
Duration of follow-up	mean=33 mos; median=30; range=9-73
Other Patient characteristics	Stage distribution, MD Anderson grades, Gleason grades, and nodal status provided.
Other Eligibility Criteria	Pts selected beginning in 1987 b/c PSA recorded.
Outcome Definitions	All outcomes limited to analyses of PSA levels, pre- and post-tx. Most results combined for RP and XRT. 4 scamples of data, best-fit regression curves & back-extrapolated PSA values in pts who developed rising PSA profile after XRT.

Appendix B. Outcomes Literature Table: Radiation Therapy

Zagars and Pollack. The serum PSA level three months after radiotherapy for prostate cancer: an early indicator of response to treatment. Radiotherapy and Oncology, 1994.

Treatment modality	XRT
Site	University of Texas, MD Anderson Cancer Center, Houston, TX
Study design	Reporting on a group of CaP pts who rec'vd definitive XRT (probably subset of above)
Sample Size	347
Accrual dates	1987-1991, inclusive
Patient stage	A2-C
Patient age	mean= median =68; range=47-84
Duration of follow-up	mean=26; median =24; range=6-67; follow-up at 3 month intervals
Other Patient characteristics	MD Anderson grade
Other Eligibility Criteria	Pts did NOT received adjuvant hormonal manipulation and had serial PSA values
Univar/Multiv Analyses (Covariates)	Log-linear fn of Cox and Oates was used in the proportional hazards model and tests of sig were based on the likelihood ratio stat. Prognostic sig of 3-monthPSA - corrected for its correlation with baseline PSA using proportional hazards model.
Outcome Definitions	Free of diseas: no clin-radio evid of metastases and no evid of loca recurrence. Local control: palpable normal prostate or one in which the abnormalities were resolving. All local recurrences confirmed by biopsy. Rising post-XRT PSA: 2 or more consecutive rising values. Composite endpt: rising PSA or relapse.
Method of Survival Analysis	Actuariral curves were calculated using the Bergson-Gage method. All times dated from completion of XRT.
Survival Curves	Actuarial outcomes according to 3-month PSA (A) Disease free; (B) Incid of rising PSA; (C) Incid of relapse and/or rising PSA.
Statistical Estimates Related to Survival Analyses	Prognostic sig of the 3-month PSA value-univar analysis (outcomes: dx freedom; rising PSA; composite endpt. Actuarial outcome at 60 mos.).

Zagars and Pollack. XRT for T1 and T2 prostate cancer: PSA and disease outcome. Urology, 1995.

Treatment modality	XRT as their only definitive initial tx
Site	University of Texas, MD Anderson Cancer Center, Houston, TX
Study design	Reporting on a group of CaP pts who had XRT as their only definitive tx, beginning when serum PSA estimation was intro at MDACC.
Sample Size	461
Accrual dates	1987-1993, inclusive
Patient stage	T1a-T2c
Patient age	median= 69; range=47-84
Duration of follow-up	mean= median=31 months; range=6-87; follow-up every 3 mos
Other Patient characteristics	grade, pre-tx PSA, 122 underwent TURP
Univar/Multiv Analyses (Covariates)	Multivar time to failure analysis done using proportional hazards model.
Outcome Definitions	Clinically free of dx: no clin or radiographic evid of local recurrence either by DRE, u/s, or sx. Local recurrence confirmed by biopsy. rising PSA: 2 or more consec rising above nadir or one higher than predecessor by 1 or factor 1.5.
Method of Survival Analysis	Actuarial curves calculated using Berkson-Gage and Kaplan-Meier methods.
Survival Curves	Actuarial surv and freedom from relapse (FFR) or rising PSA (out 6 yrs). Actuarial freedom from relapse or rising PSA according to pre-tx PSA. (out 6 yrs).
Statistical Estimates Related to Survival Analyses	Summary of univar analysis of prognostic factors (n, 5-year FFR or rising PSA; 95% CI; log-rank p value).

Zagars et al. PSA and XRT for clinically localized prostate cancer. Int J Rad Oncol Biol Phys, 1995.	
Treatment modality	Definitive XRT
Site	University of Texas, MD Anderson Cancer Center, Houston, TX
Study design	Reporting on a group of CaP pts who had XRT as their only definitive tx, beginning when serum PSA estimation was intro at MDACC.
Sample Size	707
Accrual dates	1987-1993, inclusive
Patient stage	T1a-T4b
Patient age	mean= median =68; range=47-84
Duration of follow-up	mean=31; median=30; range=6 -84
Univar/Multiv Analyses (Covariates)	Multivar time to failure analysis done using proportional hazards maodel with log-linear fn. Summary stats of factors sig for various endpts: Cox model. Hazard index by factors sig correlated with relapse or rising PSA.
Outcome Definitions	Clinically free of dx: no clin or radiographic evid of local recurrence either by DRE, u/s, or sx. Local recurrence confirmed by biopsy. Rising PSA: 2 or more consec rising above nadir or one higher than predecessor by 1 or factor 1.5.
Method of Survival Analysis	Actuarial curves calculated using Berkson-Gage and Kaplan-Meier methods. 95% CI were calculated for actuarial curves
Survival Curves	Actuarial surv curves and incid of relapse and/or rising PSA (out 6 yrs). Actuarial incid of relapse of rising PSA according to stage & Gleason. Actuarial incid of relapse of rising PSA according to pre-tx PSA. See also column R&S
Statistical Estimates Related to Survival Analyses	Actuarial 5-year likelihood of relapse or rising PSA by pre-tx prognostic factors sig in univar analysis. Actuarial 5-year likelihood of local recurr, metastatic relapse, any relapse, & rising PSA by factors sig in univar analysis.
Impotence	Actuarial incid of relapse or rising PSA by 4 prognostic groups (out 60 mos). Actuarial incid of relapse or rising PSA according to nPSA (out 5 yrs). Actuarial % relapse or rising PSA in each of 4 prognostic groups by nPSA (out 5 yrs).
Other outcomes/Results	Actuarial incid of freedom from relapse and/or rising PSA according to T-stage grouping (out 6 yrs).

Zagars et al. Prostate cancer and XRT - the message conveyed by PSA. Int J Rad Oncol Biol Phys, 1995.	
Treatment modality	Definitive XRT as only initial treatment
Site	University of Texas, MD Anderson Cancer Center, Houston, TX
Study design	This paper reports on 2 series: pre-PSA (648) and PSA (707) which have been described above.
Sample Size	648 pre-PSA; 707 PSA
Accrual dates	pre-PSA: 1966-1988; PSA: 1987-1993
Patient stage	pre-PSA: T1-T4, N0 or NX, M0; PSA: T1a-T4b
Patient age	pre-PSA: mean=65; median=66; range=44-81; PSA: mean= median= 68; range=47-84
Duration of follow-up	pre-PSA: mean=7 yrs; medan=6.5; range=20-239 months; PSA: mean=32; median=31; range=6-87
Univar/Multiv Analyses (Covariates)	Multivar time to failure analysis using long-linear relative hazard fn of Cox. Summary stats for local recurr, metastases, any relapse from proportional hazards models for pre-PSA. Summary stats for various endpts from proportional hazards models for the PSA series.
Outcome Definitions	Clinically free of dx: no clin or radiographic evid of local recurrence either by DRE, u/s, or sx. Local recurrence confirmed by biopsy. rising PSA: 2 or more consec rising above nadir or one higher than predecessor by 1 or factor 1.5.
Method of Survival Analysis	Actuarial curves calculated using the Berkson-Gage and Kaplan-Meier methods. 95% CI calculated using method of Rothman.
Survival Curves	Actuarial local recurr in pre-PSA according to stage (a) and Gleason (b). Actuarial metastatic relapse in pre-PSA according to stage (a) and Gleason grade (b). Actuarial incid of relapse or rising PSA in PSA according to according to stage (a) and Gleason grade (b). Actuarial incid of relapse or rising PSA according to pre-tx PSA.
Statistical Estimates Related to Survival Analyses	10-year results pre-PSA (n, % local control, % metastatic control, 95% CI, p value). 10-year freedom from any relapse pre-PSA (n, %, 95% CI, p value). 5-year actuarial incid of local relapse, metastatic relapse, any relapse in pre-PSA and PSA series according to T-stage and Gleason. Table 5. 5-year incid of rising PSA or relapse & rising PSA in PSA: univar analysis.
Incontinence	5-year results in PSA series: univar analysis.

Zagars et al. The role of XRT in stages A2 and B adenocaricinoma of the prostate. Int J Rad Oncol Biol Phys, 1988.	
Treatment modality	External beam megavoltage radiation
Site	University of Texas, MD Anderson Hospital and Tumor Institute, Houston, TX
Study design	Reporting on a series of pts at MD Anderson who received XRT
Sample Size	114
Accrual dates	1965-1982
Patient stage	A2 or B
Duration of follow-up	mean=5.9 yrs; median=5 yrs; range=32-188 months for all 90 surviving pts. 3 monthly eval fro 2-3 yrs; semiannually thereafter up to 5 yrs; then yearly.
Other Patient characteristics	Significant early endocrine manipulation occurred in 5 pts (3 orchiectomy, 2 estrogen).Pts either refuse RP or surgery was inappropriate
Univar/Multiv Analyses (Covariates)	Pairwise analysis of 11 prognostic factors in stage B dx. Factors potentially sig for survival and DF survival (5-year) in Stage B pts.
Outcome Definitions	Local control: persistently normal prostate by palpation even in the presence of obstrutive sx if TURP revelaed no CA. Disease-free: no disease manifestation.
Method of Survival Analysis	Actuarial methods of Berkson and Gage. All times calculated from date XRT began. 95% CI provided.
Survival Curves	Actuarial survival. Disease-free survival (out 10 yrs, n at 5 and 10 yrs.)
Statistical Estimates Related to Survival Analyses	5 and 10 year rates discussed.
Other outcomes/Results	There are several tables summarizing the results of past studies of XRT, RP, and hormonal tx.

Appendix B. Outcomes Literature Table: Radiation Therapy

Zetner. PSA density: A new prognostic indicator for prostate cancer. Int J Rad Oncol Biol Phys, 1993.	
Treatment modality	Definitive XRT using CT-guided conformal techinique
Site	Department of Radiation Oncology, Columbia-Presbyterian Medical Center
Study design	Reporting on a series of pts treated for CaP. 202 were treated during the time period identified. 86 had clinically localized dx and were tx with XRT using CT-guided conformal tech. 73 evaluable.
Sample Size	73
Accrual dates	1989-1991
Patient stage	19% A(T1), 41% B(T2), 40% C (T3)
Patient age	mean=71; range =46-83
Duration of follow-up	13 months; range=2.3-31. Follow-up period from start of XRT to last follow-up. Pts seen 1 month after completion XRT and every 3-4 months thereafter.
Other Patient characteristics	No pts rec'vd hormonal tx prior to failure. 10 pts had TURP. Gleason's and pre-tx PSA provided.
Other Eligibility Criteria	13 pts excluded b/c of prior RP, hormonal tx, or no pre-tx PSA.
Outcome Definitions	PSA failure: PSA rise above normal (4 ng/ml) or, for pts whose nadir was >4, an increase of >10% above nadir. Only one survival curve analysis.
Method of Survival Analysis	Kaplan-Meier lifetable analyses were performed over a ranges of PSA density (PSAD) levels to determine the level at which the neg predictive value declined.
Survival Curves	Actuarial disease-free surv for pts with (a) PSAD<=0.3 and >0 .3 and (b) PSAD <=0.6 and > 0.6. Curves out 36 months and p value between PSAD groups provided.
Other outcomes/Results	Results largely descriptive, looking at how patient characteristics vary by PSAD (Table 3) or how patient char. compare between disease-free and PSA failure pts.

Zietman et al. The treatment of prostate cancer by conventional radiationn therapy: An analysis of long-term outcome. Int J Rad Oncol Biol Phys, 1995.	
Treatment modality	Conventional external beam XRT
Site	Massachusetts General Hospital, Boston, MA
Study design	Reporting on 1,040 men with T1-4NxM0 CaP treated with radical radiation thearpy at MGH between 1977-1991
Sample Size	1040
Accrual dates	1977-1991
Patient stage	T2b-c 197; T2 (not otherwise specified) 87; T3 475; T4 65
Patient age	median= 69
Duration of follow-up	median=49 months; follow-up every 3-12 months
Outcome Definitions	Tx failure defined by: (1) Clinical criteria, (2) liberal biochem criteria, (3) strict biochem criteria (see p. 288 for defns of each of these 3 defns). DFS assessed using all 3 criteria. Also report on metastasis-free & dx-specific surv.
Method of Survival Analysis	Kaplan-Meier Product-Limit method with stat inferences made using Log-Rank test.
Survival Curves	Actuarial DFS (either strict of liberal biochem criteria) for T1-2NxM0 by PSA (<4, <1) and divided by Gleason (1-2, 3, 4-5; 3 figures). Curve out 10-15 yrs, # at risk at 5&10 yrs provided. Continued column Q
Statistical Estimates Related to Survival Analyses	Freedom from biochem failure (reports the 5&10 DFS % by T stage & Gleason). 10-year rates discussed.
Incontinence	MFS for T1-2 managed either by XRT at MGH or expectantly (Chodak et al, NEJM, 1994) and divided by Gleason. DSS for T1-2 managed either by XRT at MGH or expectantly (Chodak et al, NEJM, 1994) and divided by Gleason.
Other outcomes/Results	Also provide infor on PSA doubling times (Scatter plot illustrating PSA doubling times for 126 T1-2 pts relapsing following XRT).

Zietman et al. Adjuvant irradiation after radical prostatectomy for adeocarcinoma of prostate: analysis of freedom from PSA failure. Urology, 1993.	
Treatment modality	Radical prostatectomy and postop irradiation (either elective or salvage, so no clin localized dx)
Site	Department of Radiation Oncology, Mass General Hospital, Boston, MA
Study design	Reporting on 84 consecutive pts referred to MGH for either elective or salvage XRT following RP. 14 addtl med referred following development of a palpable local dx recurrence were analyzed separately.
Sample Size	84
Accrual dates	1983-1992
Patient stage	T3
Patient age	median= 65; range=47-80
Duration of follow-up	interval between surgery and XRT provided (Table 1)
Other Patient characteristics	Patient Char (includ degress of extracapsular spread and lymph node status).
Other Eligibility Criteria	No adjuvant endocrine therapy was allowed.
Univar/Multiv Analyses (Covariates)	Cox proportional hazards regression used to control for the simultaneous effect of outcome-related covar.
Outcome Definitions	Failure: detectable PSA in patient in whom it had been either undetectable postop or unknow; any rise in PSA in patient who had detectable postop levels; development of palpable local or distant dx recurr; or radiologic evid of distant metastases.
Method of Survival Analysis	Kaplan-Meier Product-Limit methods with stat inferences using the Log-Rank test. Curves out 60 months. Analyses were made from date of surgery to avoid any lead time bias resulting from varying time intervals to start of XRT.
Survival Curves	Actuarial freedom from relapse (incl PSA). Actuarial freedom from all relapse (incl PSA) of T3 receiving adj XRT according to (A) nodal status, (B) pres/abs of seminal vesicle invasion.
Statistical Estimates Related to Survival Analyses	Discuss 5-year rates. E.g., the projected freedom from total relapse (clin and biochem) of all 84 path T3 pts is 60% at 5 yrs. Those with pos nodal dx fared less well than those who were node net (43% vs 64%, p=0.021).
Incontinence	Actuarial freedom from all relapse (includ PSA) of 68 T3N0 according to (A) pres/abs of seminal vesicle invasion, and (b) degree of tumor differentiation.
Impotence	Actuarial freedom from all relapse (includ PSA) of 14 pts treated with XRT for apparentlyisolated local dx recurr following RP
Other outcomes/Results	Path stage T3N0 pts: Freedom from biochem failure following RP. Table presents the results of 3 other studies, 2 of which tx with RP alone.

Zietman et al. Use of PSA nadir to predict subsequent biochemical outcome following external beam XRT for T1-2 adenocarcinoma of the prostate. Radiotherapy and Oncology, 1996.	
Treatment modality	Definitive XRT
Site	Department of Radiation Oncology, Mass General Hospital, Boston, MA
Study design	Reporting on 314 T1-2NxM0 med with CaP treated with definitive XRT.
Sample Size	314
Accrual dates	1988-1993
Patient stage	17% T1, 29% T2a, 54% T2b-c
Duration of follow-up	median=41 months; range=25-85; follow-up every 3-12 months
Other Eligibility Criteria	No prior, concomitant, or adj androgen suppression tx allowed
Univar/Multiv Analyses (Covariates)	Cox proportional hazards regression used to control for the simultaneous effect of outcome-related covar.
Outcome Definitions	Failure: 3 successive rises in PSA following XRT.
Method of Survival Analysis	Kaplan-Meier Product-Limit method with stat inferences using Log-Rank.
Survival Curves	Actuarial freedom from biochem relapse for T1-2 grouped by nadir PSA (out 6 yrs).
Statistical Estimates Related to Survival Analyses	E.g., The overall freedom from a rising PSA for the 314 T1-2NxM0 men was 63% at 5 yrs. The 5 year actuarial freedom from failure was 89%, 73%, and 45%for those with initial PSA values of <4, 4-10, and >10.
Other outcomes/Results	%T1-2 by initial PSA & Gleason who attain designated post-tx nadir values. A case-controlled comparison between T1-2NxM0 men receiving 72Gy and 68.4 Gy irradiation was performed. Comparisons between PSA nadirs made using Chi-square test.

Abbreviations used in Appendices

adjuv, adjuvant
ADT, androgen deprivation therapy
anal, analysis
biochem, biochemical
bx, biopsy or biopsies
CA, cancer
Calc, calculated
cap, capsular
chemo, chemotherapy
CI, confidence interval
clin, clinical
Complix, complications
CRT, conformat radiation therapy
CT, computerized tomography
Cum, cumulative
DFS, disease-free survival
diff, difference
DRE, digital rectal examination
EM, endocrine management
ECE, extra-capsular extension
elev, elevated
er, endorectal
est, estimate or estimated
evid, evidence
Gl, Gleason
HRQOL, health-related quality of life
id, identify
incl, including
incont, incontinence
KPS, Karnofsky Performance Status
loc, location
LN, lymph node
LND, lymphadenectomy
mets, metastasis or metastases
MRI, magnetic resonance imaging
multivar, multivariate
NED, no evidence of disease
neg, negative
ns, nerve-sparing
PAP, prostatic acid phosphatase
path, pathological
PC, prostate cancer
pen, penetration
PFS, progression-free survival

PNBx, prostate needle biopsy
pos, positive
PSA, prostate specific antigen
PSM, positive surgical margins
pts, patients
QOL, quality of life
rad onc, radiation oncology
regr, regression
RP, radical prostatectomy
RTOG, Radiation Therapy Oncology Group
RT-PCR, reverse transcriptase polymerase chain reaction
SD, standard deviation
sig, significant or significance or significantly
sq, square
stat, statistical or statistically
surv, survival
SV, seminal vesical
SVI, seminal vesical invasion
TRUS, transrectal ultrasound
tx, treatment or treatments
undet, undetactable
unk, unknown
urin, urinary
univar, univariate
urol, urology or urological
var, variation
wk, week
wks, weeks
WW, watchful waiting
XRT, external beam radiation therapy

Appendix C

PROTOCOL FOR INTERVIEWS WITH EXPERTS

1. What information do you typically provide to patients who *are newly diagnosed* with *localized prostate cancer* regarding treatment options (surgery/radiation therapy/expectant management)

2. In your experience, what are the most important concerns expressed by patients during initial consultation? From the following list of items that may represent concerns raised by patients who've been newly diagnosed with localized prostate cancer, please indicate, based on your practice experience, whether each issue is among the most important patient concerns; how easy/difficult is this issue is to discuss with most patients; how much time you typically spend discussing this issue; and whether there are groups or types of patients for whom this issue is not a primary concern.

   a) Survival
   b) Recurrence
   c) Complications

   > Urinary functioning
   > Bowel functioning
   > Sexual functioning

   d) Bleeding
   e) Pain
   f) Anesthesia
   g) Recovery Time
   h) Coordination Of Care
   i) Financial

   > Cost of treatment
   > Time away from work

   h) Length of hospitalization

3. For each of the following items, what sources of information do you rely on when discussing treatment options with your patients? In particular, do you use data from

your own practice experience (anecdotal or database), your clinic/facility experience (anecdotal or database), the scientific literature, or other sources?

a) PSA

b) Potency

c) Rectal bleeding

d) Incontinence

e) Other morbidities

f) Recurrence

g) Mortality from prostate cancer

h) Mortality from other causes

i) Other issues

4. Do you use probabilistic language to communicate outcomes? If yes, do you use numbers or words to communicate uncertainty? (An example of using numbers would be "10%" where an example of using words would be "one chance in 10.") To what degree do you tailor the information to the individual patient (stage, age, comorbidities, marital status)? Do you use tabulated estimates (e.g. Partin tables) or other similar materials?

5. What information do you typically provide to patients regarding alternative facilities for treatment (other than your own clinic)? For radiation oncologists, in what circumstances do you recommend surgery rather than radiation therapy? For urologists, in what circumstances do you recommend radiation therapy rather than surgery?

6. Generally, what information do you discuss with a patient *during the initial consultation?* How often are follow-up visits scheduled to discuss information about treatment options and outcomes? How often do you ask the patient to return for a visit with his spouse if he has one? How many visits, if any, do you typically schedule after the diagnosis but before treatment?

7. How much time (min/hours/visits) do you typically spend with patients discussing issues related to treatment options? For what proportion of patients is this adequate, too little time, or too much time?

8. Do you provide articles, brochures, videos or computer-based information to your patients that discuss treatment outcomes? If appropriate, are brochures available in more than one language? Are there groups of patients where this information is more useful than for others? (e.g. how useful is this information for better educated vs less educated men? for high vs low income patients? for older patients?) If the patient is a managed care beneficiary, does the health plan provide specific materials for patient education?

9. What have you found to be the most challenging or difficult issues you've encountered when discussing treatment issues with newly diagnosed prostate cancer patients? (e.g., lack of data to answer definitive questions, trying to deal with patient perception, eliciting patient preferences)

10. What elements do you typically include in the following pre-treatment evaluation procedures for localized prostate cancer patients?

a) History and Physical - what do you typically assess?

i. How do you assess patient comorbidity?

ii. Do you do formal testing of potency, voiding symptoms, or continence before treatment? If yes, specify method (e.g. pt self-report?)

iii. What factors do you consider when deciding whether to recommend either surgery or radiation therapy (XRT)?

b) What clinical or pathological staging procedures do you use, and in which patients?

i. Laboratory tests: PSA, Acid phosphatase, CBC, Chemistry panel, Other

ii. Imaging: CT, MRI, Bone scan, Transrectal ultrasound, Volumetric ultrasound (radiation oncologists only), Other

iii. Are there any other procedures that you require prior to treatment, such as cytoscopy, ProstaScint, Other

c) Do you routinely recommend lymph node dissection?

d) What elements of the pre-treatment evaluation do you consider most important for ensuring successful outcomes for patients?

11. For radiation oncologists, which of the following treatment modalities do you use in your practice or refer to? What characteristics of each treatment modality ensures successful outcomes for patients?

a) External beam

b) Conformal (with or without dose escalation)

c) Brachytherapy (Iodine, Palladium, Iridium) with or without external beam

d) Proton beam therapy

e) Neutron beam therapy

f) Androgen ablation

12. For radiation oncologists, please comment on the following treatment parameters in terms of which ones you use, what characteristics ensure successful outcomes for patients?

a) External Beam

    i. Dose (time, dose, fractionation)

    ii. Target volumes (what do you treat, dose volume)

b) Technical factors

i. beam energy

ii. beam shaping ("blocking or MLC, multileaf columnator")

iii. blocking-MLC

iv. number of fields

v. fractionation (dose per fraction)

vi. localization films (ports) (frequency)

c) Equipment

    i. LINAC (what type)

    ii. Simulation (what type - conventional/CT/other)

d) Techniques

    i. External beam

        CT or MRI based planning; ultrasound, fluoroscopy, or CT guided

    ii. Implant

        CT or MRI-based planning; ultrasound, fluoroscopy, or CT guided

e) Other technical parameters that you feel are important to outcomes

13. For urologists, which of the following treatment modalities do you use in your practice, which do you refer to, and what are the characteristics that ensure successful outcomes?

   a) Surgical approach (retropubic, perineal)

   b) Nerve sparing (unilateral, bilateral, non)

   c) Average units of blood transfused from autologous or homologous sources

   d) Brachytherapy (if yes, how do you participate)

   e) Perioperative or adjuvant androgen ablation

   f) Adjuvant radiation therapy

   g) Routine autologous blood storage

14. What elements of post-treatment follow-up care do you believe are most important to ensuring successful results for localized prostate cancer patients?

15. In addition to survival, what outcome measures do you believe are most important to assessing successful treatment of localized prostate cancer?

16. Do you routinely use a care path (clinical pathway or practice guideline) for treating localized prostate cancer in your practice? If yes, is it taken from the literature or was it designed specifically for your hospital? If not from literature, how was it developed? (systematic literature review, data from institution, expert judgment)

17. Has managed care had any direct effect on the kinds or types of treatments that you are able to offer patients? Describe.

18. Final questions regarding your practice

a) About how many patients do you see in a year? (own practice/ clinic-wide)

b) About how many patients do you treat for localized prostate cancer in a year ? (own practice/clinic-wide)

c) Of your localized prostate cancer patients, what proportions are under 65, 65-74, 75+

d) Of your localized prostate cancer patients what proportions are African American, Hispanic, Caucasian, Other

e) Of your localized prostate cancer patients what proportions are educated at less than high school, high school graduate, some college or college graduate

f) Of your localized prostate cancer patients, what proportions are insured by Medicare (with or without Medigap), Medicaid only, private fee-for-service, managed care (including capitated patients and those in PPOs), self-pay, indigent, other